Feel Younger, Stronger, Sexier

The Truth About Bio-Identical Hormones

Written by

Dr. Dan Hale

Feel Younger, Stronger, Sexier
The Truth About Bio-Identical Hormones
Copyright ©2015 Dan Hale

ISBN 978-1506-908-32-8 AMAZON PRINT
ISBN 978-1622-879-27-4 TRADE PRINT
ISBN 978-1622-879-28-1 EBOOK

LCCN 2015942023

June 2015

Published and Distributed by
First Edition Design Publishing, Inc.
P.O. Box 20217, Sarasota, FL 34276-3217
www.firsteditiondesignpublishing.com

Inconjuction with Fathers Press, LLC.
www.fatherspress.com

Although the author and publisher have made every effort to ensure that the information in this book was correct at press time, the author and publisher do not assume and hereby disclaim any liability to any party for any loss, damage, or disruption caused by errors or omissions, whether such errors or omissions result from negligence, accident, or any other cause.

This book is not intended as a substitute for the medical advice of your physician. The reader should regularly consult a physician in matters relating to his/her health and particularly with respect to any symptoms that may require diagnosis or medical attention.

Edited by Dr. Henry Oursler. HenryOursler@me.com

Cover Design and Artwork by Becky Blair

My background is in Science and the complex Biochemical pathways of the sentinels of our body's wellness - The Hormones. We don't exist biologically for any other reason than to reproduce and our reproductive Hormones control every facet of our wellness. There are not hundreds of different diseases that afflict us- there is ONE thing that goes wrong, with hundreds of different possible ramifications.

We need to be treating that core value of our body's wellness, and PREVENTING the hundreds of things that result from that complex core of our sex hormones when they don't function in the harmony that nature intended.

This is what BHRT is actually about. It is correcting that core value of functioning. It is about restoring the body's biochemistry so that it runs normally.

This book by Dan Hale is the key to begin to understand how to achieve and maintain that normality. If you want to be well again, full of energy, love and life, then you must read this book!

DR. PETER TUNBRIDGE
HORMONES AND HEALTH
27 MILAN TERRACE
STIRLING, SOUTH AUSTRALIA 5152

Every pastor needs to read this book, The Truth About Bio-identical Hormones, and here is why.

I became a Senior Pastor at age twenty-one and watched as some of our best families, in their mid-forties to mid-sixties, struggled in their marriages. Some have tragically ended in divorce. Then, in hurt or shame, they leave the church.

In our forties, we began to experience difficulties, and we knew they were physically related but didn't know what to do. The antidepressants and synthetic hormones with all of their bad side effects were not an option. So our search began to find help for ourselves and the people we've pastored.

About five years ago, we began to learn about Bio-identical Hormones, and it has changed our lives physically and emotionally. Our marriage is better than ever, and we have been able to help so many people.

For so many years I have addressed these problems as being spiritual in nature, but today I tell those I counsel, "If you are a Christian with these problems, then they are probably ninety percent physical and emotional, and ten percent spiritual."

Dr. Hale's book gives you the answers to help your people have healthy lives and marriages.

Dr. G. DOUGLAS RIPLEY
DECATUR BAPTIT CHURCH
DECATUR, ALABAMA

INTRODUCTION

Every Life-Changing Journey Begins with One Significant Step

Over thirty years ago, I took an oath when I became a medical doctor. I swore to practice medicine honestly and to prescribe regimens for the good of my patients. This book is a result of that promise.

Since taking that Hippocratic Oath, I've learned more than I could have ever imagined. I was a traditionalist in my medical practice for the first thirty years. What that means is that I practiced medicine the way I had been trained – the traditional way. I prescribed synthetic hormones to hundreds of women. And I treated hundreds of men, telling them that their sexual problems were just a symptom of getting old. It was rare for me to check a man's testosterone because I believed there was not much that could be done. Injecting testosterone was *"doping"* and was something that reputable doctors did not do. Although I acted within the realm of the knowledge I had learned in medical school, I was wrong.

Today, I would approach their treatment differently – drastically different. I have come to understand that hormones are essential. They are absolutely critical to our health. They are the body's life force, necessary for the proper functioning of every cell.

But what kind of hormone therapy is best?

My passion has always been to do everything within my power as a physician to care for those who place their trust in me. That is why I was compelled to write this book. It is filled with information pharmaceutical companies do not want you to know. To withhold this information would be gross negligence at best; at worst, it would deprive people who suffer needlessly a chance at improved quality of life.

The Effects of Hormonal Loss

We lose hormones as we age. With that loss, we can expect to experience certain predictable symptoms. For women, the effects of hormonal loss can include:
- Hot flashes, night sweats, vaginal dryness, depression, anxiety, fibromyalgia, dry eyes, poor sleep, thin lips, osteoporosis, growth of facial hair, decrease in sexual interest, mood swings, body aches, bladder leakage, memory lapses, less energy, diabetes, lipid abnormalities, cardiovascular disease, restless leg syndrome, painful intercourse, arthritis, Alzheimer's, weight gain, and various

neurological problems perhaps including Parkinson's and multiple sclerosis. And the list goes on and on.

For men, the effects of hormonal loss can include:

- Decreased nocturnal (nighttime) erections, arthritis, loss of concentration, elevated lipids (cholesterol and/or triglycerides), heart attack, stroke, decreased sex drive, loss of ability to maintain a strong erection, easy fatigue, loss of muscle mass, weight gain especially around the waist, hypertension, loss of muscle tone, diabetes, decreased exercise tolerance, and stroke. Any and all of these can also lead to loss of confidence and depression.

Not All Hormones Are Alike!

The reality is that not all hormones are alike! There is a **vast** difference between synthetic hormones and natural hormones. I was wrong in my belief that synthetic hormones that are foreign to the body could attain good results. These hormones include synthetic testosterone, *Premarin* and *Provera*. I was devastated when the results of the *Women's Health Initiative Trial*, which ended in 2002, showed that these synthetic hormones cause breast cancer, heart attacks, strokes, dementia and blood clots.

As a result, the medical community, led by false information from the pharmaceutical companies, overreacted and called **all** hormones dangerous. Along with most physicians, I was reluctant to prescribe **any** kind of hormones after reading the results of this study. It made me angry to know that I had been fed the wrong information about synthetic hormones for years. The world of the medical community had been blown apart by this study, and in fear, we physicians initially lumped all hormones in the same category.

I began to research intensively, however, seeking answers. I challenged my long-held beliefs and was open to new concepts. Thousands of professional, scientific, double-blind crossover placebo-controlled studies substantiated the benefits and lack of side effects of bio-identical hormone replacement therapy. I was intrigued. Bio-identical hormones are truly natural, with plant-based ingredients whose hormonal structure is identical to that of the human body versus synthetic hormones that are chemicals with dangerous side effects.

My Change of Direction

Ten years ago, I was introduced to the world of *Pellet Bio-identical Hormone Replacement Therapy* (BHRT). The key to successful BHRT is the delivery method that most aligns with the body's natural processes that are affected by factors such as stress. It is a hormone-on-demand delivery system that I will explain later in this book. BHRT pills, creams, and injections are not the most effective delivery methods. The most effective delivery system continues to be *Pellet BHRT.*

As I studied, the enlightenment I received was monumental and life-changing for me as well as for my patients. I began to see hope restored and wellness returned to multitudes of sick people with scores of different ailments as I implemented *Pellet Bio-identical Hormone Replacement Therapy* in my practice.

Honesty involves risk. It is not easy to dispel a myth or convince a skeptic of the truth. At the cost of great personal sacrifice and censure, I have been compelled to write this book, revealing truth with integrity and irrefutable evidence. The evidence is presented here for you to examine and form your own conclusions.

Change is difficult, especially if there is a powerful financial interest involved with maintaining the status quo, even when doing so produces disastrous results. Re-educating the educated elite (medical societies) can be professionally dangerous. It has been said that it is often necessary for the present generation to die off for new concepts to be recognized and accepted. To confront the medical establishment (Big Pharma) may have major negative consequences when the legal arm of the government (the FDA) has strong political and financial ties to institutions that have self-serving interests to keep the myth alive.

Treating Symptoms vs. Providing a Cure

Major pharmaceutical companies have built an empire on the concept of equating a symptom with taking a pill. You've heard the slogans. They pummel us repeatedly at every turn. *"Ask your doctor if Lipitor is right for you." "If you have body aches, take Celebrex." "If you feel depressed, try Zoloft." "If you have trouble sleeping, the answer may be found in Ambien."*

> ### *Major pharmaceutical companies have built an empire on the concept of equating a symptom with taking a pill.*

I have no vendetta against pharmaceutical companies. Many of their discoveries are lifesaving. My problem with our present way of doing things is the resistance by Big Pharma, the FDA, and traditional medicine to incorporate natural means of preventing disease. We must not cling stubbornly to old ideas. Instead, we should search diligently and be open minded to replacing those old ideas should we find ones that are better.

It is especially disgusting that, at heart of the their resistance, is the fact that pharmaceutical companies have too much money to lose if traditional medicine embraces the most effective, safest, healthiest, and least expensive way to support hormonal balance in the body. Unfortunately, it always comes down to money. Financial profits continue to rule the day. Big Pharma intentionally promotes confusion at the cost of people's health. Synthetic hormones kill. Bio-identical hormones heal. The conjured up debate fostered by drug companies regarding BHRT is ludicrous, selfish, and scientifically unfounded.

I have devoted my second life as a physician to the cause of natural, bio-identical hormones – those that are identical to those produced by the human body. They have proven to be beneficial in thousands of reputable studies and in multiplied thousands of lives. The evidence I present in this book has come from these five sources:

- Attending medical meetings and listening to scores of lectures about hormonal balance
- Reading almost every book available on bio-identical hormones
- Reading a multitude of studies about the effects hormones have on the body—both those used by conventional medicine as well as those by doctors using

bio-identical hormones. To date, there are 360,000 articles relating to hormones on the website Medscape

- My experiences treating thousands of patients using exclusively bio-identical hormones
- Making certain that the lessons taught by the experts in BHRT and the books and studies I read correlated with what I experienced in my office using bio-identical hormone replacement therapy

New Convictions

Because of the above research, I've come to four strongly-held conclusions:

First, I affirm that there is irrefutable evidence that replacing lost hormones is essential to good health. The dying process begins with the loss of life-sustaining hormones.

Second, my further conviction is that replacing declining hormones has to be done with bio-identical hormones. This process should begin early on, not waiting until menopause or post-menopause. An individual should not wait until low hormone symptoms are so great that *"something has to be done."* You will see later in this book that damage to the body begins years before symptoms appear.

Replacing declining hormones has to be done with bio-identical hormones. This process should begin early on, not waiting until menopause or post-menopause.

Third, the goal is to increase natural hormone levels as close as possible to those of a much younger person.

Fourth, it is my strong assertion that there is no reason for an informed, caring physician to use conventional hormone-look-alike drugs which are dangerous when bio-identical hormones are readily available that are 100% identical to those produced by the human body.

The case studies presented in this book are of real patients. They are not just anecdotal stories that can be explained away as being unfounded personal encounters. They are based on facts and research. The research listed as references provides strong evidence of the remarkable transformations in my patients' experiences.

When hormones decline, our health declines. It is a fact that replacing lost hormones helps to prevent or drastically slow down many disease processes. Mainstream medicine is not revealing the truth and is deceiving people when it states that bio-identical hormones are no different than synthetic hormones. This is equivalent to saying that there is no difference in nutritious food and rat poison.

Let me clarify: I am not proposing a mythical, live-forever, utopian state of existence. Our bodies age. Death is an inevitable reality for all of us. What I am talking about here is quality of life. Health is our greatest wealth.

Let me restate that after more than thirty years of treating patients, I find it critical to look for the **reason** one feels depressed or has trouble sleeping or is tired or has body aches. We must do more than write a prescription to treat the symptoms. The self-serving medical establishment has more to gain by treating the symptoms than treating the condition that is causing the symptoms. It is faster and more financially rewarding to write a prescription for an antidepressant or a sleep-inducing narcotic or a habit-forming sedative for anxiety than to think outside the box and search for why the patient is having these symptoms now. Physicians must take the time and ask, *"What is different today in this patient's life than a year ago that would now cause these symptoms? Could it be hormonal imbalance?"*

The family care doctor should be the one most concerned about bio-identical hormone replacement as he/she is usually the first contact between the patient and the health care system. It is my hope that doctors become increasingly committed to the field of wellness and disease prevention with regard to natural hormone treatments. Your well-being depends on it. Accept no less!

How to Get the Most Out of this Book

This book is written for you. It is laid out to encourage understanding by explaining what causes loss of hormones, what hormones are lost, what the results of hormonal decline leads to, what the typical doctor will do when a patient has low hormones, and what a doctor who specializes in hormonal decline will do differently. The difference between bio-identical hormones and synthetic hormones will be explained clearly and what you can do to avoid the consequences of hormonal decline.

This book is designed to give you answers as you face the effects of aging in your body. It will give you well-researched, state-of-the-art answers to your most common questions. And most of all, it will give you hope ... hope that you don't have to resign yourself to "getting old" ... hope that you can return to a normal, active lifestyle ... and hope that your best years are still ahead of you.

One of the most damaging losses we can have is our health. All of us will have loss of important hormones as we age – especially the "sex hormones" – estradiol, testosterone and progesterone. In this book you will learn what happens to us when we lose our hormones and how to recover naturally to our optimal (best) health like we had when we were twenty years old. You will learn why we lose our sex hormones, how conventional doctors treat the symptoms of hormone loss, how doctors like my replace lost hormones naturally, and what you need to do to get your life back.

Section One is designed to help you understand bio-identical hormone replacement therapy. We'll discuss hormonal loss, how replacement therapy works, and why pharmaceutical companies are strongly influencing physicians to continue to prescribe synthetic hormones and drugs to treat only the symptoms of hormonal decline instead of treating the real problem.

In **Section Two**, we will discuss twenty-seven common symptoms and how BHRT can make a difference.

Finally, in **Section Three,** we will answer the most common questions people have about BHRT.

By reading this book,
- You will know if you have signs and symptoms of hormone loss
- What you can do to regain the vigor you once had in bed and in your daily life
- You will know how to communicate with your doctor about what is happening to you
- You will know how to find a doctor that will be able to help you with natural bio-identical hormones instead of harmful drugs

In short, this book will change your life.

All of the stories and anecdotes in this book are true. However, to protect patient confidentiality, I've taken the liberty to change names and at times to combine several scenarios. Nevertheless, they still accurately reflect the truth of what happened.

This book is written for you, the average lay-person who has questions about bio-identical hormones. Also, I hope that hundreds of physicians will read this book and come to the same conclusions I have. For both of those audiences, I've included over eleven hundred endnotes because many of you want to know the ***proven*** medical research behind these findings

I am honored that you have picked up this book and are reading it. Every life-changing journey begins with a significant step. You've made that initial step – to discover the truth about bio-identical hormones. Once you learn the truth, your life will never be the same. As you read through the following chapters, I encourage you to keep a journal of what you are learning and questions that you have.

Thank you for joining with me in this journey. You are on your way to feeling younger, stronger and sexier.

Feel Younger, Stronger, Sexier

The Truth About Bio-Identical Hormones

Table of Contents

SECTION ONE

Understanding Bio-Identical

Hormone Replacement Therapy

CHAPTER 1

Understanding Hormone Deficiency

You will know the truth ... it will set you free!

Sylvia's Story

Sylvia was fifty-three years old and in the depths of menopause when she first came to see me. On her pre-visit survey, she checked thirteen of the twenty-two symptoms of hormonal decline: *hot flashes, night sweats, vaginal dryness, poor sleep, weight gain, restless leg syndrome, no sex drive, forgetfulness, anxiety, fibromyalgia, mood swings, recurrent urinary tract infections and loss of self-esteem.*

Needless to say, Sylvia was not a happy camper when we first talked.

My marriage of twenty-seven years is falling apart. We are just living together and that's about it. We sleep in different beds because I am up and down all night. I am on two different medicines for depression and one for anxiety. My doctor stopped the hormones I was on because she said they caused breast cancer, strokes and heart attacks. She started me on Zoloft 100 mg a day. This made me gain twelve pounds in four months. I then had no libido at all. I didn't even want my husband to touch me. What you are going to do for me today will be worth the money if I can just get relief from one of my problems.

Sylvia was a very nice lady – but I could tell she was holding back tears. She had read Suzanne Somers' book, *"I'm Too Young for This! The Natural Hormone Solution to Enjoy Perimenopause."* She knew there was something out there – but her doctor would not give her bio-identical hormones. The doctor was hesitant because she knew nothing about BHRT. She did not know how much to prescribe; nor did she know what bio-identical hormones to give because she had never been trained. No pharmaceutical representative had spoken to her about BHRT.

Sylvia continued,

My doctor would not check my hormones and just changed me to a different kind of antidepressant, Prozac. She told me after a while you get used to one kind and have to change. That didn't make sense to me. Then she wanted to increase the dose of my nerve medicine. I was already like a zombie. That's why I'm here. I believe I have a hormone problem. I didn't have depression, but now with all these drugs, I do.

Sylvia was somewhat overweight at 168 pounds. She had gained thirty-two pounds in the past eighteen months. She was anxious and frustrated because she could not get the help she wanted. Sylvia's blood work revealed that her hormones were extremely low. [1]

She was given a very low dose of testosterone in a pellet form, 100 mg, to boost her energy and her sex drive. She was given a low dose estradiol pellet just under the skin to last for three months. Sylvia was to take progesterone 200 mg as a sublingual rapid dissolve tablet at bedtime.

On her return visit four weeks later Sylvia was beaming with joy. She said, *"I was hoping to get relief from at least one problem. But all the symptoms I checked on the form are now so much better. Thank you."*

Let me make four summary observations from Sylvia's case:

- Sylvia had a problem. She was not getting any better and, in fact, was suffering from severe side effects from the treatment her doctors had prescribed.
- Her traditional doctors refused to treat the root cause. Whether it was from ignorance or false facts fed from the pharmaceutical industry, they prescribed a treatment that was counter-productive.
- BHRT worked. It took only four weeks for Sylvia to see a dramatic difference in her health.
- Because of her dramatic improvement, she became convinced that BHRT was the proper treatment.

She became convinced that BHRT was the proper treatment.

Sadly, many traditional doctors refuse to check hormonal levels, especially in women. Many patients report that their doctor told them, *"It won't do any good to check your hormones. It's normal to go through menopause; it's just part of the aging process. But it is not pathological – it's not a disease."* This mindset labels the effects of aging as inevitable facts that cannot be treated. But if a doctor does not check hormone levels and believes there is no relevant treatment when hormones decline, then they simply accept the inevitable facts about gradual declining health.

How and Why Hormones Change

Aging is an age-old problem. We all get older! As we mature into puberty at age ten or twelve years old, our sex hormones rise. They blast off like rockets. Think romance. Think sexual fascination ... and at times, sexual obsession. Then somewhere between eighteen- to thirty-years-old, our hormones reach their peak and are fairly constant in men and women for the next twelve years. But when we hit thirty, those same hormones begin to diminish. In men it is a gradual decline in testosterone. In women the loss of hormones can be more dramatic and actually begin in their late twenties.

What are hormones? Hormones are chemical substances that are produced in one part of the body, such as the testicles or ovaries, and are transported to another part of the body through the blood. The function of these hormones is to stimulate an organ or group of cells to perform a certain function. Every cell in the body responds to these hormones.

Our bodies are designed by God to function best when those hormones are abundant – like we had in our youth. When there is less hormonal output, there will be a corresponding decline in the way our bodies function. This is represented by a downward spiral known as old age. As we age, hormones decrease usually around age thirty. The bad news is that without natural hormones, we can expect to experience the symptoms of old age: depression, anxiety, fibromyalgia, dryness of the eyes, poor sleep, low self-esteem, thin lips, osteoporosis, facial hair, decrease in sexual interest, mood swings, body aches, bladder leakage, memory lapses, less energy, diabetes, lipid (cholesterol and triglycerides) abnormalities, cardiovascular disease, restless leg syndrome, arthritis, Alzheimer's and weight gain. The good news is there is an answer for each of these age-related conditions.

> **The bad news is that without natural hormones, we can expect to experience many symptoms... The good news is there is an answer for each of these age-related conditions.**

Conventional Hormone Therapy vs. BHRT

Conventional doctors are told to prescribe the lowest dose of hormones for the shortest period of time possible. This is to provide relief from hot flushes. After the hot flushes (or flashes) are gone, hormone therapy can be stopped. This bizarre medical advice is a result of the *Women's Health Initiative*. This would be reasonable advice if the only alternative would be to prescribe the dangerous hormones used in the Women's Health Initiative Trial—*Premarin* and *Provera*.

In contrast to that wisdom, bio-identical hormones are a natural supplement to the body – without the negative side effects. Over and over, I have seen the three-fold power of these natural hormones:

- **They replace.** Where there was once lost hormones, BHRT replaces those lost hormones and restores them to their once prime level.
- **They repair.** Because these hormones are now at their proper level, they spread throughout the body and bring healing and repair to organs and bodily functions
- **They restore.** One of the most obvious restorations is to our sexual drive and abilities. With sex hormone levels to the point where they were in our twenties, our bodies respond accordingly.

But here is the best part of our message: all this happens **without the negative side effects!** Natural hormone replacement is both necessary for good health – and safer!

"But I Thought Doctors Were Smart"

Doctors are smart. They are highly intelligent people. But two factors are at work against their understanding of BHRT.

- The first factor is their education. They studied at some of the finest institutions in our country. But what they learned is now contradicted by more recent medical research. In essence, they learned lies.
- The second factor is even more insidious. Funded by the big money of Big Pharma, these doctors are being lied to – and led to believe that the side effects of BHRT are the same as that of synthetic hormones.

There Is a Battle Going On

Big Pharma has fought back. The medical world is totally outdated in applying the research of Bio-identical Hormones because Big Pharma can't make money on them. So doctors are speaking negatively about bio-identical hormone treatment and are prescribing synthetic hormones that cause cancer and a world of other side effects. Big Pharma is trying to stop this phenomenal natural treatment by saying the side effects of the two treatments are the same. They are not! That is why this book is so important.

"You will know the truth ... and the truth will set you free!" Those words, originally spoken by Jesus of Nazareth 2,000 years ago, are still true today. Truth has a way of opening our eyes, of breaking the chains of lies, and of restoring hope where hope has long been lost.

This book is designed to restore that hope. But to do that, the truth must be told.

You Will Know the Truth

How can responsible medical investigators use the results of a study of two synthetic drugs (*Premarin* and *Provera*) and apply its findings to natural *Bio-identical Hormone Replacement Therapy*? Is there a study that confirms BHRT as dangerous? No! Because BHRT is an all-natural replacement therapy. The body will not reject those hormones because it recognizes them as natural to itself. Nevertheless, Big Pharma has sought to convince doctors to continue to prescribe *Premarin* and *Provera* and has irresponsibly charged that BHRT has the same side effects. The lobby of pharmaceutical companies has been hurt by so many physicians using natural bio-identical hormone replacement therapies that one state, Tennessee, is trying to ban BHRT from the state.

For forty years, before the report in 2002 of the WHI, doctors were told to use synthetic hormones in their treatment. They were told that these drugs provided protection against cardiovascular disease, breast cancer, uterine cancer, osteoporosis, and colon cancer. Part of the story doctors were told by Wyeth Pharmaceuticals for all those years was that *Premarin* and *Provera* were **good** and **helpful** for mental decline or cognitive impairment and dementia.

In 2004 the results of another arm of the WHI was released—the *Women's Health Initiative Memory Study*. This study proved that not only was *Prempro* (a combination of *Premarin* and *Provera*) not protecting these women from mental decline, but it actually doubled the risk of dementia in women on these drugs. This increased incidence of dementia was evident within the first year of taking either *Prempro* or just *Premarin*. This group of women on *Prempro* was well past menopause — ages 65 to 79 — and still dementia was made worse showing brain atrophy when MRIs compared to older women who did not take these drugs. [2]

In contrast, natural estradiol, not synthetic horse estrogen, has been shown to protect against a decline in our processing abilities. [3] The younger the women were when they had their ovaries removed, the greater the risk for dementia as well as cardiovascular disease, osteoporosis, Parkinson's disease, impaired sexual function and psychological well-being, and premature death from any cause. [4] [5] [6]

Most all of the medical reasons to use synthetic artificial hormones were proven to be false. However, thousands of studies confirm that BHRT does provide more than just relief of hot flushes and night sweats.

Bio-identical Hormone Replacement Therapy provides protection against:

- Osteoporosis
- Cardiovascular disease
- Diabetes

- Depression
- Alzheimer's disease
- High cholesterol
- Fibromyalgia
- Memory decline
- Poor sleep
- Anxiety
- Hot flushes
- Night sweats
- Vaginal dryness
- Decreased libido
- Mood swings
- Urinary tract infections
- Increased skin wrinkling
- ADHD
- Arthritis
- Restless leg syndrome
- Loss of self-esteem

In 2000 a study reported in *Neuroscience* demonstrated that natural estradiol protected the nerves. *Premarin* didn't. [7] In another study of postmenopausal women, one group used *Premarin* plus a synthetic progestin (such as *Provera*) and another group of women used estradiol plus a progestin. All the women underwent a functional MRI – an imaging of brain function. Women using *Premarin* had poorer memory function than did women using estradiol or women using no hormones. [8]

Many menopausal women taking *Premarin* and *Provera* quit after a few months because they could not tolerate the side effects. However, women who used BHRT experienced the opposite: there were no side effects – they simply started feeling better and better.

The obvious conclusion: *women feel much better on natural bio-identical hormones.*

Medical studies have revealed some very interesting findings:
- A study in Sweden used a variety of estrogens topically, transdermally, and orally. (*Premarin* and *Provera* are rarely used in Europe.) Women who had the highest estrogen (either naturally produced by the ovaries or administered medically) had the least cognitive impairment. Women who used hormone replacement, primarily estradiol, saw their cognitive thinking abilities preserved by forty percent. [9]
- Multiple studies also confirm that natural progesterone and testosterone also protect the nervous system. Progesterone is an antioxidant and has the ability to regenerate nerves. *Provera* does none of that. In fact, it actually works negatively against our nerves. [10]
- Initially, *Premarin* was used by doctors to treat hot flushes. It was known that estrogen, including estrogen from a pregnant horse, would stimulate the inside lining of the uterus. Women who were taking only *Premarin* began developing uterine cancer because of overstimulation from estrogen. It was

known that natural progesterone given to women taking *Premarin* would protect the uterus from endometrial cancer.

But Big Pharma did not do the right thing, nor the sensible thing, nor the moral thing. Instead of giving women **natural** progesterone which had been available for thirty years, they came up with the idea of trying to improve on nature. *Provera* was developed by Big Pharma to protect against the disease of uterine cancer that they caused.

At this point, the options were (1) to recommend a natural hormone, progesterone, that the ovaries in women have been producing for thousands of years and functioning very effectively, or (2) to develop a patentable look-alike drug called *Provera*. The idea was to take something natural that the body produces **naturally** and make it better in a lab. Big Pharma could not patent natural progesterone, therefore there was no profit incentive to go that route. For forty years, doctors were told to use the FDA approved *Provera* for women to prevent uterine cancer.

The *Women's Health Initiative* report in 2002 demonstrated that Big Pharma had intentionally fooled doctors. *Provera* did not protect against heart attacks. It caused heart attacks. It did not prevent strokes as was advertised. It caused strokes and breast cancer in such large numbers that the FDA now had to admit that the risk was greater than the benefit. But Wyeth can still sell this drug to women! There has never been a study showing that natural progesterone causes heart attacks, strokes or breast cancer, but the FDA refuses to recommend the safer and more effective bio-identical progesterone over the synthetic dangerous *Provera*.

Synthetic *Provera* is not natural progesterone. But many doctors still believe what has been sold to them for years — that there is no difference between *Provera* and natural progesterone. To date, the company that manufactures *Prempro* (the combination of *Provera* and *Premarin*) has over 4,500 law suits to answer over these drugs.

Synthetic Provera is not natural progesterone.

Wyeth launched a massive lobbying campaign to eliminate BHRT arguing to the FDA that if *Prempro* is dangerous, BHRT must also be dangerous. This effort to eliminate the competition failed because there was not a shred of evidence that BHRT had any of the same dangerous side effects as *Prempro*. Another major reason Wyeth was not successful in banning Bio-identical Hormone Replacement Therapy was the hundreds of thousands of patients who screamed to the FDA to not take away their natural hormones.

What is so difficult to understand is that *Prempro* is still available in every pharmacy in the United States, even though it has been proven to cause cancer, heart disease, dementia, and strokes. Such is the power of Big Pharma! The only evidence Wyeth can produce that BHRT is dangerous is from studies done on FDA-approved **non-bio-identical** hormones and then try to extrapolate those side effects to BHRT. There is not the slightest evidence of any of the same dangers with the use of BHRT.

Traditional medicine has made a fatal error for decades by ignoring the thousands of studies that demonstrate the dangers of what they have used for over forty years. Traditional medicine has been exposed to nothing about the benefits of BHRT. I have found that the public usually knows more than their family doctor about natural hormones. When reading literature from traditional medicine, the same mantra will be repeated over and over: *there are no valid studies supporting the safety and efficacy of BHRT.* How ridiculous!

In this book alone, I will reference hundreds of studies that demonstrate what conventional medicine refuses to admit. Just use common sense and think about this: how could we as humans have procreated and survived for all these years if women's natural hormones caused heart disease, stroke and cancer?

It is doubtful if there will ever be another study like the *Women's Health Initiative* trial involving 160,000 women that will compare patented *Premarin* and *Provera* produced from horse urine in a lab in contrast to natural estradiol and progesterone that are found in every normally-functioning female. In other words, give one group of women synthetic hormones and the other natural bio-identical hormones and see which group fairs the best after seven years. But this will never happen because Big Pharma and the United States government know what the results would be. And they are the only ones who could afford to do such a study.

In addition to that, no major publications will showcase the contrast of synthetic vs. BHRT. These major publications depend on the money Big Pharma throws their way to publish studies of synthetic drugs. One will never see a national advertising campaign for bio-identical hormones. BHRT is not controlled by Big Pharma. And the pharmaceutical representatives and advertising industry will not expose doctors to anything but patented, dangerous, synthetic hormones.

Think about this: if we view declining hormone levels as a normal course of aging, then so is heart disease. Both can be traced back to aging. But they are treated so differently. When a patient shows signs of heart disease, treatment is readily available because pharmaceutical companies make a drug for this condition. But when a patient suffers from symptoms due to hormonal loss, traditional medicine simply calls that the normal effects of aging.

The diagnosis of "normal aging" trivializes that which will end in the death of the patient. Many of the conditions listed above—diabetes, high cholesterol, cardiovascular disease, Alzheimer's, high blood pressure—are closely related to hormonal deficiencies.

Why Not Make The Change?

Bio-identical hormones are also called "isomolecular" hormones. This is because the molecules of bio-identical hormones are structurally identical to the hormones one had in youth. There is no way of telling the difference. The molecular structure is exactly the same. This means the body cannot distinguish between bio-identical hormones and itself. The body does not see bio-identical hormones as a foreign substance. It recognizes bio-identical hormones as itself and metabolizes these hormones just as it would its own natural hormones. [11]

> *The body recognizes bio-identical hormones as itself and metabolizes these hormones just as it would its own natural hormones.*

That's why they are so safe. The body recognizes them as a *friend* rather than a *foe.*

What is so incredible is that these sex hormones can be safely and effectively administered to virtually every woman and man. The results of Bio-identical Hormone Replacement Therapy, improvement in symptoms and personality, are usually rapid ... the improvement is seen within days.

With all this understanding, why would anyone consider using synthetic hormonal treatment? Why wouldn't they go the BHRT route? What about you?

Journal thoughts and questions:

_____

_____

_____

_____

_____

_____

_____

_____

_____

_____

_____

_____

_____

_____

_____

_____

_____

CHAPTER 2

Normal Hormone Levels

*The reason you feel different and act different
than when you were younger is because ... you are different!*

A Woman's Changing Hormone Levels

**The goal of Bio-identical Hormone Replacement Therapy is to
bring those levels back to what they initially were.**

It's no secret that our hormone levels change drastically as we age. Consider these three examples:

- Testosterone levels in twenty-year-old women are typically between 70-90 ng/dL. But when women reach fifty years old, those levels drop significantly – to somewhere between 2-10 ng/dL.

**That means if you are fifty or older, you are operating on 5-10% of
the hormones you had in your body thirty years ago!**

The goal of *Bio-identical Hormone Replacement Therapy* is to bring those levels back to what they initially were.

- Estradiol in that same young female may be 200 pg/ml, but when she is fifty, it may be 5 or 10 pg/ml. That's 2-5% of the levels from thirty years earlier! She will be told by doctors that this is **"normal"** for her age. [12]
- Her progesterone when she was young ranged from 15 to 25 ng/ml, but now that she is fifty years old, it is .9 ng/ml. She will be told she is within normal range *"for her age."* Progesterone is one of the most important female hormones with many essential functions. A realistic goal is to increase her progesterone up to at least 5 ng/ml or even to 10 or 15 ng/ml.

So women, when your husband tells you *"You're not the woman I married!"* he now has medical proof!

But seriously, you knew that already, didn't you?

You knew that things were changing. You could feel it ... emotionally ... physically ... things just weren't the same. Oh, you couldn't put your finger on exactly what it was. You certainly didn't know the medical facts to prove it. But you knew something was different.

And what you were told is that these changes were **normal**, they were to be **expected**, and that there was **nothing** that could really be done about it.

A Man's Changing Testosterone Level

The question we have to ask is, "What are normal healthy levels for sex hormones?"

Men's hormone levels change also. Some hormones decline as we age. Most of us are able to maintain our normal healthy level of thyroid hormones, insulin, aldosterone, calcitonin, ACTH, melatonin, growth hormones, vasopressin, and cortisol. But our sex hormones do not remain at a normal healthy level. They drop considerably as we get older.

The question we have to ask is, *"What are normal healthy levels for sex hormones?"* We want our thyroid hormones to be normal, which implies we believe we are more likely to be healthy if our thyroid is *"normal."* Physicians and patients alike will interpret **normal** as meaning our hormones should be at the level they were when we were our healthiest, between eighteen and thirty years old.

That's true for thyroid levels, insulin levels ... everything *except sex hormones!* When a seventy-year-old man's sex hormone testosterone has declined by 90% from when he was twenty-five, doctors will tell him this is *"normal."*

"Normal?" We men know that's not true. We don't feel like real men anymore. We don't have the strength, the energy level, and especially the sexual drive and ability we once had. And that's not normal!

If a bone is broken, a doctor will set the bone back to **normal**. If thyroid levels or insulin levels are imbalanced, the proper medical practice is to seek to restore those to **normal** levels. It is odd to regard the decline of these hormones as *"normal"* when we consider that every cell in our body is programmed by hormonal messengers. The optimal function of every cell requires this hormonal programming. When we were young we had this stimulation of all our cells. Now we don't. How can anyone rationalize that the decline of hormonal activity below our youthful levels is acceptable or **normal**? [13]

Diminishing Sex Hormones

Most people don't know that their hormones begin to decline ten years or more before symptoms begin to occur.

Most of us know that our sex hormones begin to diminish with menopause and andropause (the male menopause). Think hot flashes, agitation, night sweats and decreased sex drive. Just as devastating conditions will result from the loss of thyroid hormones or insulin, the same is true when we lose our sex hormones. Apparently traditional doctors believe that maintaining all of our hormones is good – except testosterone, estradiol and progesterone. Somehow those get the *"effects of aging"* label applied to them.

The majority of people don't know that their hormones begin to decline ten years or more before symptoms begin to occur. The old adage *"Lordy, Lordy ... Joe is forty!"* holds some truth. Men are not the same at forty as we were at twenty-five.

And the worse is yet to come. By the time Joe is fifty or sixty, and certainly by seventy, he is certainly going to feel the effects of declining hormones. At seventy years old, Joe's testosterone is likely to be ten percent of what it was when he was twenty-five years old.

Perhaps we would be more conscientious about maintaining our sex hormones at normal healthy levels if we called them *"Health Maintaining Hormones"* (HMHs).

Another author, Eugene Shippen, MD, in his book *Testosterone Syn*drome picked up on this theme even more:

For instance, lower levels of testosterone and estrogen have serious deleterious effects on the proper functioning of the brain, resulting in a decrease in mental sharpness. This means that these hormones, whose functions would appear to be limited since we refer to them as "sex" hormones, turn out to be also brain hormones ... testosterone and estrogen are also muscle hormones and bone hormones, skin hormones and energy hormones, mood hormones and urinary tract hormones. [14]

What Do We Do?

Do we sit back and wait for the inevitable to happen? Do we take the chance with traditional medicine and its artificial replacements? Or do we change our thinking – and our actions – and choose BHRT?

Our choice should be based on the following three criteria:

- Is it safer?
- Is it proven?
- Is it effective?

Ask yourself those questions. Investigate the facts about *Bio-identical Hormone Replacement Therapy*. Here's what you will find:

- **BHRT is safer because it uses natural hormones that the body knows. They** are easily assimilated into the body and are not a foreign substance.
- **BHRT is proven.** In this book you will see over eleven-hundred endnote references that will tell you of the dangers of synthetic hormone replacement and the power and safety of natural hormone replacement. Many of you will want to pass over those endnotes. However, I encourage you to check them out – solid, respected medical leaders and thorough research studies prove what we are talking about in this book.
- **BHRT is effective.** It works. You will read many stories in this book of happy patients who have had their lives restored. I could tell you many hundreds more.

Journal thoughts and questions:

_____

_____

_____

_____

_____

_____

_____

_____

_____

_____

_____

_____

_____

_____

_____

_____

_____

CHAPTER 3

The Effect Hormones Have On Your Body

"You can't stop the future. You can't rewind the past. The only way to learn the secret ... is to press play." Jay Asher, *Thirteen Reasons Why*

Change is On Its Way

Physicians by the thousands are turning to the use of bio-identical hormone replacement therapy.

Fifty years ago, when a woman went to her doctor to deal with hot flashes and other symptoms, she heard the words, *"That's just a part of getting older."*

Thirty years ago, a woman would have received a treatment plan that *"Synthetic hormone treatment is the only way to go."*

But now she has options.

The way doctors practice medicine has changed dramatically. We can see it happening today. Physicians by the thousands are turning to the use of bio-identical hormone replacement therapy instead of traditional hormone replacement which is prescription drugs and synthetic hormones. Those that refuse to recognize the extremely positive benefits of bio-identical hormones often have not exerted the effort to investigate the science of BHRT, but simply accepted what is fed them by Big Pharma.

Hormones control every cell of our body and are more powerful than drugs. Hormones affect even our genes. Our health depends on hormonal balance.

How Hormones Work in the Body

Testosterone is a vital male hormone that is responsible for the development and maintenance of male attributes. Women also have testosterone, but in much smaller amounts. Testosterone stimulates the DNA in specific genes in the body to keep our genes healthy instead of going haywire. When things go haywire, they may lead to cancer, Alzheimer's, diabetes, hypertension, heart disease, decreased resistance to infections and arthritis. [15] [16]

Hormones influence the DNA of trillions of cells and genes. They stimulate DNA to produce proteins which are the building blocks for the human body. These proteins affect how we grow, our sexual traits, our brain function, our strength, our circulation, our ability to fight infection and stress and even cancer. With the hormonal deficiencies of aging, our cells cannot function to maintain health. [17]

The word hormone is derived from a Greek word that means *"to set in motion."* Hormones pass through the blood stream communicating messages from the brain to the DNA in each of the trillions of cells. The membranes of each cell have receptor sites that function as a lock to a door. Hormones are powerful chemical messengers that control vital organs in the body. In order for the hormone to enter into a cell to pass on the biochemical messages from the brain, it has to unlock the receptor sites on specific "target cells."

As the hormone comes in contact with the target cells with its message from the brain, the hormone binds to the receptor site. A particular receptor site will respond only to a particular *"key"* that *"opens that particular door"* to that cell. Once inside the cell, the hormone sets in motion the DNA in the cell to perform its function—making more hormones or producing proteins.

If a target cell is a muscle, the hormone may cause the muscle to relax or contract. Another target cell may be a gland. The hormone may cause that gland to produce a particular hormone (for example, estradiol or progesterone or testosterone) or it may cause the gland to stop producing such hormones.

You can see that these actions by a hormone secreted by the brain can have great effect over vital functions in the entire body.

The problem occurs when the target cells stop responding to the stimulus from the hormone secreted by the hypothalamus and the pituitary gland. The target organs might be the testicles. When they stop responding to the hormone "luteinizing hormone," they cannot produce as much testosterone as they did 30 years ago. The result causes andropause in men.

The same is true with the ovaries in women. When they cannot produce enough testosterone or progesterone or estradiol in response to follicle stimulating hormone, it causes the typical menopausal symptoms in women.

> ***"Hormones are our life force; the decline of hormones is the hallmark of aging. Without hormone replacement, we will end up mere shells of our former selves."***

But all is not hopeless. The hormones that are no longer produced in the testicles or ovaries can be replaced with bio-identical hormones that have the EXACT molecular structure that matches exactly the natural hormone it is replacing. Anything else that is a pseudo hormone – an almost-the-same hormone – is dangerous as seen in the results of the *Women's Health Initiative Trial*.

As noted by Suzan Somers in her book *Ageless: The Naked Truth about Bio-identical Hormones,*

"Hormones are our life force; the decline of hormones is the hallmark of aging. Without hormone replacement, we will end up mere shells of our former selves." [18]

It is not just a coincidence that the increased incidence of late life illnesses that cause so much disability and death results at the same time in life as the decline of hormones.

Without hormones, proteins are not produced. Instead of repairing and regenerating our bodies, there is a continued breakdown of body processes. Proteins help prevent the disease processes of aging such as cognitive (brain function) decline, osteoporosis, depression, atherosclerosis, immune dysfunction, and even loss of libido. These are chronic diseases that require life-long drug therapy. But if our hormones are functioning correctly, our bodies maintain the building blocks necessary for good health naturally.

The list of what hormones do is extensive. But here is a sample list of what hormones do in our bodies:

- Helps us sleep
- Keeps our energy high
- Regulates heartbeat
- Helps undo stress
- Regulates respiration
- Helps preserve memories
- Prevents fatigue
- Keeps us calm
- Keeps bones strong
- Keeps muscles of heart strong
- Maintains proper growth
- Helps to fight infection
- Keeps muscles strong
- Helps prevent allergic reactions
- Keeps control blood pressure
- Helps pain relief
- Stimulates sex drive
- Keeps joints stable
- Regulates body temperature
- Provides for fertility
- Helps our body burn fat
- Regulates energy
- Maintains virility
- Maintains menstrual cycle
- Helps prevent cancer
- Provides proper immune system
- Maintains brain function
- Provides and maintains pregnancy

It is easy to fall into the trap of thinking that all these problems are just inevitable. You may think you're going to die because you are tired. But you have to consider *why* you are so tired all the time. *Why are things so different from a year ago?* When our memory lapses, we wonder if we'll ever remember anything again. When our sex life diminishes or ends, we imagine the worst. But we don't have to settle for low energy. But memory lapses do not mean the end of our life. And our sex life doesn't have to end just because we get older.

The reason you cannot remember well is because something is happening to your brain. Perhaps it is due to poor blood circulation or a lack of production of neurotransmitters such as serotonin. Instead of passing it off as aging or prescribing an antidepressant, a doctor should ask, *"Why is this patient having poor memory or depression or has decreased resistance to infections?"* Your body is sending you a signal that something is wrong. You and your doctor need to respond to it.

A physician caring for a patient who is having anxiety should not automatically write a prescription for an antianxiety medication. The question should be, *"Why is this patient now so anxious? Three years ago she was happy and carefree."*

Emotional Health

It is no secret that hormones play a major role in our physical health. They also affect our emotional health. Hormonal imbalance has been the cause of much emotional trauma. Marriages and relationships have suffered because of it.

When someone experiences major changes in their body, they know something is happening ... but they can't explain it. Emotional symptoms might include:

- Fear of the future
- Fear of the unknown
- Anxiety
- Depression
- Anger
- Disorientation
- Loss of focus

They end up taking their anger and fear and frustration out on others, especially on the ones they love.

And, of course, it's become the subject of much humor as well. To say that men need help in understanding their wives is a classic understatement. The following chart says it all:

THE HORMONE GUIDE *How To Speak to Women*			
Dangerous	**Safer**	**Safest**	**Ultra Safe**
What's for dinner?	Can I help you with dinner?	Where would you like to go for dinner?	Here, honey, have some wine!
Are you wearing that?	You sure look good in brown!	Wow! Look at you!	Here, honey, have some wine!
What are you so worked up about?	Could we be overreacting?	Here's my paycheck.	Here, honey, have some wine!!
Should you be eating that?	You know, there are a lot of apples left.	Can I get you a piece of chocolate with that?	Here, honey, have some wine!
What did you DO all day?	I hope you didn't over-do it today.	I've always loved you in that robe!	Here, honey, have some wine!

We laugh at things like that ... but hormonal imbalance is no laughing matter.

Understanding the Symptoms

In a recent study in the United Kingdom, it was shown that anxiolytic, hypnotic medications may triple mortality risk. [19] A study of more than 100,000 age- and sex-matched patients showed that those who used nerve medicines and/or hypnotics were 3 times more likely to die prematurely during the 7-year follow-up period than those who did not use these drugs. Clearly we can recognize that such medical treatment is suspect. When such symptoms are so very common to women at this exact age, the treating physician should see a pattern. The problem with women in this age group is **not** that they have a **Valium** deficiency, but a **hormone** deficiency. Doctors, please check their hormones!

Symptoms of a perimenopausal or menopausal patient should be a flashing red warning light of what is happening inside. When your doctor says, *"Tell me, how you are doing? How do you feel?"* he or she is not asking those questions to be social.

How you feel is a representation of how your body is performing. Every physician knows full well that when a patient says she is feeling much better after being treated for pneumonia the chest x-ray is more likely to show improvement. When a patient says she is worse and feels like she may not survive, the doctor should be very concerned. Symptoms are signals trying to say something is wrong.

When a woman begins experiencing symptoms that were not present two years earlier, and now describes a list of ten problems that she is feeling, something has happened. She may be told, *"You are just getting older."* But that doesn't help anyone. Many women see their doctor and report that they are irritable, tired, have lots of stress, irregular menstrual cycles, vaginal dryness, no orgasms or lackluster orgasms at best. Some women have even been known to say they would rather clean the toilet than have sex. Folks, that's drastic!

Women at times have the impression that their doctor feels like they are just nuts or a hypochondriac. Because of these negative vibes from their doctors, many women just suffer in silence.

What's needed is understanding, compassion – and, above all, insight into proper treatment.

Journal thoughts and questions:

_____

_____

_____

_____

_____

_____

_____

_____

_____

_____

_____

_____

_____

_____

_____

_____

_____

_____

_____

CHAPTER 4

The Women's Health Initiative And Synthetic Hormones

"The first indication of menopause is a broken thermostat."

Glenda's Story

Glenda was a forty-nine-year-old mother of three who worked in a government office as a computer engineer. She was very well educated ... but suffering terribly. She called our office to tell her story:

I have been having hot flashes so bad that I had to take three changes of clothes to work with me every day. When I enter my work place I have to go through three different clearances. It was so embarrassing to have three changes of clothes to be inspected. I had the pellet hormone treatment done last week on Friday. After three days, I have not had one hot flash. Now I take no change of clothes to work. I can't believe what has happened. I've been using hormone creams for two years without hardly any help. I'm telling everyone I can what happened to me!

Glenda's story is not unusual. Thousands of women have been helped by BHRT. It's a known fact.

The Medical Scoop

In this chapter, we're going to look at some of the medical facts and research behind hormone treatment. I must warn you ... this is one of those deep "medical-speak" chapters. If you're not one who is drawn to all the medical facts and research, feel free to skip this chapter.

But for the rest of you, I think you will see the importance of knowing the medical research behind this treatment. That is especially true for those of you in the medical community who are reading this book. Knowing the truth is essential to accurately understanding the hormone battle.

Most of the conversation so far has been about women. There is a reason for that. It is not fair, but women suffer much more than men as they age. Doctors are ill-equipped to handle most of these kinds of problems. In medical school before 2002 when the *Women's Health Initiative* study reported its devastating results, doctors-to-be were taught to prescribe *Premarin* and *Provera* (also known as *Prempro* when both are in the same pill) to all women going through menopause who complained of the typical symptoms of hot flashes, night sweats, hair loss, poor sleep, anxiety, and depression.

The *Women's Health Initiative* (WHI) was a very large study of 160,000 women who were healthy and menopausal between age fifty and seventy-nine. The study was planned for eight and a half years but terminated after five years for ethical reasons. The risks outweighed the benefits. [20]

For years doctors were told that *Prempro* would reduce the chance of heart disease and strokes, prevent cognitive (brain function) decline, improve mood and promote more sexual satisfaction. This recommendation was based on a faulty study. It was not a double-blind placebo controlled cross-over scientific study. We now know that *Prempro* is a bad drug actually causing atherosclerosis and cognitive decline (brain fog and poor memory).

Other Side Effects of Premarin Include:
- Vaginal bleeding
- Uterine fibroids
- Endometriosis
- Blood clots
- Fluid retention (edema)
- Tender breasts
- Headaches
- Gall stones
- Leg cramps
- Nausea and vomiting
- Heart attacks
- Strokes
- Diabetes
- High blood pressure
- Endometrial cancer
- Breast cancer

Prempro actually caused an increase in breast cancer by twenty-six percent after four years. The cancers found in the *Prempro* group compared to non-users were larger, were at more advanced stages when found, and were more likely to have spread to nearby lymph nodes. Heart disease also increased with the use of *Prempro* by twenty-nine percent and an increase by eighty-one percent during the first year of use. *Prempro* caused a doubling of the risk of dementia including Alzheimer's disease. Blood clots in the lungs and legs doubled with the use of *Prempro.* Strokes increased by forty-one percent. Urinary incontinence also increased with *Prempro.* [21]

Using natural human hormones for humans – instead of horse hormones for humans – just makes sense!

It was in the 1970s that the cancer rate of menopausal women began to escalate dramatically by over three hundred percent—with 200,000 new cases per year. This trend continued to steadily incline until 1999 when some began to question the dangers of traditional hormone therapy. In 2003 the rate of breast cancer began to decline by eighteen percent. Because of the findings of the WHI, the sales of *Prempro* dropped by seventy-four percent. The number of women who were on *Prempro* – eighteen and one-half million – declined to 7.6 million, a drop of sixty-nine percent. [22]

This was the first time since 1945 a decline in breast cancer was seen as women were stopping their *Prempro*. The reason, of course, was the results of the federally funded *Women's Health Initiative* study in 2002. In the next six months sales of *Prempro* dropped by fifty percent and have continued to decline since.

The public has spoken—pseudo hormones are not what women want. Instead, BHRT has dramatically increased. How could Big Pharma be so wrong? Using natural human hormones for humans – instead of horse hormones for humans – just makes sense! [23] [24]

There was another arm of the *Women's Health Initiative* study that involved women who had no uterus. It was thought that if a woman had no uterus, she did not need *Provera*. So this group took only *Premarin*. *Premarin* without *Provera* did not increase the risk of heart attacks as it did when *Premarin* was combined with *Provera*. *Premarin* did cause more strokes by a significant margin. However, there was less risk of hip fractures and perhaps a lower risk of breast cancer when *Provera* was not used. [25]

The Response of the FDA

With the above disastrous findings showing the dangerous, even deadly, effects of *Prempro*, the Federal Drug Administration issued a warning — an especially strong warning. They mandated a "black box" warning that stated all estrogen replacement products should have the same.

...increased risks of myocardial infarction (heart attack), stroke, invasive breast cancer, pulmonary emboli (blood clots in the lungs), and deep vein thrombosis (blood clots in the legs), in postmenopausal women during 5 years of treatment with conjugated equine estrogen (Premarin) combined with medroxyprogesterone (Provera) relative to placebo. [26]

The *Women's Health Initiative* trial found dangers when *Premarin* was used in combination with *Provera*. No study was done confirming that when bio-identical hormones were used the same dangers would be found.

Think of it this way: If Toyota Camrys were found to have brake problems, the Camry is identified as having the defect. The warning is not that all automobiles have brake problems. But this is exactly what the FDA did. In the WHI Study *Premarin* plus *Provera* caused heart attacks, strokes, breast cancer and dementia.

But the conclusion pushed by Wyeth toward the FDA was that ***all*** hormones must do the same.

Traditional medicine recognizes only patented (manufactured by a drug company) synthetic hormones as viable hormone treatment. The usual traditional doctor barely recognizes that bio-identical hormones even exist and believes that bio-identical hormones have the same side effects as synthetic hormones. Fortunately, through education and books like this, that is in the process of changing in America!

It is usual for the FDA to remove a drug from the market when the medication causes cancer and has no redeeming life-saving benefits. But in this case, the FDA allowed *Premarin* and *Provera* to continue being used – as long as the dose was decreased. This approval of a lower dose of *Prempro* was made by the FDA without any further studies providing evidence that a lower dose was safe – and it clearly has no lifesaving benefits. Eventually, a study released in 2003 concluded that Premarin was not safer with a lower dose. [27]

In Conclusion

The medical community must step up and face the facts. The reality is that synthetic hormone replacement is dangerous and has terrible side effects. But many studies have shown conclusively that bio-identical hormones are safe and effective. It is obvious that BHRT is very effective in relieving hot flushes and vaginal dryness, but also protects against heart disease, cancer, mental decline, and osteoporosis. FDA approved drugs can never claim this. [28]

Journal thoughts and questions:

_____

_____

_____

_____

_____

_____

_____

_____

_____

_____

_____

_____

_____

_____

_____

_____

_____

_____

_____

_____

CHAPTER 5

The Writing Is On The Wall

"It's Tough to Make Predictions ... Especially about the Future!"

Can We At Least Run The Tests?

"I just want to know!"

That's all patients want – to know the truth. They have a right to know what is going on inside their bodies.

Sandy was a forty-two-year-old patient who reported to us, *"I begged my doctor to check my hormones."* But his response was, *"Checking your hormones won't do any good. I believe your problem is depression. Here is a prescription for Lexapro. Try it for a month and tell me how you are feeling."*

She said she knew that she wasn't depressed and refused to take the medication.

Sandy knew something was wrong ... but her doctor wouldn't run the tests. His instant diagnosis and treatment was to put her on medication for something he *thought* was wrong. But Sandy, an untrained lay person, knew her body. She knew something was wrong – but she also knew she wasn't depressed.

> ***When your body needs hormones, the signals will be anxiety, hot flashes, night sweats, irritability, poor sleep, decreased mental acumen, depression and low sex drive.***

That doctor took the easy way out in prescribing *Lexapro.* No patient, male or female, should be denied having their hormones checked and interpreted by a knowledgeable doctor.

The writing was on the wall – the doctor just refused to read it!

The body is constantly searching for proper balance or equilibrium. When your body needs water, you feel thirsty. When you are cold, you will have the urge to put on a coat or turn up the thermostat. When your body needs hormones, the signals will be anxiety, hot flashes, night sweats, irritability, poor sleep, decreased mental acumen, depression and low sex drive.

Getting to the Root Cause

It is important to identify the root cause of what's wrong – and not settling for treating the symptoms. It is not good for the doctor to automatically reach for the prescription pad and write for a drug that tries to suppress the symptoms without searching for why she is this way.

When someone is short of breath or has chest pains when they exercise, there is a reason why. Something is wrong – and the pain is our body's way of letting us know. It is known that middle-aged men with symptoms of low testosterone are at risk of increased narrowing of the carotid artery that leads to the brain. Studies have shown that normal testosterone levels offer protection against atherosclerosis. [29]

Many studies point to low hormones contributing to the development of the metabolic syndrome (obesity, elevated blood pressure, elevated fasting plasma glucose, high serum triglycerides and low HDL—high-density cholesterol) which increases the risk for coronary vascular disease. [30]

It is not surprising to know so many diseases develop as hormones diminish with aging when it is so often seen that those between the ages of thirty and forty have very few of the symptoms listed above. The difference between those under forty and those above forty is hormone levels. Estrogen increases HDL (good cholesterol) and decreases the bad cholesterol (LDL). Estrogen also reduces overall risk of heart disease by forty to fifty percent in men. [31]

Doctors are Stuck Today

Very few physicians understand the interplay between testosterone, progesterone and estradiol, especially in women, but also in men. In the next few chapters you will learn more about hormones than the majority of doctors have learned with years of medical education and practice.

I must admit that I was in their same position. As I said earlier in the book, it wasn't until I started investigating the facts, reading the medical studies, and coming to my own conclusions (apart from the influence of Big Pharma) that I understood what natural hormones can positively do for our bodies and how synthetic hormones can affect us negatively.

The sad truth is that traditional or mainstream medicine is stuck. Doctors today do not see the need to address sexual concerns which affect quality of life as high a priority as other medical issues. When mainstream medicine does not recognize sexual problems as important, women will suffer. They will continue to be untreated and will suffer adverse health consequences and will experience unnecessary personal relationship problems and have a poor quality of life as a result of not having hormonal issues treated properly.

Are we getting to the root of the problem …
or are we just treating symptoms?

Since the discovery of penicillin two generations ago, the medical education of doctors has told them:

- If their patient has a strep bacterial infection, use penicillin
- If they have an infection in the bladder, use trimethoprim sulfa
- If they cannot sleep, prescribe Ambien
- If they have anxiety issues, give them Valium
- If they have heartburn, write a prescription for Nexium.

And ... if the patient has lost interest in things that used to bring them pleasure, they must be depressed. So pull out the script pad and write a prescription for an antidepressant.

You can see the trend.

The difficulty is ... are we getting to the root of the problem ... or are we just treating symptoms?

What Needs to Be Done?

The problem in treating women's hormonal issues is much more difficult than the above treatment plan of giving drugs to treat only symptoms. The treatment plan should involve:

- Taking a very detailed history of all related symptoms, a family history of hormonal issues, medications the patient is using, treatments doctors have tried in the past, and the results from those treatments.
- A complete physical exam should be performed including an evaluation of the mental status of the patient, of the cardiovascular system including appropriate blood work for lipids, the respiratory system, the orthopedic system looking for evidence of osteoporosis, the genitourinary system looking for genital atrophy, vaginal dryness, uterine fibroids, looking for fibrocystic breast disease and evaluating the thyroid. A pap smear is mandatory as well as a mammogram. Men should also have a PSA and perhaps a digital rectal exam. (Many doctors now question if performing a PSA and a digital rectal exam are necessary.)
- Detailed blood work should be done such as the following:
  - Lipid Panel with a breakdown of sub-particles
  - Vitamin B12
  - Complete Blood Count with a differential
  - Comprehensive Metabolic Profile
  - C-Reactive Protein
  - Homocysteine
  - Cystatin C
  - Cortisol
  - DHEA—dehydroepiandrosterone
  - Estradiol (E2)
  - Folate
  - Follicle Stimulating Hormone (FSH)
  - HbA1c
  - Iron Metabolism Study
  - Luteinizing Hormone (LH)
  - Phosphorus
  - Magnesium
  - Progesterone (P4)
  - Free Testosterone
  - Bioavailable Testosterone
  - Total Testosterone
  - T3 and T4
  - Thyroid Stimulating Hormone (TSH)

o   Reverse T3

Men should have the same tests run plus:
    o   PSA
    o   Sex Hormone Binding Globulin (SHBG)
    o   Prolactin

A FSH is not necessary in men.

How to Interpret Lab Studies

A major problem occurs when the treating physician does not recognize the meaning of the results of each of the above tests. It has been said, *"Don't do a test if you don't want to know the results."* The reason for this warning to doctors is if you do not want to handle the problem a test may show, don't order the test.

What happens if a doctor knows very little about hormone replacement therapy and the patient asks the doctor's advice after the lab reports that she has low hormone levels?

The doctor with limited knowledge of hormones will now have to decide what to do about these very low results. The doctor may say, *"These results look normal for your age."*

Intuitively the patient knows this is not true because of the way she feels. The obvious response by the patient is going to be, *"So, why do I feel this way? Why am I having hot flashes, and night sweats? Why am I so irritable and depressed? I am not normally a depressed person."* The patient who has read any of the many books on bio-identical hormones will know the doctor is wrong when she says, *"You will just have to live with it."* The patient will go elsewhere looking for help.

Numerous patients report that they cannot get their doctor to check hormone levels. The real reason may be that the doctor doesn't know what to do when the results come back. And so they follow the dictum: *"Don't check her hormones if you don't know how to interpret the results."*

What's the Prescribed Course of Action?

What should you do as a patient? Let me suggest a few courses of action:
- **Know yourself.** To the best of your ability, write down what is going on inside of you, both physically and emotionally.
- **Read about the issues.** You are already doing that by picking up this book. Don't go into a medical appointment blind. By reading and studying the issues, you may very well know more than the doctor you are going to see.
- **Interview your doctor.** Is he/she up-to-date on bio-identical hormone treatment? Will they treat the real problem, or will they simply cover up the symptoms? What educational training has he/she had in bio-identical hormone treatment?
- **Don't settle for old, outdated information.** The study of medicine is constantly progressing – yet your doctor may be stuck with the information he/she got thirty years ago in medical school.

Remember, it's tough to make predictions ... especially about the future. But if you are armed with the right information, it surely makes it a lot easier!

Journal thoughts and questions:

_____

_____

_____

_____

_____

_____

_____

_____

_____

_____

_____

_____

_____

_____

_____

_____

CHAPTER 6

Millions Of Women Suffer Without Hormones

"You Don't Know What You've Got Till It's Gone"

Demographic Realities

There are more than 144,000,000 women in the United States. Thirty-three million of them are fifty-five years old or older. These thirty-three million women will live another twenty-eight years, fully one-third of their lives, without hormones. There are approximately 65,000,000 women who are menopausal and an unknown number who are perimenopausal. These women will spend more than half of their lives without live-giving hormones. [32]

Wrong Thinking: *You can be just as healthy without sex hormones (or health hormones).*

That just isn't true. We need sex hormones for a healthy lifestyle.

Dr. Thierry Hertoghe, a very well respected, internationally known third-generation endocrinologist, said, *"Lack of hormones is what is truly dangerous."* [33]

Please read that sentence again: *"Lack of hormones is what is truly dangerous."*

What Dr. Hertoghe is saying has two very significant implications:

- **First**, if you have hormone deficiencies, you must get treatment. Your life literally depends on it.
- **Second**, if you are a medical professional, it is your *responsibility* to treat patients who have hormone deficiencies. To simply prescribe pills that mask those symptoms is not responsible treatment.

The problem physicians faced after the *Women's Health Initiative Trial* was that many wrongly interpreted the dangers associated with traditional hormone replacement using *Premarin* and *Provera* to apply to all types of hormone replacement. The thought of *"hormone replacement"* has developed such a negative connotation that the majority of physicians have turned away from any kind of hormone replacement treatment.

Terry's Story

When Terry came to us for treatment, she reported,

After my hysterectomy I told my surgeon that he had to do something. I can't live like this. He told me he could not give me Premarin because it causes cancer. But here is a prescription for Lexapro, an antidepressant. After taking that I started to gain weight and it killed my sex drive completely. I am forty-five and my husband is thirty-seven. He told me sex once every four months ain't going to get it. But it hurts so bad when we have sex because I am so dry. I'm afraid of losing my marriage.

Terry was treated with Pellet Bio-identical Replacement Therapy. When she returned for follow-up in 1 month she was crying with happiness. Her words were, *"This saved my marriage."*

There are thousands of women suffering because they are not able to take advantage of hormone replacement therapy because their doctor is afraid to give them anything after the results of the *Women's Health Initiative Trial*. But there are women who are also afraid to take any kind of hormones because of this same fear. Traditional doctors are now beginning to realize that bio-identical hormone replacement is safer and more efficacious that traditional hormones.

"This saved my marriage."

Foreign or Identical? Synthetic or Natural? Your Choice.

The three sex hormones are testosterone, estradiol and progesterone. All of these hormones can be found as bio-identical hormones used to treat hormone deficiencies.

Your body does not know how to handle foreign chemicals.

The Endocrine Society has defined bio-identical hormones as *"compounds that have exactly the same chemical and molecular structure as hormones that are produced in the human body."*

This means that the body "sees" bio-identical hormones as it sees itself. They are **identical**. This is extremely important. Traditional hormone replacement therapy uses drugs. Drugs are medically defined as therapeutic substances whose structure and nature are **foreign** to the human organism. Hormones, then, are not drugs. Hormones are molecules produced by our own glands and therefore do not come with the undesirable side effects of traditional hormone drugs — as long as the hormones prescribed are **identical** to those made by the body. [34]

The human body has natural enzymes made to process natural hormones. When a drug is introduced to the human body whose structure and nature are foreign to the human organism, there are side effects. Many of these bring negative consequences.

Just read on a package insert or listen to an advertisement and notice the long list of consequences to using drugs. The reason for these side effects is the body does not know how to handle foreign chemicals. A splinter in your finger is that recognized by the body as something that is foreign and harmful. Your body reacts by forming pus, trying to get rid of the foreign body.

When you take a drug that the body does not recognize as itself, it reacts with side effects. These might include nausea and vomiting, blood clots, fluid retention, breast cancer, heart attacks, or weight gain.

Listen to what your body is telling you: *something is not right!*
Common Side Effects of Premarin:
- Blood clots
- Breast tenderness

- Fluid retention
- Gall stones
- Headaches
- High blood pressure
- Impaired glucose tolerance
- Increased risk of diabetes
- Increased risk of endometrial cancer
- Increased risk of breast cancer
- Increased risk of stroke
- Increased risk of stroke
- Leg cramps
- Nausea
- Vomiting
- Worsened uterine fibroids
- Worsened endometriosis [35]

A Closer Look at the Two Hormones Used in the Women's Health Initiative Trial

The first hormone used in the *Women's Health Initiative Trial* was *Premarin.* It is conjugated equine estrogen (CEE). Do you see the word "equine?" That should set off a warning alarm in itself – it comes from a horse! In other words, it's not natural to the human body. But it gets worse: it comes from the urine of a pregnant horse.

I always wonder, *"Where do scientists come up with these things?"*

The other hormone used in the *Women's Health Initiative Study* was *Provera*, a progestin. *Provera* is a synthetic chemical. The word "synthetic" used in the context of hormones could mean *"not having the same chemical formulation as found in the human body."* Later, many studies will be presented demonstrating the extreme danger of taking this artificial hormone. When *Premarin* and *Provera* are combined in the same pill it is called *Prempro*. Instead of using a dangerous synthetic hormone, a safe, bio-identical progesterone can be used. It is bio-identical to what the ovaries naturally produce.

Multiple studies demonstrate that the medroxyprogesterone acetate (MPA) part of *Prempro* is a very bad actor causing an elevation in cholesterol and cardiovascular disease.

The Suffering Must Stop!

I shudder to think how many women today suffer through hormonal loss. Their health is damaged, their quality of life is shattered, and their hope is lost. For those who turn to synthetic hormones, the side effects may be worse than the symptoms they originally had.

"Modern science" and Big Pharma have sold us a bill of goods that is a lie. It must be exposed. These women must hear the truth about bio-identical hormone replacement. It literally can save their lives!

Journal thoughts and questions:

_____

_____

_____

_____

_____

_____

_____

_____

_____

_____

_____

_____

_____

_____

_____

_____

_____

_____

_____

CHAPTER 7

Understanding Bio-Identical Hormones

"The first and most necessary part is to understand."

Where Do Bio-identical Hormones Come From?

Let's address the term *"Bio-identical Hormone Replacement Therapy."* What does it mean? What are bio-identical hormones, and where do they come from?

Bio-identical hormones are made from wild Mexican yams or occasionally soy. From these plants diosgenin is extracted. Your compounding pharmacist (we'll talk more about who they are in the next chapter) converts diosgenin to the bio-identical hormones testosterone, estradiol, or progesterone by adding an enzyme. Over-the-counter progesterone that can be bought without a prescription usually does not contain this enzyme and should be avoided. Some bio-identical hormones are manufactured by pharmaceutical companies that are FDA approved.

To understand bio-identical hormones, we first have to know about traditional hormone replacement. What most physicians use for hormone imbalance are *Premarin* (the one made from horse urine) and *Provera*. There are other pills, vaginal creams, vaginal rings and injections.

Bio-identical Hormone Replacement Therapy (BHRT) describes supplementation of hormones that are molecularly identical to those hormones produced in the human body. Unlike manufactured Conventional Hormone Therapy, the hormones used in BHRT do not contain extra structural elements which may alter hormone receptor binding and function in the human body.

Compounded bio-identical hormone replacement therapy is a form of personalized medicine whereby the dose, regimen, and dosage forms are customized based on the patient's symptoms, hormone levels, and preferences. Compounded bio-identical hormone replacement therapy is perceived to be more effective, better tolerated, with fewer health risks than its conventional hormone therapy counterpart.

What Should I Expect from My Physician?

Physicians specializing in BHRT will listen to your complaints, do a physical exam and check your blood for a variety of substances including hormones, complete blood count, blood sugar, thyroid hormones, lipids (cholesterol and triglycerides), etc.

From these tests, a prescription is written for the hormone or hormones you need and the strength (the milligram dosage) that is required to bring your hormones back to a healthy level. No two people are going to be the same and neither will they have the same hormone needs. This requires a great deal of expertise in administering bio-identical hormones. ***"One-size-fits-all" medicine is easy, but practicing good medicine requires more skill.***

A prescription is written for the hormone(s) you need and the strength (dosage) required to bring your hormones back to a healthy level.

Most physicians who use bio-identical hormones use compounded hormones. The advantage is the doctor can order the exact strength of each hormone that the patient needs. Traditional medicine uses the "one-size-fits-all" approach. The pharmaceutical company makes *Prempro* so everyone gets exactly the same thing – *Prempro* – in exactly the same dosage. It is unlikely that any patient will have a *Prempro* deficiency; but she may very well have a deficiency of testosterone and/or estradiol and/or progesterone. Each patient has her unique needs.

Continued monitoring needs to occur.

Not only does the initial treatment need to be tailored to that particular patient, but continued monitoring needs to occur. When the patient returns for a follow-up visit, she will again have blood tests done to see what her hormone levels are after she has been on the treatment. The doctor will also ask probing questions and listen to her as she describes how she has felt. At this point she may need a little more of one hormone and not another.

What are the Benefits of BHRT?

There are a myriad of benefits from bio-identical hormone replacement therapy. We'll discuss these throughout the remainder of the book. This chart summarizes many of those benefits:

Various benefits will be discussed as we learn more about bioidentical hormone replacement therapy including:	
Improved sleep	Improved mood
Better concentration	Sharper memory
Better health of the urinary system	Better lipids (cholesterol and triglycerides)
Less chance of uterine cancer	Reduced risk of breast cancer
Marked reduction of hot flushes	Reduced night sweats
More vaginal moisture	Less thinning of the vaginal mucosa
Reduces chance of osteoporosis	Providing for stronger muscles
Protection from heart attacks	Protection from strokes
Less depression	Less anxiety and stress
Prevention from dementia	Prevention of Alzheimer's disease
Stronger libido	Enhancing orgasms

What Would a Traditional Doctor Do?

This is completely different from the experience a patient would receive when taking *Prempro*. It is inconceivable that a doctor, after giving a patient *Prempro*, would say, *"I am going to check your Prempro blood level to see if you need more or less Prempro."*

Think about it this way: a doctor would not treat high blood pressure without checking your blood pressure. Nor would your cholesterol be treated without a blood test to determine cholesterol levels. Your doctor is always going to check your blood sugar if you are a diabetic. But to check your sex hormones, many doctors will tell you ... *"You don't need to have your hormones checked; what you are experiencing is just part of aging."*

There is a Difference

We have entered a new age in medicine where we are able to treat people more naturally and more effectively. Doctors today who specialize in BHRT are thoroughly equipped to help you restore the energy and passion in your life that you so desperately want.

I hope you can tell by now that there is a difference – ***a world of difference*** – between conventional hormone replacement and bio-identical hormone replacement treatment.

Journal thoughts and questions:

_____

_____

_____

_____

_____

_____

_____

_____

_____

_____

_____

_____

_____

_____

_____

_____

_____

_____

_____

CHAPTER 8

What Is A Compounding Pharmacy?

"We're all different. We are not the same.
So why does traditional medicine treat us all the same way?"

Different Strokes for Different Folks

How many times have you been talking to someone about the medication you are on and found out that the person you are talking to is taking the exact same pill, the same color, the same size, the same name brand, the same milligram strength and maybe from the same doctor?

The reason this happens is obvious: people are different, their medical history is different, their symptoms are different, and therefore they need a different type or dose of medication.

This allows the doctor to have literally hundreds of variations of different hormone dosages that can be tailored to fit any one particular patient.

For example, in treating high cholesterol, a particular medication may require only two or three dosages. But a doctor who is treating someone for low hormone levels using bio-identical hormones may have seven different milligram dosages of testosterone with various combinations available, and eight different milligram dosages of estradiol with various combinations and five different milligram dosages of progesterone with various combinations.

This allows the doctor to have literally hundreds of variations of different hormone dosages that can be tailored to fit any one particular patient.

The practice of doing that is called ***"Compounding."***

What Is Compounding?

Compounding is a practice in which a licensed pharmacist or a licensed physician combines, mixes, or alters ingredients of a drug to create a medication tailored to the needs of an individual patient.

Why do some patients need compounded drugs? Sometimes, the health needs of a patient cannot be met by an FDA-approved medication. For example:

- If a patient has an allergy and needs a medication to be made without a certain dye

- If an elderly patient or a child can't swallow a pill and needs a medicine in a liquid form that is not otherwise available [36]

In the bio-identical hormone replacement treatment, the drug and its dosage are tailored specifically for the needs of the individual patient. Rather than a "one-size-fits-all" drug like we talked about in the previous chapter, a compounding pharmacy can produce, according to the doctor's prescription, the exact strength of each hormone. The prescription will be made just for you and no one else.

***The prescription will be ... bio-identical,
an exact copy, to your own hormones.***

The prescription will be prepared from plant extracts that are bio-identical, an exact copy, to your own hormones. The variation from one patient to another may be extensive. One may need just testosterone with many different dosage options. Another may need just progesterone with an infinite variability in dosages. Another may need estradiol with many different milligram dosages. This prescription can be filled only at a compounding pharmacy.

What Is a Compounding Pharmacy?

Perhaps you have never heard of a Compounding Pharmacy. Your local pharmacist that compounds your medications especially for you should be represented by *The International Academy of Compounding Pharmacists* (IACP). This is an association representing more than 3,600 pharmacists, technicians, students, and members of the compounding community who focus upon the specialty practice of pharmacy compounding. Compounding pharmacists work directly with prescribers including physicians, and nurse practitioners to create customized medication solutions for patients whose healthcare needs cannot be met by manufactured medications.

Patients and Professionals for Customized Care is an advocacy group which brings together patients and practitioners who know firsthand that compounded medicines are a vital part of modern, individualized health care. P2C2 now has 164,000 members working to ensure that access to personalized medication solutions remains possible.

Who Oversees Compounding Pharmacies?

Generally, state boards of pharmacy have primary responsibility for the day-to-day oversight of state-licensed pharmacies that compound drugs in accordance with the conditions of section 503A of the FDCA, although the Federal Drug Administration retains some authority over their operations. However, outsourcing facilities that register under section 503B are regulated by FDA and must comply with CGMP requirements and will be inspected by FDA according to a risk-based schedule.

Compounded bio-identical hormones are regulated by each state medical regulatory agency. Compounding pharmacies use FDA approved ingredients. The FDA does not regulate each compounding pharmacy, but leaves this to the more closely monitored state authorities. Compounded pharmacies are licensed by the state just as each state regulates doctor's license through the medical licensing board or driver's license through the department of transportation in that state.

Are Compounding Pharmacies Safe?

Only drugs that are safe to be compounded are used by the local Compounding Pharmacy.

Some may question if compounding pharmacies are safe. That is a very valid concern. But let's think about it this way: how does their "record" of safety compare to FDA approved medications? How many medications have been recalled and taken off the market that were initially approved by the FDA? These were medications that the FDA said, *"After many thorough tests on animals and then humans, this is a good safe drug."* But after three or four years on the market, it was found to be very dangerous and even cause death.

The fact is that Compounding Pharmacies are much more closely supervised at the local state level. Because of this close supervision, only drugs that are safe to be compounded are used by the local Compounding Pharmacy.

Becky's Story

Becky had never heard of a Compound Pharmacy. When her doctor prescribed a compounded hormonal supplement for her, she had questions. Living in Nashville, a very large city in the South, she found out that there were only two Compound Pharmacies in the entire city. This raised questions of legitimacy, safety, and supervision in her mind.

But when she went there, she saw the professionalism of the staff, the safety procedures that were in place, and the competency of the compound pharmacists. This dispelled her fears and gave her confidence that her medications were in good hands. *"The people at the pharmacy were so kind and helpful. They answered all my questions and took the time to help me understand all that was going on."*

If you have ever used a Compound Pharmacy, I'm sure your experience is similar to Becky's. Take a moment to Google where the nearest Compound Pharmacy is to you. Go by and ask them questions. Interview their staff – and you will understand what many do about the role of a Compound Pharmacy.

Journal thoughts and questions:

_____

_____

_____

_____

_____

_____

_____

_____

_____

_____

_____

_____

_____

_____

_____

_____

_____

CHAPTER 9

The Three Sex Hormones

"Sex was intended to give us mutual pleasure ... for a lifetime."

The Sexual Dimension of Our Lives

Sex is a very important part of our lives. God designed the sexual dimension of our lives, not simply for procreation and having children, but also so that we would experience oneness and maximum pleasure together.

Physical changes in our bodies rob us of sexual pleasure in our later years.

We were designed to experience sexual pleasure and enjoyment for a *lifetime*. However, for many men and women, physical changes in their bodies rob them of this pleasure in their later years.

Is There Any Hope?

One such woman was Barbara. Listen to her story ...

You are my last hope. If you can't help me, there's no place else to go. I've seen fifteen doctors. You are number sixteen. My husband said, 'Here's the money to see this doctor, but that's it. No more.'

I'm a school teacher. But I have to push myself every single day to get out of bed and go to work. And I love my work, but I am so tired it's like I've worked eighteen hours and it's only 9:30 in the morning. I'm forty-seven years old and overweight. I don't have the energy to exercise. I try to eat right but everything I eat turns to fat.

My husband is so upset with me because I never want to have sex. I sometimes fake it to please him. I'm not lazy. I worked hard through college and have a master degree, but things fell apart when I turned forty. I have hot flashes so bad that I have a small fan beside my desk at school. I have to use it even in the winter. My students have asked what was wrong with me. I don't know what to do.

Barbara's mother died at fifty-two of a stroke and her father died at fifty-seven from a heart attack. She brought a bag full of medicines with her to our appointment. Barbara said, *"Each doctor gave me something different. I tried each one, but nothing helped. They just made me feel worse."* She had five different antidepressants and four kinds of pain medicines. She was placed on *Xanax* for nerves by one doctor and *Ambien* for sleep by another.

Barbara was clearly desperate. It was so distressing to know that fifteen previous doctors would not even think about checking her sex hormones before telling her she had chronic fatigue syndrome. I applauded her optimism. After all the disappointments she had been through, it would have been easy to give up and be depressed. But a friend had told her about bio-identical hormones and how she had been helped. So Barbara came to see us.

The physical exam revealed some remarkable things. Her blood pressure was borderline at 142/88. She weighed 203 pounds and was 5'4". She was pleasant – but her eyes demonstrated her desperate emotional desire for help. She had moderate vaginal dryness. Her last period was five years earlier. Her uterus was small – consistent with menopause.

Barbara's blood work revealed the problem. Her testosterone was very low. Her estradiol level was 2% of what it should have been. Her follicle stimulating hormone (FSH) was very high. An increase in FSH indicates a deficiency in estradiol. Her progesterone was extremely low and her blood sugar was higher than it should have been.

This was a classic presentation of the metabolic syndrome. Barbara had central obesity, elevated blood pressure, elevated blood sugar, elevated triglycerides, and her HDL was low.

As I discussed these findings with her, she was relieved just to know what was causing her to feel so bad. Barbara actually smiled and said, *"Thank you for finding my problem. I was beginning to think it was just in my head."*

A low glycemic index diet was discussed and a low impact exercise program suggested. Barbara was treated with bio-identical testosterone pellets beginning with a low dose because her blood pressure was some borderline. She was given a bio-identical estradiol pellet subcutaneously and we started her on natural progesterone at bedtime. To help her sleep, she was to take melatonin at bedtime and try to wean herself off the *Ambien.*

In one month Barbara returned to the office so excited. She said,

In four days my hot flashes were gone. I've not had one since. My husband and I are having so much fun now. When I get home after school I sometimes call him at work asking when he'll be home. He knows why I'm asking. My vaginal dryness is gone. I've started walking around the track at school every day. I'm up to four miles a day now. I've lost fourteen pounds because my husband and I have changed our eating habits so much. I sleep like a baby now.

Barbara's blood pressure went down. Her blood sugar returned to normal levels, along with her triglycerides. And her cholesterol showed signs of dropping.

Barbara has continued on the above plan for one year. She lost sixty-one pounds. Her blood pressure, cholesterol, triglycerides and blood sugar are now all normal. She enjoys her work and has energy to go all day and still exercise. She and her husband just had a special ceremony at their church to renew their vows after fifteen years of marriage.

Don's Story

Don was fifty-eight years old. On his first visit he said,

I feel so bad by three in the afternoon that I have to take a nap. I actually had a sofa placed in my office under the guise of a place for business associates to sit. By five

o'clock, I was ready to go home. At home I would prop my feet up on the ottoman and just sit and watch TV. I would fall asleep, wake up, and fall asleep again until I dragged myself to bed at ten o'clock. The next morning I would get up as tired as I was when I went to bed the night before. I had my testosterone checked and it was 258.

My doctor gave me testosterone pellets and now my testosterone level is over 1100. I go in about every three months and have more pellets inserted. Now I have energy all day. I never need to take a nap. When I go home from work, usually after six or seven, I play with the dog outside and take a walk every evening. I feel great. And my wife and I are on our second honeymoon after forty-two years of marriage.

To put it bluntly, BHRT works!

Let's take a look in this chapter at the three sex hormones in our bodies.

Sex Hormone #1: Testosterone

Testosterone is a very important hormone in our body. It does many things:

- It helps memory, maintains muscle mass, increases motivation and self-confidence, and heightens our interest in sex. Testosterone is the hormone of vitality and self-confidence.
- Bio-identical testosterone replacement may help to reverse changes in body composition in both men and women (weight gain, fat going to the abdomen and buttocks, loss of muscle tone) and associated diseases or illnesses. [37]
- Testosterone treatment has been shown to decrease body fat and increase lean body mass. [38]
- Bio-identical testosterone in much smaller doses may be beneficial in women who are perimenopausal, menopausal or postmenopausal by improving circulation and reducing blood pressure in those with hypertension. [39]
- Testosterone has shown to aid in weight loss, muscle loss, fatigue, weakness, and significant loss of appetite especially seen in patients undergoing treatment from cancer [40] or other inflammatory diseases such as asthma, irritable bowel syndrome, or rheumatoid arthritis. [41]
- Declining testosterone seen with aging is a strong a way of predicting the mortality in older men. Knowing one's testosterone level is a stronger indication of how long he will live than knowing his cholesterol. [42]
- Men with low testosterone are prone to frailty, weak bones and muscle loss. Low testosterone is also linked to premature death and to a number of other diseases such as sexual disorders, diabetes, and visceral obesity, elevated blood sugar, high blood pressure, and blood clots. [43]
- Testosterone deficiency is associated with insulin resistance and may predispose older men to the metabolic syndrome or type 2 diabetes mellitus. Cardiovascular disease, hardening of the arteries, heart attacks, strokes, blood clots, angina, congestive heart failure are related to low testosterone seen in male aging as all these metabolic processes are all likely linked. [44]

- Testosterone in men and women increases our sense of well-being, as well as reducing fatigue.
- Osteoporosis results from loss of testosterone and is substantially improved with testosterone supplementation. There is less breast cancer, improved dementia and an increase in lean body mass with less fat resulting from an increase in natural testosterone.

What Does Testosterone Do?

Testosterone is the energy hormone. It is like gasoline for your car. Without fuel, your car won't move. It would have no power or energy. Do you sometimes feel as if you have to push yourself to get through the day? Chronic Fatigue Syndrome is frequently diagnosed when nothing specifically wrong can be found.

> *We cannot live without testosterone, and we will not live well when we have diminished testosterone.*

The doctor doesn't know what is causing the fatigue, so the diagnosis of chronic fatigue syndrome is made. This is more commonly diagnosed in women. Many women have seen numerous doctors searching for the reason for their chronic debilitating fatigue having many tests done, but the physician probably has never checked the fuel tank for testosterone.

Testosterone is not just a sex hormone. It affects every part of the body. Testosterone helps our cells to manufacture protein, which helps us build bones and control our sugar and cholesterol. It help us to concentrate; it protects us from Alzheimer's; it helps our immune system to fight infection; it heals and builds muscles. It is easy to see that we cannot live without testosterone, and we will not live well when we have diminished testosterone.

Women Need Testosterone Also

Testosterone is the first sex hormone to begin declining in females and males. Testosterone is produced in the testicles and the ovaries. It is much higher in men … but women need testosterone also. Men have ten- to twenty-times more testosterone than women. A woman's ovaries produce more testosterone than estrogen. A woman's testosterone will be twice as high at twenty-one years old than when she is forty. It will continue dropping – and after menopause it will be only ten percent of its previously high level.

For good health it is essential to maintain normal hormone levels of all three sex hormones. In some, testosterone begins to decline in the mid- to late-twenties, but most will begin to notice a difference by age thirty-five. The patient notices the tendency to gain a little weight. The sex drive may not be as strong when testosterone begins to decline. There usually is a slight decrease in energy at first with more dramatic changes with time. As testosterone declines, we experience more anxiety and low self-esteem. Often there is mild depression, fatigue and a decrease in muscle tone. Women notice thinning of the upper lip and sagging cheeks. Pubic hair thins with a decrease in sex drive.

It is so unfortunate that physicians ignore the well-documented and prolific medical science with thousands of medical studies demonstrating the benefits of testosterone for women. This information has been readily available to physicians for over fifty years. Women frequently report that when they asked their physician about testosterone therapy they hear the retort, *"You don't want to look like a man, do you?"*

Physicians are more likely to check a man's testosterone than a woman's. Perhaps the reason is from years of misguided teaching most physicians had in their medical training. Even in this era of enlightenment, doctors believe that women who have sexual problems at an early age must have psychological/emotional problems. Why else would a physician prescribe a medication for psychological or emotional problems or refer her for counseling? The possibility of psychological or emotional problems being caused by loss of hormones is seldom considered.

Donna, a woman in her late forties, said,

I really do love my husband. He is a good man and deserves a good wife like I used to be. I used to enjoy sex but I feel empty inside. When he touches me, I am afraid he will want to have sex. I asked my family doctor what was wrong with me and she told me this was normal. 'It happens to every woman.' She gave me the antidepressant Lexapro. I told her I did not feel like depression was my problem and wanted my hormones checked. She refused and told me to just take the medication. The antidepressant killed what little libido I had, and I was not able to have an orgasm. It also caused weight gain, which was the last thing I needed as I had already put on twelve pounds in the last year. I stopped my antidepressant. I just want to be my old self again.

Men's testosterone also drops with aging – but it is much slower. A man's testosterone may drop fifty percent over ten years and he will still have an acceptable sex life. However, women will drop eighty percent of their testosterone two to four years after going through menopause. Women are given an antidepressant, which kills their waning sex drive. Men are given *Viagra*. Do you see the potential for problems?

Beatrice was a thirty-eight-year-old patient who suffered from endometriosis. She was told she needed a hysterectomy and, while they were inside, they would also remove her ovaries because *"they weren't doing you any good anymore."* She reported,

Before I left the hospital, I knew something was wrong. I felt like I was going to die. When I saw my gynecologist, I asked her to check my hormones. She would not. I asked her for help. She gave me Prempro. I am a pharmacist. I know how bad this drug is, so I refused to take it. I knew from my reading that Prempro actually decreased my already low testosterone.

I researched bio-identical hormones and found a doctor who administered Pellet Hormone Therapy with a progesterone sublingual tablet at bedtime. It was amazing! Within three days, I knew I had done the right thing. Within three weeks, I was my old self. My husband is thrilled to have his wife back.

Even women in their seventies may experience a reversal of the above symptoms with testosterone supplementation to appropriate blood levels. Rae, a sixty-six-year-old grandmother of fifteen, said, *"I always feel bad about myself."* She had no self-confidence, believing that others were smarter and had more personality than her. After Pellet Hormone Replacement Therapy, she was talking to a small group of women and said, *"After the hormones I feel so much better about myself."*

"My husband is thrilled to have his wife back."

Testosterone provides self-confidence and well-being. Most women will feel more motivated. Rae went on to say that her sex life was more like it was when she was twenty-five. She lost fifteen pounds in six months. This is a very common response by women using very small doses of testosterone – just enough to bring their testosterone level back up to the level of a young woman who has at least one orgasm a day.

A very large percentage of women have a decreased interest in sex at menopause often beginning as early as the mid-thirties.

Charlene, a very memorable seventy-two-year-old lady, whose husband died nine months earlier, had an impish smile on a regular three-month visit. The week before, her fifty one-year-old daughter, Brenda, who was also a patient using BHRT, was smiling when she told the story that her mother had a boyfriend. *"Now, they haven't done anything ... but he visits her a lot."* A week later when Charlene came in with a new hair style and make up and jewelry, we asked her how things were going. She proceeded to say, *"I have a boyfriend. He is a mechanic. He says he's had his eye on me for a long time. He wants me to keep doing the hormones."* She could have passed for fifty-five years old that day.

Testosterone deficiency can cause both men and women to have difficulty with memory. The response to bio-identical testosterone supplementation is almost universal—one can remember better. Muscle mass is lost with testosterone deficiency – but men and women who have testosterone replacement see an increase in muscle mass and strength.

Natural testosterone not only helps a fifty-year-old man feel like he is thirty again, it protects his overall health.

Men have a much more gradual loss of testosterone. They will usually complain of being tired and not having the interest or ability to perform in bed or the gym. Men are more likely to complain of not having the emotional energy to maintain concentration at work.

Natural testosterone not only helps a fifty-year- old man feel like he is thirty again, it protects his overall health ... including diabetes, high lipids, cardiovascular disease, depression, and loss of muscle mass.

Sex Hormone #2: Progesterone

The second sex hormone in our discussion is progesterone. Progesterone is made in the ovaries just as is testosterone and estradiol. Progesterone begins to decline in women after testosterone declines. It is common for this to begin by age thirty-five. Women may notice a change in their periods such as prolonged bleeding or a shorter time between the menstrual cycles. They also may experience mood swings and may have more trouble sleeping. This seems to be the time of life when women see their doctors about anxiety, sleeping medication and depression.

Progesterone may be thought of as the anti-stress hormone.

Antidepressants and stress can cause progesterone deficiency. Progesterone may be thought of as the anti-stress hormone. When one has low progesterone for a long period, cortisol may become low due to excess stress. Progesterone functions as a natural antidepressant and a natural diuretic. Progesterone is a calming hormone that regulates the menstrual cycle, promotes a sex drive and helps maintain bladder control. It helps with sleep, helps prevent bladder problems, protects against endometrial carcinoma, and helps prevent osteoporosis. Progesterone is probably just as important to bone health as estradiol, and perhaps even more so. This is why osteoporosis actually begins to develop very early in the life of women—even by age thirty, when estradiol may still be plentiful.

Most patients like to use a rapidly dissolving tablet under the tongue at bedtime. Some prefer the topical cream applied to an area of thin skin once a day. Your doctor should check your progesterone level regularly every three months.

Premenstrual syndrome is a condition of low progesterone.

Progesterone may be given to menstruating women cyclically for fourteen to twenty-four days of the cycle and stopping for one to two weeks. Some women who are menopausal wish to continue having a period for the rest of their lives as this replicates nature. Some doctors recommend stopping all hormones three days per month. Many patients report that the symptoms are too dramatic to do without hormones for three days. Another option is to stop all hormones one day a week. However, there is very little scientific evidence in support of these protocols.

Premenstrual syndrome (PMS) is a condition of low progesterone. Bio-identical progesterone replacement may be very beneficial in preventing PMS. Some patients who suffer from PMS symptoms are low in estradiol also and benefit from the addition of both bio-identical progesterone and estradiol. This combination will increase circulating dopamine and norepinephrine and serotonin, helping to relieve depression.

Progesterone is an *"antiestrogen."* This means progesterone keeps estrogen in balance. Without progesterone, women may have *"estrogen dominance."* In other words, they will have more estrogen than progesterone. Estrogen dominance can affect eighty percent of women usually in their perimenopausal years.

Low Progesterone can cause:

- PMS
- Bloating
- Fibrocystic disease
- Heavy periods
- Panic attacks
- Increased risk of uterine cancer
- Uterine fibroids
- Water retention
- Migraine headaches

There is also a higher risk of breast cancer if one has estrogen dominance—more estrogen than progesterone. Some women may need progesterone treatment instead of estrogen supplementation during this period from the mid-thirties.

Remember, testosterone begins to diminish in the late twenties followed by progesterone levels declining. But estradiol continues to be produced by the ovaries until the late thirties and often well into the forties. Progesterone and estradiol may be visualized as a seesaw, with progesterone keeping estradiol intact. If there is low production of progesterone and estrogen is still high, one may develop estrogen dominance.

Excess estrogen in the face of low progesterone may result in nervousness, mood swings, poor sleep, depression, loss of sex drive, migraine headaches, and irregular and heavy menstruation. This is estrogen dominance: too much estrogen and too little progesterone to counter balance estrogen. This may lead to infertility, irregular bleeding and an increased chance of breast or uterine cancer.

The Effects of Progesterone:
- Protects the breasts, endometrial and probably the ovaries from cancer
- Helps keep blood levels normal
- Helps maintain sex drive (libido)
- Is Anti-Inflammatory
- Inhibits Breast Tissue Overgrowth
- Lowers Cholesterol and Increases HDL cholesterol
- Decreases Coronary Artery Spasm
- Helps to maintain sex drive
- Antidepressant
- Thins Blood, Prevents Blood Clots
- Promotes Osteoblasts
- Mobilizes Fluid/Decrease Swelling
- Reduces breast tenderness
- Increases Metabolism/Weight Loss
- Reduces craving for carbohydrates and sweets
- Increases the breakdown of fat into energy
- Decreases PMS symptoms and menstrual flow
- Acts as a natural diuretic
- Enhances Action of Thyroid Hormone
- Protects against fibrocystic breast disease
- Promotes proper cell oxygen levels
- Converts to other sex hormones
- Normalizes zinc and copper levels
- Maintains the lining of the uterus [45]

Side Effects of Provera Include:
- Birth defects if taken during pregnancy
- Increased risk of breast cancer
- Menstrual irregularities
- Breast milk production
- Breast tenderness/pain
- Depression
- Mood changes
- Nervousness
- Sudden severe headache
- Dizziness

- Changes in vision
- Eye inflammation and lesions
- Chest pain
- Numbness or tingling in the arms or legs
- Fluid retention (edema)
- Formation of blood clots, especially in the lungs and brain
- Hair loss, or unwanted facial hair grown
- Acne
- Impaired glucose tolerance (pre-diabetic effects)
- Skin rashes
- Weight gain
- Nausea
- Jaundice
- Shortness of breath
- Swelling of the hands or feet
- Pain in legs [46]

Twenty-nine-year-old Nina was having some irregular menstruation and severe migraine headaches that incapacitated her for at least two days a month. *"My marriage is fine. But my husband says I have been very irritable and hard to live with."* Her hormone levels were all reasonably normal except progesterone. This would be expected from her symptoms. Also her mother went through menopause at thirty-eight. This patient did not need estradiol or testosterone, but she did need progesterone sublingual tablets – one at bedtime twenty-one days per month. One month later she said, *"I have not had even one migraine since starting the progesterone. And I am not bitchy like I was. I'm afraid to stop progesterone because I know my migraines will return if I do."*

Sex Hormone #3: Estradiol

The third sex hormone we want to look at is estradiol. Most women usually still have enough estradiol into their early forties, but eight percent will experience natural menopause by age forty. Menopause is defined as a woman not having a period for twelve consecutive months, representing her end to fertility. The estimate is that there are between 3,500 to 4,000 women entering menopause daily in the United States. Your doctor will check for several hormones, but the most conclusive is follicle stimulating hormone (FSH). This is a hormone excreted from the pituitary gland which sits at the base of the brain.

As an ovary produces a follicle and this follicle matures to the point of releasing an egg, there is marked release of estradiol. As long as estradiol is produced in sufficient quantities, your FSH will remain low. But with menopause, there are no longer viable follicles left in the ovaries. From that point on, estradiol will no longer be produced in the ovaries. Without sufficient estradiol, FSH begins to rise. Some physicians use a rise of FSH above 23 as a marker for diagnosing menopause. Estradiol is also produced in the adrenal glands, but insufficient to inhibit follicle stimulating hormone from rising. Of course, those who have a hysterectomy will see dramatic menopausal changes immediately after surgery.

Estradiol transmits signals across a synapse from one nerve cell to another in the brain to help serotonin to decrease anxiety.
Estradiol is a hormone that:

- Helps prevent depression
- Helps prevent irritability
- Protects against heart disease
- Protects the eyes from macular degeneration
- Protects the eyes from cataract
- Helps maintain collagen in the skin to prevent small wrinkles
- Promotes thicker skin
- Keeps bones strong by maintaining calcium
- Prevents blood clots
- Helps maintain concentration
- Improves insulin sensitivity
- Functions to open arteries
- Decreases bad cholesterol (LDL)

Estradiol exerts a wide range of biological effects throughout the body in men and women.

Estradiol is an anabolic steroid like testosterone, but much weaker. It helps build muscles. It deposits fat around the hips and breasts and thighs, giving the natural female figure. Estradiol helps prevent Alzheimer's disease, regulates your body temperature, regulates blood pressure, improves your mood and maintains your interest in sex. Estradiol stimulates the production of serotonin in the brain, a neurotransmitter which keeps you happy and not depressed. Estradiol, the form of estrogen produced in the ovaries, lowers the production of lipoprotein lipase, an enzyme in fat cells, which helps lower body fat.

Estradiol exerts a wide range of biological effects throughout the body in men and women. [47] It will help prevent disruption and inflammation in tissue after an injury. [48] It may also prevent muscle damage because of its antioxidant and membrane-stabilizing properties, repair, and inflammation. [49]

A woman entering menopause will lose eighty percent of her estradiol in the first twelve months. Because of the loss of testosterone, progesterone and estradiol beginning in perimenopause, carrying through into menopause and then postmenopause, women will exhibit an accelerated decline in muscle mass and strength. [50]

Muscle weakness in women occurs at an earlier age than in men, but strength is preserved by hormone replacement therapy, [51] which is related to the loss of estradiol [52] and causes subsequent decreases in ability to function. [53] Higher natural estradiol levels cause more muscle strength and fewer falls which prevents fractures of the limbs and spine because of greater bone mineral density in women 75 years old. [54] Estradiol may also aid in the repair of damaged muscles and regenerate new muscle cells.

Estradiol also is essential in keeping our bones strong with the kind of bone makeup that would prevent fractures in aging women. Estradiol deficiency in older men leads to osteoporosis, an inability to metabolize carbohydrates and lipids, and premature coronary atherosclerosis in men. [55] Low estradiol levels in both men and women are associated with an increased risk of heart attacks, strokes and blood clots as well. [56]

Postmenopausal women with acute cardiovascular disease have a significantly higher probability of death than men of the same age. The quality of life of a postmenopausal woman can predict how long she is likely to live. [57] Bio-identical hormone replacement therapy maintains healthy levels of these essential hormones to preserve quality of life in the postmenopausal years.

- *Increase Sex Drive*
- *Stimulates Growth of Uterine Lining*
- *Slows Bone Breakdown*
- *Acts as a natural calcium channel blocker which opens arteries*
- *Protects against macular degeneration*
- *Aids in the formation of serotonin—a neurotransmitter—which lowers lipoprotein A*
- *Decreases depression, irritability, anxiety and pain sensitivity*
- *Maintain collagen in the skin*
- *Lowers LDL*
- *Increases HDL*
- *Increases bone density*
- *Decreases plaque in the arteries*
- *Increases metabolic rate*
- *Decreases chances of colon cancer*
- *Increases insulin sensitivity*
- *Helps to maintain memory*
- *Helps to maintain water content in the skin—fewer wrinkles*
- *Reduces homocysteine*
- *Less risk for cataracts*
- *Decreases platelet stickiness*
- *Decreases total cholesterol*
- *Helps absorb calcium, magnesium, zinc*
- *Improves sleep*
- *Improves endorphins*
- *Acts as an antioxidant*
- *Decreases triglycerides*
- *Increases growth hormones*
- *Helps maintain potassium*
- *Improves orgasms*
- *Reduces palpitations*
- *Thickens the vaginal wall* [58]

Estrogen performs over four hundred vital functions in a normally functioning female that affects 9-10,000 genetic codes. These genetic instructions are necessary for the body to maintain balance.

Could This Be What You Need?

When looking at the above list, you have to ask, *"How can I be expected to function well without such an important hormone?"*

Donna was in that situation. She had severe menopausal symptoms after her hysterectomy. Donna was a television producer in Florida who had many responsibilities at work. Her hysterectomy turned her life upside down. When she told her gynecologist how miserable she was after the surgery, Donna was told by the doctor, *"Don't worry. You'll get over it in six months."* With estrogen receptor sites in every part of the body from the brain to the feet, how can one expect to *"get over it"*?

At forty-eight years old, she experienced every symptom of menopause including a twenty-pound weight gain, a divorce, decreased breast size, fibromyalgia, facial hair, decreased memory, low energy, poor sleep, and vaginal dryness resulting in painful intercourse.

Donna said,

I told my doctor that I thought my hormones were out of whack. Can you check my blood to see what my hormones are like? When I asked my doctor about my hormones, the one that did my hysterectomy, she said, 'This is just part of what you are going through. It won't do any good to check your blood. Don't worry. You'll be OK.' Then she said, 'Here is a prescription for something to help.' She gave me a prescription for an antidepressant—Cymbalta. This caused me to gain even more weight and killed what little sex drive I had. On Cymbalta I had even more dulling of my ability to remember and concentrate. I stopped the antidepressant.

Donna told a story about a community get-together where she had a chance to talk to her ex-husband. She said, *"I asked him if he wanted to talk sometime and see if we could work things out. He said, 'You have a hormone problem.' Even my ex realized it was my hormones – but my doctor refused to admit it."* Donna started Pellet Bio-identical Hormone Replacement Therapy with phenomenal results. She began losing weight and was able over the next four weeks to stop her use of Cymbalta. Her hot flushes stopped within four days and she regained the vaginal moisture as she had in her twenties.

This has been a longer-than-usual chapter. And it is replete with endnotes and references. But the reality is that everything we have talked about here is well-documented, scientifically and medically tested, and reliable.

If the message in this chapter resonates with you, I invite you – now, today – to talk with a BHRT specialist and begin the process of regaining your sexual life.

Journal thoughts and questions:

_____

_____

_____

_____

_____

_____

_____

_____

_____

_____

_____

_____

_____

_____

_____

_____

_____

CHAPTER 10

A Brief Overview Of How

The Hormonal System Works

"The knee bone's connected to the ... Oh, you know how the song goes!"

Biology 101

Biology class. You remember it. Perhaps ninth or tenth grade in High School. Some of you loved it; some probably dreaded it. But the reality is ... most of you have forgotten all but the most basic information. And you were probably more concerned with who was going to ask you to the prom than you were about the biological make-up of human beings.

I'd like to take you back to that biology class.

Only this time, let's focus on how the hormonal system works. After all, it's your body we're talking about. And now that you're older, and it's more personal to you, you really need to understand the basics of how it all works together.

Our bodies are designed with the utmost intricacies. ***It all starts with the hypothalamus***, a gland located at the base of the brain. Just below the hypothalamus is a very small gland known as the pituitary gland, weighing one-fourth of an ounce.

The hypothalamus and the pituitary glands are interconnected
and designed so they act as one.

The hypothalamus senses the levels of hormones circulating throughout the body. It knows how much testosterone, estradiol, progesterone and thyroid hormones should be present. When the hypothalamus senses that the ovaries are not producing enough estradiol, it sends a message to the pituitary gland to release hormones. Gonadotropins pass through the pituitary stalk from the hypothalamus to the pituitary signaling that the ovaries need to be encouraged to produce more estradiol. The same action occurs to maintain proper levels of testosterone, thyroid, growth hormone, insulin, etc.

The pituitary then produces a messenger, a hormone known as the follicle stimulating hormone (FSH), which flows through the blood stimulating the ovaries to produce more estradiol. This process is duplicated every second of the day and night, maintaining equilibrium throughout the body. When the ovaries slow down the production of estradiol, this is called *Perimenopause* — a time when the woman's body begins to make a transition from fertility and menstruation to infertility and no periods. With a further decrease of estradiol and eventually a complete halt in the production of estradiol, the pituitary increases the production of FSH trying to encourage the ovaries to produce more estradiol.

The increase in follicle-stimulating hormone signals the ovaries to work harder to produce more estradiol. FSH rises, constantly stimulating the ovaries every second of the day, but to no avail. No matter how hard the pituitary works producing more and more FSH, the ovaries are no longer able to produce more estradiol because there are no more eggs in the ovaries. There is evidence that this over-stimulation of the ovaries may be a cause of an increased risk of ovarian cancer in menopausal women.

When the hormone estradiol is given to women in menopause, the effectiveness of this treatment can be measured not only by symptom relief but also by testing the blood level of follicle-stimulating hormone. The goal should be to alleviate symptoms of estradiol deficiency. A lowering of FSH will be a positive sign that estradiol is increasing, ultimately getting to the healthy levels that a woman had when she was younger. As estradiol declines in menopause the FSH increases, but with estradiol treatment supplementing with natural estradiol, the FSH will drop back to normal levels.

How does it work? Listen to Irene's story.

Irene's Life Was Changed!

Irene was forty-seven years old and miserable. She was having hot flashes, night sweats, vaginal dryness, loss of sex drive and depression. She was on two different kinds of antidepressants. Irene said,

I am miserable. I have gained eighteen pounds since turning forty years old. I believe the antidepressants I was taking caused that. I have absolutely zero sex drive—none! When my husband begins to make sexual moves toward me, it makes me cringe. I never was this way before. I talked to my doctor about checking my hormones.

After threatening to see a different doctor, she finally agreed. She called me, actually her nurse called, and told me my hormones were normal for my age. I was so disappointed because I knew something was not right.

Irene was right. Her estradiol level was very low. And her FSH was very elevated. Both numbers demonstrated that she needed estradiol. Her testosterone was also low, giving reason why she had no sex drive. Her progesterone was virtually non-existent. Irene had all these very low hormones replaced with bio-identical hormone pellets. She returned in one month with a completely different story.

I have a sex drive now like I did when my husband and I were dating. I've not had a hot flash since the first week.

I know I was supposed to gradually decrease my antidepressants, but after doing that for the first week, I decided to stop both. I had a little tremor for two days but this went away and I don't take any medicines at all now. I have a sex drive now like I did when my husband and I were dating. I've not had a hot flash since the first week. I used to have to get up at night and change my gown but not anymore. My husband says I have as much vaginal moisture now as I did when we were first married. I know this sounds crazy but I was so miserable I would sometimes think about hurting myself. But not now. Life is great!

Journal thoughts and questions:

_____

_____

_____

_____

_____

_____

_____

_____

_____

_____

_____

_____

_____

_____

_____

_____

_____

_____

_____

CHAPTER 11

How Physicians Are Strongly Influenced By Pharmaceutical Companies

"There are Lies, Damned Lies, and Statistics"
(most often attributed to Mark Twain)

Intense Rhetoric

Let's be honest. There are battles going on out there. We see it in weight-loss programs, where one company accuses another of not being effective. Then they tout their product, giving you reasons why you should choose them. You see the same thing happening on TV commercials with automobile insurance companies, financial investment firms, and a myriad of other products.

The media – whether it be television, printed materials, or the internet – is a great place to "pitch" ideas. Unfortunately, it's often hard to tell who is really telling the truth, and who is simply putting a biased "spin" to their message.

And there is a battle between those of us who understand the benefits of bio-identical hormone replacement therapy and those in the *"established"* medical practices and pharmaceutical companies.

What is the truth?

Three Statements to Put Things in Perspective

Before we get into an analysis of how pharmaceutical companies work, let me make three statements that I hope will put things in perspective:

One, there are many wonderful drugs that have been produced by pharmaceutical companies that have saved lives and helped patients. It is not my intention here to paint a broad stroke saying all pharmaceutical companies are evil and do no good. That certainly is not the case. However, the second statement is equally important.

Two, all pharmaceutical companies have an agenda. Of course they do. Their agenda is to promote their products, putting them into the hands of as many doctors as possible, who will prescribe these drugs to as many patients as possible. The bottom line: all pharmaceutical companies are in business to make as much money as possible and to capture as much market share as possible. If I were a stockholder in those companies, I would expect nothing less.

Three, this agenda often clouds what is really best for patients. Let's face it, a lot of money has gone into the research and development of all of these drugs. And these large companies must realize a significant return-on-their-investment. This often means that if research numbers must be fudged, if other courses of treatment must be disparaged, or if personal attacks on those with new and fruitful treatments must be made, so be it. If history has taught us anything, it has taught us that leaders are territorial and always protective of themselves and their turf. Anything that gets in the way of their agenda is seen as the enemy.

All pharmaceutical companies have an agenda ... and this agenda often clouds what is really best for patients.

So, What's the State-of-the-Industry?

Each year the President of our country goes before Congress and delivers a State-of-the-Union address, where he tells the country, from his perspective, of course, what is going on in the United States.

I would like to do the same in this chapter. I would like to tell you the truth about what is going on and how physicians today are influenced by Big Pharma.

First, it has been said that ninety-five percent of what doctors learn after medical school is taught to them in one way or the other by pharmaceutical companies.

Actually this process of influencing doctors begins before graduation. Medical schools are strongly supported financially by pharmaceutical companies. Medical schools have a vested interest to teach young doctors that pharmaceuticals are the first line of treatment for most everything that ails their patients.

After medical school, pharmaceutical representatives visit doctors regularly in their residency training, educating them on their new-latest-best-miracle drug. When the doctor is in his own medical practice, multiple pharmaceutical representatives continue the educational program by paying weekly visits to the doctor.

After the pharmaceutical representative delivers a presentation of their particular drug to the doctor, the pharmaceutical company can then monitor through pharmacies how many prescriptions that doctor writes for any particular drug, be it their drug or a competitor's drug. If the busiest doctors are not responding as hoped, they are visited again and again to bring them on board. The doctors that are not as busy are not visited as often.

Second, doctors listen to television just as their patients do. Advertisements for pharmaceuticals are all over the networks. Your physician is not immune to this constant bombardment of information presented in a very positive manner. "Patient actors" smile and give glowing reports of how wonderful they feel on this particular drug. However, the side effects are glossed over quickly – ending again with everyone smiling. Every doctor will have patients who say, *"Doctor, I saw on television about a medicine for the pain like I have in my feet. Do you think that would work for me?"*

Third, your doctor is required in order to maintain his or her certification to attend so many hours of CME (continuing medical education). Pharmaceutical companies play a major part in sponsoring these events. They have direct face-to-face interaction with many physicians at booths where their wares are displayed.

Pharmaceutical companies have a paid *"speakers list"* of doctors who are trained to talk about a particular disease process with a treatment that includes a drug manufactured by a particular pharmaceutical company. The doctor lecturing may be influenced by the pharmaceutical representatives to present certain medications in a more favorable light.

Fourth, medical magazines are full of advertisements. The magazine depends on this advertising to pay their bills. A typical medical journal may have two-thirds of their one hundred pages dedicated to advertising. These magazines are influenced to place reports of studies favoring a particular drug and discouraged to not report a study demonstrating the advantages of a bio-identical trial using a product not manufactured by Big Pharma.

Fifth, the internet is prolific with medication advertisements as popups. They are difficult to ignore. Some talk to you. They are professionally produced to catch your attention and remind the physician of this particular drug. And all the while, they are presenting their product in the best light possible.

Pharmaceutical Representatives Talk Mostly About the Advantages of Their Drugs

There has never been, nor will there ever be, a pharmaceutical representative visiting your doctor demonstrating the benefits of pellet bio-identical hormone replacement therapy.

Pharmaceutical companies make a profit when they are able to patent their drugs and sell them for a certain number of years before they enter the market as generic drugs, which as we all know, are sold at a drastically reduced rate. Therefore, they have to make their profit quickly before others can produce these drugs and then sell them for much less.

This means doctors are going to be visited often by pharmaceutical representatives. Pharmaceutical companies are going to advertise in magazines (not just medical magazines) as well as on television. Doctors are going to see large display booths at their medical conventions and hear lectures praising these drugs. None of these events will occur with bio-identical hormone replacement medications. Bio-identical hormones are compounded by your local pharmacist specific for you as prescribed for your particular deficiencies.

There has never been, nor will there ever be, a pharmaceutical representative visiting your doctor demonstrating the benefits of pellet bio-identical hormone replacement therapy.

The Reality of Bio-identical Hormones

In chapter nine, we discussed the three sex hormones: testosterone, estradiol and progesterone. These three hormones are molecularly similar as one evolves from one hormone to another and then can revert back to the original hormone as the body calls for that particular one. All three of these sex hormones can be found as bio-identical hormones used to treat hormone deficiencies. The Endocrine Society has defined bio-identical hormones as *"compounds that have exactly the same chemical and molecular structure as hormones that are produced in the human body."* [59]

This means that the body recognizes bio-identical hormones as itself. This is extremely important. Traditional hormone replacement therapy uses drugs whose structure and nature, actions and reactions in the body are foreign to the human organism. Hormones, then, are not drugs. Hormones are molecules produced by our own glands and so do not come with the undesirable side effects of traditional hormone drugs—as long as the hormones prescribed are identical to those made by the body. [60]

I am sure you can see where I am going with this: ***if bio-identical hormones are not drugs, they cannot be made and patented by Big Pharma.***

The human body has natural enzymes made to process natural human hormones. When a drug is introduced to the human body whose structure and nature are foreign to the human organism, there are consequences in the form of side effects.

Think about it this way: the gasoline that you pump into your car's fuel tank is a petroleum fuel. So is diesel fuel. But there will be side effects if you use diesel fuel in an engine that is made to use gasoline.

Anyone can read a package insert or listen to an advertisement and see the long list of consequences to using drugs which are foreign to the body. The reason for these side effects is the body does not know how to process foreign chemicals, drugs. But these drugs continue to be promoted by Big Pharma – with little or no regard for the consequences.

What is the consumer to do?

Be Informed!

It's that simple: be informed. Learn the truth. Listen with discernment when the side effects and consequences of manufactured drugs are listed. And know the truth about bio-identical hormones.

Journal thoughts and questions:

_____

_____

_____

_____

_____

_____

_____

_____

_____

_____

_____

_____

_____

_____

_____

_____

_____

_____

CHAPTER 12

A Deeper Look At The Dangerous Synthetic Hormones Used In The *Women's Health Initiative Trial* As Compared With Bio-Identical Hormones

"You Can Fool Some of the People Some of the Time ..."

Warning!

Bill O'Reilly's show on FOX News channel, *The O'Reilly Factor,* has become a very popular and successful news show. Maybe you've seen the show. Bill always begins with these words: *"Warning! You are about to enter the no-spin zone."* It's become his identifying mark.

As we begin this chapter, I would also like to issue a similar statement: *"Warning! You are about to enter a chapter that is filled with medical research and studies."*

For some of you, that makes you salivate! You can't wait to see what the experts and studies are showing. You are so glad there are all those endnotes! For others, this chapter might represent the solution to those sleepless nights: *"Read one page and you'll be asleep in no time!"*

For those of you in the second camp, I hereby give you permission to skip this chapter and move on to the next one. But for those of you who are motivated to read the medical research, here we go – complete with all the endnotes!

The Effects of Foreign Substances on the Human Body

An example of the results of intruding a foreign substance – a drug – into the body was found in the *Women's Health Initiative Study.* As we said earlier, this study involving over 160,000 menopausal women was the largest ever designed to investigate the benefits and the risks of traditional hormone replacement therapy using the most commonly used hormones *Premarin* and *Provera.* Women with a uterus received *Prempro*—a combination of *Premarin* and *Provera.* Women with no uterus received only *Premarin.* The study was designed to last eight-and-a-half years. However, in 2002 after 5.2 years, the arm of the study using *Prempro* was terminated because of the deadly side effects. [61]

The *Premarin* only arm of the study did not demonstrate an increased risk of heart attacks, as the *Prempro* arm did, but there was a significant increased risk of stroke in women taking *Premarin.*

Premarin is a type of animal-derived estrogen. The source of estrogen is from the urine of a pregnant horse known as conjugated equine estrogen or CEE. How does the human body metabolize this drug? Natural 17beta estradiol found in young, normally functioning women is metabolized in twenty-four hours by natural human enzymes. By contrast, the synthetic estrogen made from horse urine, *Premarin*, requires thirteen weeks to be completely processed and eliminated from the body. [62]

The study designed to last eight-and-a-half years was terminated after 5.2 years because of the deadly side effects.

What does this mean? Women who have healthy ovaries will have continuous fresh estradiol every day. They will never have horse urine in their circulation. For women with no ovaries secondary to a hysterectomy or women who are menopausal, the natural 17beta estradiol produced by the ovaries can be replaced with natural bio-identical 17beta estradiol instead of a foreign horse hormone, *Premarin*.

Premarin, conjugated equine estrogen, contains 12 different estrogens that should never be given to a woman. None of these twelve are ever found in a normally functioning woman.

The other hormone used in the *Women's Health Initiative Study* was *Provera*, a progestin. A progestin such as *Provera* is a synthetic look-alike progesterone. In other words, it is a **synthetic** chemical. *Provera* is not progesterone. Later, many studies will be presented that demonstrate the **extreme dangers of taking this artificial hormone.**

There is an alternative! Instead of using a dangerous synthetic hormone, *medroxyprogesterone acetate,* a natural bio-identical progesterone can be used. Natural progesterone is bio-identical to what the ovaries produce.

But the *Women's Health Initiative Trial* did not study natural bio-identical estradiol or progesterone. Thousands of studies have demonstrated the advantages of using natural hormones in humans instead of a hormone from a pregnant horse. Doctors who use natural hormones prove daily that BHRT is safer and more effective than artificial hormones. To compare the combination of *Premarin* and *Provera* (*Prempro*) to natural progesterone and estradiol would confirm once and for all that any sane physician should use *Bio-identical Hormone Replacement Therapy* instead of the cancer causing *Prempro*.

Please understand, *Premarin* and *Provera* were studied in the WHI and found to be dangerous. Bio-identical hormones were not studied in the WHI. To condemn BHRT as bad because the synthetic Big Pharma drug is dangerous is ludicrous. There is absolutely no correlation to the two.

So, what was the FDA's response to the WHI Trial? It was to put a *"black box"* warning label on ALL estrogen replacement products even though only ONE estrogen was studied.

Why hasn't Prempro been removed from the market? ... Why has there been an effort to condemn a bio-identical product that the FDA has never studied and has never caused death?

It is usual for the FDA to remove a drug from the market that causes cancer when there are no life-saving benefits. Why hasn't that drug been removed? We don't know for sure ... but it is easy to understand that there is a close relationship between the FDA and Wyeth Pharmaceuticals. Could there be a cover-up, or perhaps a political payback involved? Why has there been an effort to condemn a bio-identical product that the FDA has never studied and that has never caused death?

Millions of women stopped their hormones after results were released from *Premarin* plus synthetic *Provera* arm of the *Women's Health Initiative Trial* that revealed an increased risk of breast cancer, cardiovascular disease, dementia, stroke, and blood clots in women taking *Premarin* and *Provera* compared with those in the placebo group.

Keep in mind, traditional medicine uses a synthetic progestin, *Provera*, instead of bio-identical progesterone to counterbalance estrogen. Why would bio-identical progesterone not be used? Could it be that the drug company manufacturing *Provera* knew from previous smaller studies that natural bio-identical estradiol and progesterone were safer and more efficacious than the synthetic *Prempro*?

In *The Journal of the American Medical Association* in 2003, a study using information from the *Women's Health Initiative Trial* showed a significant twenty-four percent increase in breast cancer risk among women, age 50–80 years, who were given conjugated equine estrogen *Premarin* .625 mg per day plus *Provera* 2.5 mg/day for almost six years. [63]

Most all trials report that there is an increase of two- to four-times greater risk of breast cancer associated with *Provera* compared to the use of estrogen alone. [64]

There is strong evidence that progesterone may reduce estrogen-stimulated growth of breast cells in which bio-identical estradiol or progesterone gels or a combination of both were applied daily to the breasts of postmenopausal women for fourteen days prior to surgery not for malignancy. The use of natural progesterone for fourteen days reduced the estradiol-stimulated overgrowth of normal breast cells. This shows that bio-identical progesterone provides protection from the breast stimulation of estradiol. This is part of the balancing of hormones that is necessary for optimal health. [65]

Why does traditional medicine continue to push unnatural, synthetic Provera onto unsuspecting women patients when it is known to cause breast cancer?

It was demonstrated fifty years ago that bio-identical progesterone protected the breast from cancer. Women who chronically do not ovulate due to lack of progesterone are at increased risk of breast cancer. When it is well known that abundant progesterone in premenopausal women may be protective against breast cancer, why does traditional medicine continue to push unnatural, synthetic *Provera* onto unsuspecting women patients when it is known to cause breast cancer? [66]

In the United States, the use of *Provera*, unlike in Europe where it is rarely used, is by far the most commonly used non-natural progestin which is endowed with androgenic (male-like) properties. The increased breast cancer risk found with the use of *Provera* might be related to its 'non-progesterone' activities. [67]

When synthetic *Provera* is taken by mouth, the liver processes this unnatural hormone. Consequently the side effects are increased because it has to pass through the liver before being absorbed into the circulation. This process changes *Provera* to a more dangerous form. This is why natural, micronized progesterone used as a sublingual rapid dissolve tablet is beneficial as this method of administration avoids this first pass through the liver. These changes of *Provera* as it passes through the liver might explain why there is an increase in breast cancer with the use of this traditionally used dangerous hormone. [68]

Natural progesterone does not have a cancer-promoting effect on breast tissue. This provides a biological reason that sublingual micronized progesterone added to estrogens in sequential or cyclic-combined regimens does not increase the risk of breast cancer. [69]

The greater breast cancer risk related to the use of hormone replacement therapy containing estrogen and synthetic progestins is due to the kind of progestin used. *Provera*, a key ingredient in *Prempro*, increases the stimulation of estrogens on breast tissue and estrogen-sensitive cancer cells. When hormone replacement therapy is indicated, preparations containing bio-identical progesterone and not a synthetic *Provera* should be used. In this way the risk of endometrial (inside lining of the uterus) cancer is minimized without increasing the risk of breast cancer. [70]

Natural progesterone is bio-identical to the progesterone that the ovaries produce. While it is true that synthetic medroxyprogesterone acetate, a progestin, can have similar actions as natural bio-identical progesterone such as protecting against osteoporosis, endometrial cancer, aiding proper function of the thyroid, and may help prevent fibrocystic breast disease, the list of negative effects of *Provera* is long.

Dr. Pamela Smith, MD, MPH, has written an insightful book entitled *"What You Must Know About Women's Hormones."* She lists some side effects of progestins. Here they are, in alphabetical order:

- Acne
- Bloating
- Breakthrough bleeding, spotting
- Breast tenderness
- Counteracts many of the positive
- effects estrogen has on serotonin
- Decrease in energy
- Decrease in sexual energy
- Decreased HDL (good cholesterol)
- Depression
- Fluid retention
- Hair loss
- Headaches
- Inability to help produce estrogen and testosterone
- Increased appetite
- Increased LDL (bad cholesterol)
- Insomnia
- Irritability
- Nausea
- Protects only the uterus from cancer (not the breasts)
- Rashes
- Remains in your body longer than bio-identical progesterone
- Weight gain which can prevent it from balancing with the other
- Hormones [71]

It is fair and responsible to ask: *Why do women continue to take these dangerous synthetic drugs?* It is even more important to ask: *Why do doctors continue prescribing them?* And finally, it is the responsible thing to ask: *Why does Big Pharma continue to promote them?*

Journal thoughts and questions:

_____

_____

_____

_____

_____

_____

_____

_____

_____

_____

_____

_____

_____

_____

_____

_____

CHAPTER 13

A Deeper Look At Bio-Identical Hormone Replacement Therapy

"The Proof Is In the Pudding."

A Startling Contrast

What would your doctor say if you were taking *Prempro* and you asked, *"Doctor, you checked my iron and told me I needed iron. Now can you check my Prempro blood level to see if I'm taking the right dose?"* You may be laughed out of the office.

Horses have equine estrogen. Humans use human estrogen.

Why? Because there is no normal blood level of conjugated horse estrogen in your body. There is no *Provera* found in a female unless she is taking this drug. Your doctor can draw blood to check the level of estradiol of an eighteen-year-old that has never used a non-human hormone treatment – and your doctor can check the level of estradiol of a fifty-five-year-old woman who is using BHRT. The same chemical, estradiol, can be found in both individuals naturally. The blood levels may be the same in both. Here's the key point: **Horses have equine estrogen. Humans use human estrogen.**

Your doctor will never draw blood to check your level of *Provera*. It does not exist naturally. A doctor treating a patient with synthetic drugs has no way of monitoring in the blood what dose to use or what dose is too much – or even if the patient needs that drug. At the conclusion of the *Women's Health Initiative Trial* the authors of the study concluded that the danger of using traditional hormone replacement, *Premarin* and *Provera*, was greater than the benefits of using them.

Melissa's Story

Fifty-year-old Melissa had been on *Prempro* for eight years. She described her bouts of depression:

I had never been depressed before but when I turned forty-and-a-half I started feeling like life was empty. I just didn't want to do anything. I was never this way before. I even thought about how I would kill myself if I ever got the courage. I knew this was not normal. My husband told me to see my doctor. When I saw her, she placed me on Zoloft 50 mg daily.

After three weeks on this medicine, I saw her again, telling her I could not sleep. She gave me a prescription for Ambien 10 mg at bedtime. After three months, I was still depressed, maybe even worse than before. My doctor changed Zoloft to Cymbalta 30 mg twice a day. What little sex drive I had completely disappeared and when we had sex it was impossible for me to have an orgasm.

Unfortunately her marriage did not survive. *"I know it was mostly my fault, but I didn't know what to do. I don't blame my husband for leaving me. I gained thirty-two pounds on Cymbalta. I was like a zombie."* Even though she had vaginal dryness, she said she did not have painful intercourse because she was now divorced for over five years and had no interest in having a relationship with a man again.

When asked if her doctor had told her of the dangers of *Prempro* she replied, *"No, she just told me I needed it. She has been my doctor for almost twenty years so I trusted her to tell me if there was any danger in taking Prempro."* It was interesting to note that her mother died at fifty-six years old of breast cancer after taking the combination of *Premarin* and *Provera*.

Melissa's lab values showed dramatic loss of hormones. [72] All other blood work was within normal limits. She was encouraged to change her diet to eat more fruits and vegetables decreasing her intake of sugar, especially soft drinks. She was drinking six to eight Cokes a day to help her energy. Melissa was encouraged to begin a walking program daily, even if it was just for fifteen minutes.

Melissa was started on *Pellet Hormone Replacement Therapy* using a small amount of bio-identical testosterone, estradiol and under-the-tongue progesterone. In one month she reported,

I've completely stopped the Cymbalta. I just cut back on my own. And I haven't needed to take my Ambien any more. I sleep all night without it. And, by the way I've been noticing a man at work and I think he's been looking back. My husband has remarried so he's not in play for me. I now have the energy to exercise after work. I walk three miles a day and I've lost eight pounds so far. I don't need Cokes any more for energy.

A One-Size-Fits-All Approach – Versus a Tailored, Personal Regimen

You will never hear someone say, "Prempro makes me feel healthy, with vitality, and I feel physically attractive. I'm so glad my doctor put me on Prempro. This has saved my life."

Each of the three hormones discussed earlier plays an important part on its own in our physical and emotional health. The key is to have proper balance and alignment between all three of them. When all three are functioning together at their height of what each can do, the patient will have health and vitality. They will feel very physically attractive and self-confident. You will never hear someone say, *"Prempro makes me feel healthy, with vitality, and I feel physically attractive. I'm so glad my doctor put me on Prempro. This has saved my life."*

Mainstream medicine has a one-size-fits-all approach. The traditional doctor will write the same prescription, no matter what the woman's symptoms are, without considering blood levels, hormones, and various symptoms that may be in play. Can you imagine your doctor saying, *"I'm going to check your Premarin level to see if you need this drug"?* The women who are taking *Premarin* all take the same strength of *Premarin* – its prescription is not personalized or tailored to the needs of the individual. In contrast, the doses of bio-identical hormones are adjusted regularly according to the patient's symptoms and the results from the blood work.

Most physicians who use bio-identical hormones use compounded hormones instead of those manufactured by Big Pharma. The advantage is that the doctor can order the exact strength of each hormone the patient needs instead of the "one-size-fits-all" manufactured by pharmaceutical companies. The doctor listens to the patient's complaints, does a physical exam and checks the blood for a variety of substances including hormones, complete blood count, blood sugar, thyroid hormones, lipids (cholesterol and triglycerides), etc.

It is common on the interview and physical exam of perimenopausal and menopausal women to find:

- Early bone loss even before age fifty on a DEXA scan
- Muscle weakness by age forty-five
- Decreased muscle size
- Thin pubic hair a sign of low estradiol
- Thinning scalp hair especially after age fifty-five
- The clitoris to be smaller than when she was younger
- The labia (lips of the vagina) are beginning to hang loose instead of up against the vaginal opening
- The vaginal mucosa is dry and irritated
- The breasts are not as large as they were ten years before
- The breasts are beginning to sag
- The patient reports that the nipples are not as sensitive during sex play
- Often the patient exhibits a flat mood
- Loss of memory – the patient may not be able to remember what she had for breakfast or the birthdates of her children
- Most commonly, women lose interest in sex when going into menopause
- Many report the loss of sexual fantasies
- There is usually less sensitivity to sexual stimulation of the breasts or clitoris
- Women will report that their orgasms are more difficult to obtain, require more effort to achieve, are less intense and are few and far between
- Menopausal women are often not happy with the changes they see in their body
- Perimenopausal and menopausal women will usually masturbate less
- These women will often have diminished desire for sex

From this a prescription is written for the bio-identical hormone she needs and the strength (the milligram dosage) that is required to bring the hormones back to a healthy level. The prescription is taken to a compounding pharmacy to be filled.

Choosing a Compounding Pharmacy

Where do I go to get my bio-identical hormone prescription filled?

Pharmacy compounding is the art and science of preparing personalized medications for patients. Compounded medications are *"made from scratch"* – individual ingredients are mixed together in the exact strength and dosage form required by the patient. This method allows the compounding pharmacist to work with the patient and the prescriber to customize a medication to meet the patient's specific needs. *The Professional Compounding Centers of America* (PCCA) estimate that one in four compounded products in the United States are a form of Hormone Replacement Therapy.

Your compounding pharmacy should be a member of PCAB (*Pharmacy Compounding Accreditation Board*). This is an accrediting agency of pharmacies that assures that the pharmacy you are using has the highest standards in compounding. As the demand for compounded medications has increased, the pharmaceutical profession saw a need for a system of standards by which each compounding pharmacy can test its quality processes. Compounding pharmacists also wanted a mechanism to allow them to know that they are producing a high quality compound, and in doing so, providing the best quality to their patients.

PCAB Accreditation gives patients, prescribers and insurance companies a way to select a pharmacy that meets or exceeds *U.S. Pharmacopeial Convention's* high quality standards. USP's mission is to improve global health through public standards and related programs that help ensure the quality, safety, and benefit of medicines and foods. Eight of the nation's leading pharmacy organizations joined together, contributing their time, money and leadership, to create PCAB: a voluntary quality accreditation designation for the compounding industry.

The Dollars and Sense of Hormones

You may wonder how the manufacturer of synthetic hormones, Wyeth, can continue selling medications that have been proven to cause so much disease, including death, when the FDA says the risks outweigh the benefits. The answer may be found in **political and economic connections** between Wyeth and the medical societies who show support for *Premarin* and *Provera* to their membership.

In his book *Stay Young & Sexy with Bio-identical Hormone Replacement: The Science Explained,* Dr. Jonathan V. Wright states,

Wyeth endows a $200,000 lectureship fund named for NAMS (North American Menopausal Society) President Dr. Wulf Utian and was named a "Partner in Menopause Education" (requiring a contribution of at least $8,000) for the NAMS's 2007 Annual Meeting. Additionally, half of NAMS's Board of Trustees for 2007-2008, including Dr. Utian, received "consulting fees" or "research support" from Wyeth.

The list goes on and on, whether it be *The American Medical Women's Association, The American Society for Reproductive Health, The Association of Reproductive Health Professionals, The Black Women's Health Imperative, The Center for Women Policy Studies* or a host of other endowments, the message is clear: Big Phama has its hands in a lot of places.

Choices of Treatment Plan — Synthetic or Bio-identical?

Choosing the right treatment plan for you is crucial to your feeling better. Some may be ineffective and others may be extremely effective.

You have to consider the choices.

Why would you want to take a synthetic chemical that has been shown to cause breast cancer, cardiovascular disease, stroke, and thromboembolic events when the alternative is natural bio-identical testosterone, progesterone and estradiol readily available that have not been shown to cause these untoward events?

To demonstrate the marked differences in traditional hormone replacement, *Premarin* and *Provera*, read the following quote. It comes from an article entitled *MPA Medroxy-Progesterone Acetate Contributes to Much Poor Advice for Women.*

This trial, the Women's Health Initiative trial, which used Premarin alone, or in conjunction with MPA to reduce the chance of cancer of the uterus Prempro, has turned women's health at menopause into a minefield. It is old news, but the combined hormone arm was ended prematurely because of increased incidence of breast cancer and the eleven-year follow-up study found increased mortality attributable to breast cancer. Increased risk of dementia, stroke, and cognitive decline was also present in both arms relative to placebo in women aged sixty-five years and older.

While the Women's Health Initiative trial made a valuable contribution in revealing the risks associated with conjugated equine estrogens plus MPA treatment in postmenopausal women, it unfortunately generated considerable controversy in the field because it was interpreted as an indictment of postmenopausal hormone replacement, when in fact, it did not study hormone replacement at all: that would have required use of the natural hormones, estradiol and progesterone. The actions of the natural hormones are significantly different from those of Premarin and MPA. [73]

> **Thousands of studies have confirmed that BHRT is safer and more efficacious than traditional dangerous synthetic hormones.**

That article makes a significant point when it said that there was considerable controversy *"because it was interpreted as an indictment of postmenopausal hormone replacement"* encouraged by Big Pharma and those supporting Big Pharma.

If they had been honest, the interpretation would be *"This trial was ONLY an indictment of Premarin and Provera."* Since that time, there have been thousands of studies that have confirmed that BHRT is safer and more efficacious than traditional dangerous synthetic hormones.

In Conclusion

In Section One of this book, I have sought to build a very clear case:

- Traditional synthetic hormones are dangerous and deadly.
- Bio-identical hormone replacements are safer, healthy, necessary, and completely beneficial to needy patients.
- Upon taking BHRT, a patient's quality of life improves dramatically and stays that way as long as they continue treatment.

In Section Two, we will discuss twenty-seven common symptoms and how BHRT can make a difference.

Journal thoughts and questions:

_____

_____

_____

_____

_____

_____

_____

_____

_____

_____

_____

_____

_____

_____

_____

_____

_____

_____

SECTION TWO

How Bio-Identical Hormone

Replacement Therapy

Makes A Difference

CHAPTER 14

Testosterone In Men

The Onslaught of Advertising

You've heard all the ads: *"Cialis ... Be ready when the moment's right." "Viagra helps guys with erectile dysfunction (ED) get and keep an erection." "Ask your doctor if Viagra is right for you."* You never heard that fifty years ago! Treatments for erectile dysfunction have become big business since *Viagra*, *Cialis* and *Levitra* hit the market beginning in 1998.

How Does Testosterone Work?

Testosterone plays a key role in the development of male reproductive tissues such as the testis and prostate as well as promoting secondary sexual characteristics such as increased muscle, bone mass, and the growth of body hair. In addition, testosterone is essential for health and well-being as well as the prevention of osteoporosis.

A man's testosterone levels start decreasing after age 30.

A baby boy begins to produce testosterone as early as seven weeks after conception. Before a boy is even born, testosterone is working to form male genitals. Those testosterone levels rise during puberty, peak during the late-teen years, and then level off. After age thirty, those testosterone levels begin decreasing every year.

During puberty, testosterone is responsible for the development of male attributes like a deeper voice, beard, and body hair. It also promotes muscle mass and sex drive. Testosterone production surges during adolescence and peaks in the late teens or early twenties. After age thirty, it's natural for testosterone levels to drop by about one or two percent each year.

Testosterone is a vital male hormone that is responsible for the development and maintenance of male attributes. Women also have testosterone, but in much smaller amounts. Testosterone stimulates the DNA in specific genes in the body to keep our genes healthy instead of going haywire which may lead to cancer, Alzheimer's, diabetes, hypertension, heart disease, decreased resistance to infections and arthritis. [74] [75]

Testosterone is what makes a boy become a man. When fifteen-year-old boys talk to each other, it is often a game of one-upmanship. They boast, brag, talk big, and feel invincible. That's men-talk. Men like feeling strong and virile. Men like making decisions and winning. Men like having erections and they really like having sex. Testosterone plays a role in all of this. Testosterone causes the penis to become muscular and firm. And when hormones are flowing in a young man's body, he is on top of his game.

What Happens When Testosterone Decreases?

Loss of testosterone in men is called andropause. ***Andropause is a gradual loss of testosterone that begins in the late twenties to the mid-thirties and continues on a gradual decline for the next fifty years.*** This decline is so gradual that most men hardly notice the changes caused by this deficiency. Menopause in women is dramatic exemplified by hot flushes, vaginal dryness, weight gain, depression, mood swings, poor sleep, just to name a few symptoms. Men are different, as we all know.

One of the first signs of testosterone deficiency in men is erectile dysfunction. Erections are more difficult to achieve and maintain with less fullness of erections. Even *Viagra* does not help all the time. Marked decrease in spontaneous early morning erection is a hallmark for low testosterone. There is less volume of semen in ejaculation. There is not as much strength of a climax and decreased muscular pulsations. Too often, this is just pushed off as stress. Men are told they are just getting older or are overworked.

There's a bit of truth to the *"use it or lose it"* theory. A man with low levels of testosterone may lose his desire for sex. Sexual stimulation and sexual activity cause testosterone levels to rise. Testosterone levels can drop during a long period of sexual inactivity. Low testosterone can also result in erectile dysfunction (ED).

Men may notice an increase in tiredness, diminished sex drive, weight gain especially around the abdomen, decreased mental clarity, arthritis, depression, osteopenia and osteoporosis, loss of self-esteem, decreased exercise tolerance and loss of vitality. Men are more likely to notice a decrease in athletic performance, sore joints and muscles with stiffness, less flexibility, decrease in muscle size and tone, and a decrease in stamina.

The Effects of Testosterone on the Body

As you can see in the diagram to the right, [76] testosterone levels affect everything in men from the reproductive system and sexuality to muscle mass and bone density. It also plays a role in certain behaviors.

Men may be told by their doctor that their cholesterol is too high and their HDL cholesterol is too low. There may be an increase in sugar in the blood or insulin resistance suggesting pre-diabetes. His blood pressure probably will be a little higher than it was five years ago. If there is fat accumulation around the abdomen, the doctor may suspect an increased risk of heart disease. A carotid ultrasound may find a narrowing of an artery in the neck.

But the man had none of these signs and symptoms five years earlier. So why now?

If you have your testosterone levels checked, you will most likely find the answer. In the last ten years, your testosterone dropped 67%! But your doctor will tell you, *"This is within normal limits,"* or *"This is normal for a man who is your age." "It happens to all men."* Don't believe it! ***Please remember that the above signs and symptoms are like a flashing red light that says, "Warning! Your health is deteriorating. It will continue to decline – unless you do something about it."***

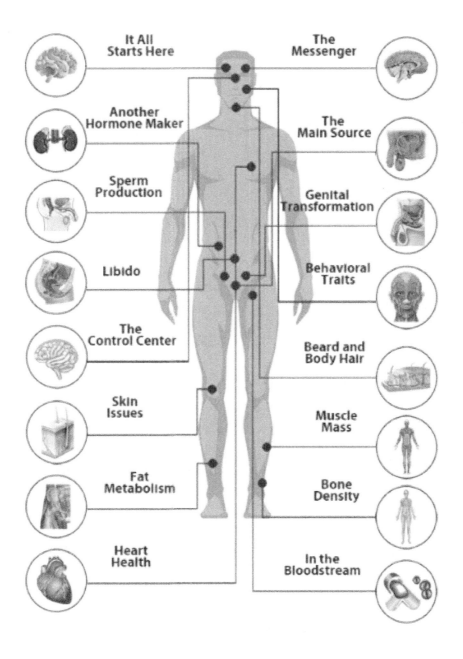

Remember, symptoms are an indication something is going on in your body. When you have recurrent heartburn, it may be the sign of an ulcer. When you have sneezing, burning and itching eyes while mowing the lawn, you may have allergies. You understand the point: the changes you see at age forty-eight were not there when you were thirty-two. Something is happening, and it is probably decreased production of testosterone.

It is very important to know the hormone blood levels – but it is equally important to know the symptoms of the patient. Many years ago a physician, Sir William Osler, said, *"Listen to your patient, he is telling you the diagnosis."*

***When men say they are tired, have no sex drive, and when they do
have sex, staying erect is difficult, the ejaculation is less, the
orgasm is short and not as strong ... there is a reason and it is not
"just getting old."***

When men say they are tired, have no sex drive, and when they do have sex, staying erect is difficult, the ejaculation is less, the orgasm is short and not as strong, they have trouble concentrating, they are not able to exercise as much, their muscles are getting flabby, they have weight gain around the abdomen—there is a reason and it is *not "just getting old."* The patient just told you by his symptoms what his diagnosis is: *"My testosterone is low."*

Now think this through with me: when a young man is twenty years old, his eye sight is normal if it is 20/20. Now that he is sixty, he may have a reading of 20/60. How would he respond if his ophthalmologist tells him, *"Your eyesight is now 20/60, that's normal for your age. Nothing needs to be done. Just try to find books with large print"*?

In the same way, it is difficult to understand how a physician can say to a man who is symptomatic of low testosterone, *"Your problem is not low testosterone. Your testosterone is 275. That's within normal range for a man your age. Now that you're older you don't need as much testosterone."* It is so emotionally rewarding to treat such a man who was told he was normal for age with *Pellet Hormone Replacement Therapy,* because virtually every time he will notice a remarkable difference within the first two weeks.

Some Success Stories

Jim was a fifty-nine year old patient who was told by his family doctor that his testosterone of 263 ng/dL was normal for a man his age. Jim saw his physician because he was tired all the time. *"I used to work out almost every day. I have tried to keep it up, but I can't do exercise for more than ten minutes without having to rest. That's not me."* But when his testosterone increased to 985 ng/dL after treatment with testosterone, he said, *"This changed my life in one month. I have so much more energy ... and I don't use Viagra anymore."*

John was seventy years old. His wife, Mary, was sixty-seven. Mary had been a patient of ours for the last six months. Prior to seeing us, she was tired, had absolutely no sex drive, had gained fifty pounds over the last thirty years, and had most of the signs and symptoms of being postmenopausal. Six months earlier she said, *"I'm just getting old but my friend told me it was my hormones and I would have more energy if I had this treatment."* She was obviously low in testosterone, progesterone and estradiol.

Mary was treated with the appropriate hormone replacement based on her age, weight, symptoms and her lab results. She was started on oral vitamin B12 1000 mcg a day. She was given a prescription for Armour Thyroid 30 mcg each morning before eating. She was given a low glycemic index diet to follow.

After six months she had lost twenty-three pounds and had a remarkable turnaround. *"I walk three to four miles a day. I could never have done that before. I think about sex again. I want to be intimate with my husband."* Now Mary brought John in to have his hormones checked. She said, *"I told John I want to have sex again. We have tried but he needs help."*

John was a very pleasant man, still working at age seventy, but not as much as he used to. He was embarrassed that his wife was so blunt. *"I just don't have the energy I used to. Mary brought me in, but I don't know if I need hormones or not. I've tried Viagra and Cialis, but they don't help enough. It won't stay hard enough to do any good."*

John's testosterone was miserable at 173 ng/dL. John was interested in just one thing: he wanted to be able to have sex with Mary. His lab work otherwise was normal. He had no diabetes or anemia. His blood pressure was unremarkable, even at seventy years old. John thought he was doing okay physically ... until Mary discovered BHRT.

John had an insert of testosterone 2000 mg pellets. To help John even more, I gave him a bottle of *Revive TCN* one capsule a day for one week, then one every other day. [77] He was asked to come back in one month.

He was able to have fun with Mary *"like we had when we were first married forty-six years ago."*

On recheck one month later, it was so much fun to watch John and Mary. They were smiling, giggling like teenagers, and sharing inside jokes with each other. John's testosterone was now 1160 ng/dL. He was able to have fun with Mary *"like we had when we were first married forty-six years ago."*

Seeing smiles like John's and Mary's brings so much happiness and personal edification to know that these two older patients are healthier and able to enjoy the quality of life they desire.

Treating Low Testosterone in Men

There are three problems with the errant treatment of men with low testosterone by telling them, *"You are normal for your age."*

- **First, medical students are taught from day one, *"Treat the patient, not the lab."*** In other words, *"Listen to the symptoms of the patient. He will tell you what is wrong."* It is wrong to just look at the lab report and tell the patient, *"Everything is okay. Your lab work is normal."*
- **Second, the results of blood work may be reported as normal for age.** Obviously, most men who are going to have their blood tested are older. Young men do not have their testosterone levels checked. Therefore this eschews the number calling a low testosterone normal for most men. When looking at what most men have and calling that *"normal"* is inaccurate. The better word would be if we called it *"average"* for that age group. But it is not "normal" for any age. Most men sixty-five years old don't want to feel like all the other men who are sixty-five. They want to feel like they felt when they were thirty-five!

You don't want to feel like a thirty year old, do you?

Patrick was a sixty-four-year-old diabetic who was being treated for hormone deficiency with bio-identical testosterone pellets. On his regular visit to his endocrinologist, the doctor said with some alarm, *"Patrick, your sugar and HgA1c are fine, but you have a real problem."* Patrick responded, *"What's wrong?"* The doctor said, *"Your testosterone is like a thirty-year-old man. That can't be normal."* Patrick asked, *"So what's wrong with that, doctor?"* His doctor questioned, *"But Patrick, you don't want to feel like a thirty-year-old, do you?"*

If only all of us had that problem! But the truth is that it is possible.

- **Third, forty years ago it was very acceptable to tell a patient normal systolic blood pressure (the top number) is *"100 plus their age."*** For someone seventy years old, a normal blood pressure would be 170/90. This patient would be told, *"Your blood pressure is normal for your age. No treatment is necessary."* But now we know that a patient is far more likely to suffer a stroke or heart attack with numbers that high. It is now known that men with low testosterone are far more likely to have coronary artery disease leading to a stroke or heart attack. It is wrong to tell these men *"Your testosterone is normal for your age. No treatment is necessary."* One day doctors will check a man's testosterone just like they do his blood pressure and cholesterol levels today to assure he has the best chance of having good health.

What Are You Going To Do About It?

Every man I know wants to feel young again. Many of you identified with Jim's and John's stories earlier in this chapter.

I know it is hard for men to admit they need help. It's hard for many of us to admit that our bodies can't do what they used to be able to do. But what if there was help? What if BHRT could reverse the symptoms you are experiencing? What if it could help restore testosterone levels to the level they were when you were twenty-five? I encourage you to check it out. Make an appointment to see a BHRT specialist today. You'll be so glad you did.

Journal thoughts and questions:

_____

_____

_____

_____

_____

_____

_____

_____

_____

_____

_____

_____

_____

_____

_____

_____

_____

_____

CHAPTER 15

Estradiol In Men

What? Men Have Estrogen?

Do men really have estrogen? Yes, they do. Without a small amount of estrogen, men might be brain dead. (*Yes, I know ... the women are tempted to insert a joke here ... but let's move on.*)

Testosterone is the predominant hormone in men. Estradiol is the predominant hormone in women. Men naturally have lower levels of estradiol than women. Women naturally have lower levels of testosterone than men. So the questions are: If men need some estradiol, how much is good for them to have? What good does estradiol do? And, if you have too much of it, what harm does it do?

What Does Estrogen Do in a Man's Body?

It is possible for a man's testosterone level to not be terribly low, and yet he may still have symptoms of fatigue, weight gain around the abdomen, decreased sex life, depression, etc. Why is that? What's going on?

You might remember that early on we discussed the conversion of one hormone to another and back to the original hormone. Testosterone in men may be converted to estradiol naturally by an enzyme known as aromatase. That's normal. Also, as mentioned in the last chapter, the sex hormone binding globulin has a tendency to increase as we age, binding more of the total testosterone and leaving men with less free and usable testosterone.

The levels of aromatase gradually increase with age. The body's conversion of testosterone to estradiol can become a bad thing if estradiol levels are too high in men. This conversion occurs easily, as these two sex hormones are chemically similar.

It's a Balancing Act

Estradiol is important to certain functions in men.

Estradiol is important to certain functions in men. Certainly estradiol is extremely necessary to brain function. Just the right amount of estradiol is essential for certain sexual functions. Too much estradiol may neuter a man, but also too little may have the same effect.

A woman's estradiol may be as low as 40 pg/ml at certain times of the month and may be as high as 800 pg/ml two weeks later. But in men, the window of opportunity is much smaller. Estradiol in men should be approximately 35 pg/ml give or take 10 pg/ml. Your liver processes and eliminates excess estradiol. But as the liver loses its ability to function (through aging, excess alcohol, or drugs), it may allow excess estradiol to accumulate. Also, fat cells manufacture estrogen. Men and women who are obese may have excess estrogen.

Because testosterone and estradiol are so similar chemically, estradiol may occupy the receptor sites of testosterone on trillions of cells throughout the body. Even the hypothalamus receptor sites (the part of the brain that controls our hormones) may be occupied by estradiol instead of testosterone. This tricks the hypothalamus by signaling there is plenty of testosterone circulating in the blood, when it really is estradiol instead. Remember, the hypothalamus is constantly monitoring the blood for testosterone. The occupation of testosterone receptor sites by estradiol in the hypothalamus causes the pituitary gland to decrease the production of luteinizing hormone which is intended to stimulate the testicles to produce more testosterone.

Too much estradiol occupying testosterone receptor sites will switch off some activity designed to perform male functions.

- Muscles in men depend on testosterone to become stronger.
- Receptor sites to testosterone are abundant in the muscles in the penis.
- The heart has more receptor sites to testosterone than any other muscle in the body.

Because aromatase increases with age, this process of estradiol stimulating more testosterone receptor sites becomes more problematic causing erectile dysfunction, dull concentration, and loss of muscle mass.

The ratio should be fifty (testosterone) to
one (estradiol) as seen in a young man

The important number to function well is the ratio of testosterone to estradiol. The ratio should be fifty (testosterone) to one (estradiol) as seen in a young man. As we age, this ratio changes to seven or eight to one. There is far more testosterone than estradiol in a young man – fifty times more. There may be only seven times more testosterone than estradiol in older men. That is why you see the symptoms of erectile dysfunction, fat accumulation, muscle loss, etc.

The liver processes hormones, including estrogen. This process is slowed down with aging and alcohol abuse. This allows for a buildup of excess estrogen in the body. As the liver ages, its ability to process zinc decreases. This is significant, as zinc aids in the elimination of excess estrogen. If a man's estradiol is too high, he may be told to take zinc 50 mg twice a day for two weeks and then once a day following that. He may also take a supplement DIM (diindolymethane) twice a day to lower his estradiol level.

Fat cells produce estrogen, but not estradiol. With a smaller amount of testosterone, men have a tendency to gain weight, especially around the waist. This causes more production of estrogen – especially the most undesirable form of estrogen: *estrone*. Obese men and women have higher levels of estrogen, usually estrone. Estrone is the type of estrogen that is more likely to cause breast cancer in women.

Too much alcohol causes a significant increase in estrogen. It is known that in women, estrogen can increase threefold with just one drink. Heavy use of alcohol in men can result in high estrogen levels. The physical evidence of this is seen in man-boobs, spider veins (which are small widened blood vessels on the chest and abdomen), a large abdomen, and testicular atrophy.

Some drugs may increase estrogen in men. Hydrochlorothiazide (fluid pills, or diuretics) may be used as a solo treatment for high blood pressure, but are also frequently a part of another antihypertensive medication. Studies have shown that diuretics lower blood pressure effectively, but the long-term effects may be dangerous and lower life expectancy. Diuretics cause the kidneys to excrete potassium and the liver to eliminate zinc. As zinc is removed, aromatase is increased which increases estrogen in the body. This results in cardiovascular disease in men.

When a man has too little testosterone in his body – along with too much estrogen – it adds up to a danger in his life.

In summary: Because SHBG (sex hormone binding globulin) increases with age, this protein binds more testosterone allowing less free (active) testosterone. As we age, the liver cannot eliminate estrogen as easily. Aging allows more fat accumulation in our bodies, as there is less testosterone to encourage exercise. Zinc aids in the elimination of excess estrogen in men, but when the liver is not functioning at full capacity, estrogen builds up. Drinking alcohol, especially in excess, also promotes estrogen accumulation. When a man has too little testosterone in his body – along with too much estrogen – it adds up to a danger in his life.

All of these factors contribute to a metabolic disaster for men: male menopause, otherwise known as andropause. Just giving men testosterone may not be effective. More testosterone may just convert to estradiol, causing an even greater problem. This is why a doctor should be aware of all the intricacies of the male menopause and how to prevent the loss of testosterone and the accumulation of too much estrogen.

Why is Elevated Estrogen Such a Disaster for Men?

If estradiol is so good for women, shouldn't the same be true for men? Well, here's some stunning information: *men and women are different!*

In men, if estrogen is too high, the risk of coronary artery disease increases. This is the opposite effect in women. Estrogen in men increases clotting factors which leads to blood clots. Estradiol in women increases substances that dissolve blood clots. Estradiol in men constricts coronary arteries that can cause heart attacks, while in women, estradiol dilates the arteries around the heart and protects the heart.

Elevated estradiol in men also causes fatigue, erectile dysfunction and poor concentration. Elevated estradiol may result from the administration of testosterone. Too much estradiol is not good. Most men feel good with a level of estradiol of 35 pg/ml. A range of 25 pg/ml up to 45 pg/ml is acceptable. This is why having your estradiol checked with each office visit at least every three months is important.

What Can Be Done to Prevent Too Much Estrogen and Too Little Testosterone in Men?

The doctor taking care of your hormone deficiency should do a variety of lab studies. **A detailed history** of your symptoms will tell the caregiver much about what is happening inside your body. Your doctor will ask questions such as:
- What is your diet like?
- Do you exercise regularly?
- Are you under undue stress?

A physical exam will determine your BMI (body mass index). If your BMI is high (too much fat), you have a much greater chance of having excess estrogen, both in women and men. In men, if you have excess estrogen there is a greater chance you have low testosterone because estrogen can occupy receptor sites in the hypothalamus which tricks the brain to appear that you have sufficient testosterone when actually it is estrogen.

From this information the doctor can encourage life-style changes:
- If your weight is above what your doctor considers safe for you according to your BMI, you may be encouraged to lose weight. Of course, if your testosterone is low, it will be more difficult to lose weight.
- If your cholesterol and triglycerides are too elevated, you may be placed on a lipid-lowering diet.
- If you do not exercise, you may be encouraged to begin an exercise program.
- If you have undue stress at work or at home, you may need some counseling about how to reduce your stress.
- If you smoke, STOP! There are some very good stop-smoking programs your doctor can recommend.
- If you drink too much alcohol, STOP! There are some very good programs to help you stop drinking.
- If your estradiol is too high, your doctor should be careful about administering testosterone because your body will attempt to convert the testosterone to estradiol. There are two possible dietary supplements that may be helpful:
  - You may be encouraged to take the dietary supplement DIM—3,3'-Diindolylmethane. DIM is a compound derived from the digestion of indole-3-carbinol, found in cruciferous vegetables such as broccoli, Brussel sprouts, cabbage and kale. This supplement aids the liver in the excretion of excess estrogen. The dosage is usually one capsule twice a day.
  - Also adding Zinc, 50 mg once a day, may be beneficial in reducing estrogen in your body.

Though it sounds very counterintuitive, a man's estradiol level is very important. Keep an eye on it. Check it regularly!

Journal thoughts and questions:

_____

_____

_____

_____

_____

_____

_____

_____

_____

_____

_____

_____

_____

_____

_____

_____

_____

_____

_____

CHAPTER 16

Alzheimer's Disease And Dementia

An Introduction to Alzheimer's Disease

Alzheimer's – it's that dreaded disease that now afflicts more than five million Americans. It's hard to ignore it anymore.

One in three seniors will die of Alzheimer's or another type of dementia.

The Alzheimer's Association states that someone in the United States develops Alzheimer's every sixty-seven seconds. It is the sixth leading cause of death in America today. One in three seniors will die of Alzheimer's or another type of dementia.

Hormonal changes affect the brain. Is it possible to avoid brain atrophy with hormonal replacement therapy? The evidence says *"Yes!"*

Dementia is a general term indicating loss of brain function that is seen in certain diseases. Alzheimer's disease is one form of dementia that gradually gets worse over time. It affects memory, thinking, and behavior. One is more likely to get Alzheimer's disease if they are older. But some people develop Alzheimer's before they get old. Developing Alzheimer's disease, however, is not an inevitable part of normal aging.

Having a close relative, such as a brother, sister, or parent with Alzheimer's increases the chance of having this disease. A certain gene, APOE epsilon4 allele, increases one's odds of developing Alzheimer's disease. Trauma to the brain may cause one to have Alzheimer's later in life. Women are more likely to develop Alzheimer's than men especially if they have had high blood pressure for a prolonged time. The brain of an Alzheimer's patient shrinks in size. Neurons of their brains die and develop tangles and plaque forms.

Medications containing the drug *memantine* may temporarily help the patient remember things and better manage their daily tasks. This drug may slow down the worsening of mental abilities, but Alzheimer's disease continues to progress, even on medication.

"Early onset Alzheimer's disease" occurs before age sixty. This type is much less common than late onset, and it tends to get worse quickly. "Late onset Alzheimer's disease" occurs after age sixty and is the most common type. It is not clear if this type runs in families or not. The cause of Alzheimer's disease is not clear, but genes and environmental factors may play a role.

One Satisfied Patient

A very sweet eighty-six-year-old widow named Mary reported that she had lost the energy she used to have. She wanted it back. She was well-to-do and did not want to go to an assisted living facility. On exam, she was alert but had to search for answers. She could not remember names of family members and could not remember her phone number without some help.

Mary complained that she had trouble sleeping, but she was afraid to take sleeping pills because she feared she might fall when she got up. She did not have signs of Alzheimer's disease but did have some early dementia. She was on no medications but did take a multivitamin.

Mary's physical exam was what would be expected for a slim, elderly, 118 pound lady. Her lab work showed her testosterone was almost nonexistent and her progesterone was low, with elevated FSH. All other studies were acceptable.

She was treated with bio-identical hormone pellets of estradiol 6 mg and testosterone 50 mg. She was given a prescription for bio-identical progesterone 100 mg to be taken at bedtime. She was instructed to get good quality melatonin 5 mg and take one or two at bedtime. She was to continue her multivitamin, but was asked to take oral chewable B12 1000 mcg tablets once a day.

Three months later she said, *"I am so very happy because now I can play Gin Rummy with friends that are much younger than me. I drove myself here today. I walk almost daily at the mall and I met a friend there. He likes to walk with me. I clean my own house without anyone coming in to help, and I'm sleeping all night."* In talking with her, she was much quicker to answer and seemed to have a different glow about her. Lab studies performed two days before her visit showed all her levels were significantly better.

In talking with her, she was much quicker to answer and seemed to have a different glow about her.

After four years, she is continuing the therapy. Obviously, bio-identical hormone pellets helped her tremendously!

Alzheimer's Symptoms

The symptoms of Alzheimer's disease include:
- Changes in emotional behavior or personality (blank stare on the face)
- Slowing of language
- Recent and long-term memory loss
- Changes in perception (seeing people looking through the window)
- And loss of thinking and judgment (cognitive skills)

One early sign is forgetfulness. Mild thinking (cognitive) impairment is one stage worse than normal forgetfulness due to aging ... but this may not be Alzheimer's disease. People who suffer from dementia with mild cognitive impairment may have problems with thinking and memory that do not interfere with everyday activities. Usually these people are aware of their forgetfulness. This is not a sure sign of developing Alzheimer's disease.

People who have mild cognitive (brain function) impairment commonly associated with aging have symptoms of difficulty performing more than one task at a time, difficulty solving problems, forgetting recent events or conversations, and taking longer to perform more difficult activities.

However, patients who have early Alzheimer's disease will be significantly different. They will have difficulty performing tasks that take some thought but used to come easily, such as balancing a checkbook, playing complex games such as bridge, learning new information or routines, getting lost on familiar routes, language problems (such as trouble finding the name of familiar objects), losing interest in things previously enjoyed, flat mood, misplacing items, personality changes and loss of social skills.

As Alzheimer's disease worsens, the symptoms become more pronounced. The signs are now obvious and interfere with the person's ability to take care of their personal needs. The symptoms of more advanced Alzheimer's disease include:

- Change in sleep patterns, often waking up at night
- Delusions
- Depression
- Agitation
- Difficulty doing basic tasks, such as preparing meals, choosing proper
- clothing
- Difficulty driving
- Difficulty reading or writing
- Forgetting details about current events
- Forgetting events from their own life
- Losing awareness of who they are
- Hallucinations
- Arguments
- Striking out physically
- Violent behavior
- Poor judgment
- Loss of ability to recognize danger
- Using the wrong words
- Mispronouncing words
- Speaking in confusing sentences
- Withdrawing from social contact

Patients with severe Alzheimer's disease can no longer understand language, recognize family members, or perform basic activities of daily living, such as eating, dressing, and bathing, may have incontinence and problems swallowing.

A physician should be able to diagnose Alzheimer's disease by performing a complete physical exam, including neurological exam, asking questions about their medical history and symptoms, and a mental status examination. In diagnosing Alzheimer's, there are other causes of dementia that have to be ruled out such as anemia, brain tumor, chronic infection, intoxication from medication, severe depression, stroke, thyroid disease, and vitamin deficiency. A CT scan or MRI of the brain may be done to look for these other causes of dementia.

In the early stages of dementia, brain image scans may be normal. In later stages, an MRI may show a decrease in the size of different areas of the brain. While the scans do not confirm the diagnosis of Alzheimer's disease, they do exclude other causes of dementia (such as a stroke and tumor). However, the only way to know for certain that someone has Alzheimer's disease is to examine a sample of their brain tissue after death. [78]

Help for Alzheimer's Patients

There is no cure for Alzheimer's disease. Current medicines approved by the FDA may slow down the rate at which symptoms become worse. The benefit from these drugs is usually small. One should know the many potential side effects before instituting therapy using these drugs. Supplements may help prevent or slow down Alzheimer's disease, but there is no current evidence to support this view.

It is probably wise to consume a low-fat diet, eat cold-water fish such tuna, salmon, and mackerel that are rich in omega-3 fatty acids at least two to three times per week, reduce the intake of linoleic acid found in margarine, butter, and dairy products, increase antioxidants such as carotenoids, take vitamin E and vitamin C, by eating plenty of darkly colored fruits and vegetables, maintain a normal blood pressure, stay mentally and socially active throughout life, consider taking nonsteroidal anti-inflammatory drugs like ibuprofen (Advil, Motrin). Statin drugs, a class of medications normally used for high cholesterol, may help lower the risk of Alzheimer's disease. However, there is no hard scientific evidence that the above common-sense, healthy practices will prevent Alzheimer's disease. [79]

Bio-identical Hormone Replacement Therapy can help prevent degeneration of the central nervous system during menopause and aging. It may even be protective against neurodegenerative diseases such as Alzheimer's disease. [80]

Hormone replacement therapy is advantageous to the central nervous system as estradiol affects cells in the brain, including protection against strokes, reduces the risk of Alzheimer's disease, and improved brain function. [81]

The Benefits of Estradiol

Estradiol protects the nervous system from the body's fight against the body's effort to detoxify and free radicals that damage all components of the cell, including proteins, lipids, and DNA. This stress is increased without estradiol, causing the toxic effects of free radicals, and is dangerous to the central nervous system. The consequences of being without the protection of estradiol may be neuro-degenerative diseases including gene mutations, chronic fatigue syndrome, heart and blood vessel disorders, heart failure, heart attack and inflammatory diseases. Further insults on the body come from disruptions in normal mechanisms of cellular signaling, which may cause cancer, Parkinson's disease, Alzheimer's disease, atherosclerosis, fragile X syndrome, Sickle Cell Disease, lichen planus, vitiligo, autism, and chronic fatigue syndrome. [82]

"Estrogen replacement therapy is associated with improvement of cognitive deficits and reduced incidence of Alzheimer's disease."

The beneficial effects of bio-identical estradiol was touted in an article published by *The Endocrine Society in 2002: "Estrogen replacement therapy is associated with improvement of cognitive deficits and reduced incidence of Alzheimer's disease."* This study noted that bio-identical estradiol, and natural progesterone, alone or in combination, protected against glutamate toxicity. Without becoming too complicated, glutamate is a neurotransmitter. It is especially important in the brain to keep us thinking and remembering. Having just the right amount is paramount. Too much glutamate is toxic to the brain and results in memory loss and eventually Alzheimer's. Estradiol and progesterone that are natural to humans protect the brain from excess glutamate. [83]

The Dangers of *Provera*

In contrast, the synthetic hormone *Provera* does not protect against glutamate toxicity. **Not only does *Provera* not protect the brain, it actually makes things worse.** Estradiol by itself protects the brain, but when *Provera* is given with estradiol, the protection of estradiol is lost. The findings from this study are important in that hormone replacement with bio-identical estradiol and progesterone is beneficial in the maintenance of brain function during menopause and aging and for protection against diseases such as Alzheimer's disease, whereas the use of synthetic Provera is harmful to the brain. [84]

Not only does Provera not protect the brain,
it actually makes things worse.

Provera has been shown to block the stimulating effects of estrogen in uterine cells and to inhibit estrogen-stimulated uterine proliferation. That is a good thing. [85] Because of the anti-estrogen effects of progestins such as *Provera*, these drugs have been added to hormone replacement therapy over the years to reduce the risk of uterine cancer secondary to unopposed estrogen. Reducing the risk of cancer is also a good thing. [86] Synthetic progestins such as *Provera* have been added to hormone replacement therapy, not only to prevent endometrial hyperplasia, an over-growth of the inside lining of the uterus, but *Provera* was thought to diminish estrogen's effects in the breast that caused breast cancer. This is where things go wrong. [87] This long-held belief has been found to be just the opposite. The combination of estrogen and *Provera* **INCREASED** cancer risk more than just estrogen alone. [88]

The Proof IS in the Testing

Hormone replacement therapy has shown a significant reduction in the risk of developing Alzheimer's disease. Epidemiological studies have demonstrated that *women who receive estrogen replacement therapy are less likely to develop Alzheimer's disease or develop Alzheimer's disease with a later onset*. [89]

In four different studies, the risk reduction of developing Alzheimer's dementia was from between 29 to 44 percent in the group using hormone replacement versus those patients who had never used hormones. The neuroprotective effect of bio-identical estradiol treatment was better than that with *Premarin*, and **when Provera was added, patients actually did worse.** Also the risk of developing Alzheimer's disease decreased the longer the patient was on estradiol, but did not help unless used for more than ten years.

This suggests that there is an optimal time to begin hormone replacement therapy — during perimenopause (just when hormones begin declining before menopause) usually around age thirty-five. Some of the benefit of hormone replacement therapy may be lost if one waits until menopause.

There is an optimal time to begin hormone replacement therapy — usually around age thirty-five.

There was a two-fold increase of the risk of probable dementia when *Premarin* and *Provera* were used. The more recent large random control trials used only oral conjugated equine estrogen with continuous *Provera*, whereas natural steroid hormones are probably more beneficial regarding protection of the nervous system or side effects, due to their distinct pharmacokinetic properties. [90]

A study involving men with Alzheimer's disease or mild brain function impairment was performed at *University of Washington School of Medicine* in Seattle. Their goal was to determine if testosterone supplementation was effective in these conditions. Testosterone injections were administered to one group and placebo injections to another. Serum testosterone levels were raised 295 percent in the treated group. Improvements in spatial memory, constructional abilities and verbal memory were evident in the testosterone treated group. Prostate specific antigen did not significantly change during this brief treatment. *The investigators found benefit of testosterone supplementation in men with cognitive impairment and with Alzheimer's disease.* [91]

A study that evaluated the effects of testosterone therapy on brain function, neuropsychiatric symptoms, and quality of life in male patients with Alzheimer's disease and healthy elderly men was reported in *Neurology* in 2006. Patients with Alzheimer's disease were treated with testosterone and healthy male controls were treated with a placebo gel daily. *Patients receiving testosterone had significant improvement in quality-of-life scores and the treatment was well tolerated.* Testosterone had minimal effects on cognition (brain function) and the treated group showed more numerical improvement and less decline in visuospatial functions. [92]

In this chapter, we have seen that BHRT may be helpful in preventing deterioration of the central nervous system during aging. It also may help protect against neurodegenerative diseases such as Alzheimer's disease.

Journal thoughts and questions:

_____

_____

_____

_____

_____

_____

_____

_____

_____

_____

_____

_____

_____

_____

_____

_____

_____

_____

CHAPTER 17

Anemia

What Is Anemia?

Anemia is a condition in which a person does not have enough red blood cells. This results in fatigue and damage to the body. If you are chronically tired, you may be anemic.

Anemia is a frequent feature of menopausal women and male hypogonadism and anti-androgenic therapies (drugs that lower testosterone after surgery for prostate cancer in which the testicles are removed). Older men and women with low testosterone are far more likely to be anemic than those with normal testosterone. [93]

Bio-identical Testosterone Hormone Therapy stimulates the production of red blood cells which carry oxygen to every cell in the body, providing energy.

Louis's Story

Louis was seventy-seven years old and in reasonably good health, except for well controlled atrial fibrillation. Louis complained,

I am always tired. I give out so quickly when I try to do anything. My heart doctor told me it was my heart. But a friend of mine told me hormones helped him. My wife is not living, and I'd like to meet a woman – but I don't have enough energy even if I was with a woman.

I read a lot about keeping healthy. I know that low testosterone could cause all kinds of health problems. I know I'm not going to be young again, but I just want to have enough energy to enjoy the years I have left.

Louis's CBC showed a hemoglobin well below normal. His hematocrit was also low. His testosterone was predictably low. He probably was not losing blood from his gut, but just not manufacturing enough in his bone marrow or spleen. With this type of anemia, the body may produce too few red blood cells or the blood cells may not function correctly. In either case, anemia can result.

It is interesting to see the reason a patient may have anemia listed as due to *"old age"* – as though getting old is a disease. Louis's doctor knew he was anemic. He was told that his anemia was a result of aging. If his anemia were due to aging, the reason for anemia in old age was most likely due to the body not producing enough testosterone to stimulate the bone marrow to produce enough red blood cells.

When bio-identical testosterone is administered, the anemia of old age is cured. But, it is doubtful you have ever heard a doctor say that the reason a patient has anemia was secondary to testosterone deficiency. It would be almost impossible to find that an investigation for anemia in an older patient would include checking his testosterone level.

Louis was treated with bio-identical testosterone pellets. He felt much better within one month – but the real changes were evident by his third month. His hemoglobin and hematocrit were completely normal. His testosterone was 862 ng/dL at one month but still up to 527 ng/dL at three months. Louis noted, *"I have more energy now. I walk each day and am beginning to do my own yard work. And I've been seeing a lady. We are spending more and more time together."*

> **"I have more energy now. I walk each day and am beginning to do my own yard work. And I've been seeing a lady. We are spending more and more time together."**

Louis was given a small dose of testosterone pellets to keep his blood level up for the next three months. In more conversation Louis said, *"Actually, I have proposed to the lady I told you about."* He was given a bottle of *Revive* to give him a boost of confidence in the bedroom.

It is so interesting to note that a common list of causes for anemia includes: *Sickle cell anemia, iron-deficiency anemia, vitamin deficiency, bone marrow and stem cell problems, abnormal uterine bleeding, bleeding from the stomach (ulcers or stomach cancer), anemia of old age, bleeding from the colon, pregnancy, Crohn's disease, advanced kidney disease, Hypothyroidism, chemotherapy, alcohol abuse, lead poisoning, and a myriad of other disease processes.*

But absent from the list is anemia caused by low testosterone. To doctors specializing in *Bio-identical Hormone Replacement Therapy*, the production of red blood cells is obviously directly related to testosterone. This is why with each visit a Complete Blood Count is done, especially in men. It is not healthy to have a hemoglobin or hematocrit (H&H) too low or too high. If the H&H is above normal, the patient should not have a treatment with testosterone until he donates blood or has blood removed in a lab and discarded.

What We Have Seen in this Chapter

In this chapter we have seen that:
- Older men and women with low testosterone are far more likely to be anemic than those with normal testosterone.
- The production of red blood cells is directly related to testosterone.
- *Bio-identical Hormone Replacement Therapy* helps with anemia.

Journal thoughts and questions:

_____

_____

_____

_____

_____

_____

_____

_____

_____

_____

_____

_____

_____

_____

_____

_____

_____

_____

CHAPTER 18

Anti-Aging

The Inevitability of Aging

Death is inevitable. But the quality of life during the years one lives is a choice.

Surveys will always list "the fear of death" at the top of their "fears" lists. However, more and more people are afraid they will not be able to enjoy a healthier quality of life in their later years. In this chapter, you will see that bio-identical hormones play an essential part in providing a longer and healthier life.

How Hormones Affect the Aging Process

Changes in hormone levels contribute to the process of aging because the endocrine system plays a major role in cellular interactions, metabolism, and growth. [94] The endocrine system refers to our glands that secrete hormones directly into the circulation to be carried to some other gland to stimulate it. The major endocrine glands include:

- The pineal gland
- Pituitary gland
- Pancreas
- Ovaries
- Testes
- Thyroid gland
- Parathyroid gland
- Hypothalamus
- Gastrointestinal tract
- Adrenal glands

More specifically, there is a strong clinically important relationship between decreases in testosterone and estrogen with age, age-related decline in muscle and bone mass and strength, and eventually health span in humans. In aging women, hormone replacement is the first line and most effective treatment for menopausal symptoms and improvement of low quality of life due to estrogen deficiency.[95]

There is a strong clinically important relationship between decreases in testosterone and estrogens with age, age-related decline in muscle and bone mass and strength, and eventually health span in humans.

Studies clearly demonstrate that you can trace hormone deficiencies and from these measurements predict the health and longevity in older persons. Aging is not dependent on just one factor (such as hormones) but is multidimensional. It involves physical, psychological, and social changes, which as a whole affects life span. However, our hormones can powerfully influence the physical, psychological and social changes seen in aging.

It is helpful to examine the physical mechanisms by which loss of hormones impairs healthy aging. This may aid in the treatment of physical deficiencies and extend life span. An important impairment of aging is loss of physical ability. This is seen with the loss of skeletal muscle mass that accompanies aging. Far too often, the role that hormones play in the regulation of metabolism of muscles and bones and their influence on physical function is overlooked by care givers. [96] Loss of the three sex hormones (testosterone, progesterone and estradiol) is the initiating trigger that results in muscle loss, muscle weakness, decreased functional performance, and decreased life span.

Aging Women and Testosterone

"Testosterone! You don't want testosterone in women! Do you want to look like a man?" This is a very common comment by physicians when women ask about hormone replacement therapy using testosterone. *"But, doctor, didn't I have testosterone when I was a young woman?"* The answer to that is yes – significantly lower levels, but they do have testosterone.

Women in their forties will lose fifty percent of the testosterone they had in their thirties.

Here are some facts about aging women and testosterone:
- Women have twenty to twenty-five times lower levels of testosterone compared with men. [97]
- As women age, the loss of testosterone causes decreased libido, lean body mass and physical function, brain function, emotions, bone loss, and frailty. [98]
- Women in their forties will lose fifty percent of the testosterone they had in their thirties. [99]
- In just ten years, women will have half as much testosterone as they did at age thirty. By the time women complete menopause, for most just over fifty years old, they will have just fifteen percent of the testosterone they had in their thirties. By age fifty, most women will lose eighty-five percent of the testosterone they had when they were thirty. [100] Some women will lose another sixty percent more testosterone within two to five years following menopause. Most women by age sixty to sixty-five will have just five percent of the testosterone they had in their prime. [101]
- Women who have their ovaries removed will see a dramatic reduction in their sex hormones almost immediately, most within a few days after surgery. Even if the ovaries are preserved, most will have a decline in hormones within two years of a hysterectomy.

Aging Men and Testosterone

There is so much information available about testosterone supplementation in men that they are becoming more knowledgeable than doctors about hormone replacement. They had to. So many doctors tell their male patients, *"Your testosterone level is normal for your age."* Doctors say this even when the lab shows his testosterone to be only twenty or twenty-five percent of what it was when he was twenty-five years old. Most physicians know a lot about how to treat blood pressure, sore throats and arthritis, but little about how to treat men (or women) with natural bio-identical testosterone.

> *By age seventy, most men will lose ninety percent of their youth testosterone. Almost all men seventy years old will be well below the testosterone level they were at when they were younger.*

Here are some facts about aging men and testosterone:
- Testosterone declines at a rate of one to two percent per year in men beginning around the mid- 30s.[102] Twenty percent of men over age sixty will have testosterone that is classified as low. [103]
- By age seventy, most men will lose ninety percent of their youthful testosterone. Almost all men seventy years old will be well below the testosterone level they were at when they were younger. These are not just theoretical considerations, but carry very serious health consequences to aging men.
- Aging in men is associated with decreases in bone mineral density, [104] lean body and muscle mass, [105] strength, [106] capacity to exercise, [107] an increase in abdominal fat, an increase in the bad low-density lipoprotein cholesterol, an increase in the worse low-density lipoprotein, and a decrease in the good high-density lipoprotein cholesterol. [108] All of this happens in nonelderly hypogonadal men also if their testosterone is low. [109]
- These changes in men that have declining testosterone will lead to muscular and skeletal frailty, and osteoporotic bone fractures causing major disability and limitations in elderly men. [110] It will eventually lead to cardiovascular disease. [111]
- The most obvious clinical signs of relative deficiency in older men are a decrease in muscle mass and strength, a decrease in bone mass, and an increase in central body fat. Lowering serum testosterone concentrations in healthy volunteers decreased fat-free mass, muscle strength, and mixed muscle fractional synthetic rate, [112] but testosterone supplementation increased fractional synthetic rate in young hypogonadal men [113] and older men. [114]
- Administration of supplemental testosterone to youthful levels increases the production of long protein chains in muscles, total body cell mass, and muscle strength. [115] As testosterone levels decline with aging, there is an increase in fat and redistributed to the abdomen in men and throughout the body to the point there are fewer areas where there is no fat. [116]
- This decline in muscle mass and increase in fat mass obviously causes decreased muscle strength, and this leads to limitations in activity. This is

seen in the elderly as loss of balance causing a higher chance of falling with serious injuries such as fracture. But other chronic conditions are seen such as type 2 diabetes mellitus, obstructive sleep apnea, obesity, liver failure, depression, chronic obstructive pulmonary disease, kidney failure, [117] decreased quality of life, and overall failure of multiple body systems and increased death rate with aging. [118]

- The influence of testosterone on protein metabolism is well known, [119] but testosterone also is essential in proper regulation and to maintain stability of glucose and lipids, [120] and bone growth. There is an increased prevalence of osteoporosis in men over sixty years who have low total testosterone levels as well as an increased rapid bone loss at the hip, [121] followed by an increase in hip fractures and fractures in various other bones. [122]

- Osteoporosis is thought of as a disease in postmenopausal women. There are 3 times more women with osteoporosis than men. However, there is an increased incidence of osteoporosis in men as longevity increases our life span. Because of this comes an increased rate of fractures and associated morbidity and mortality. Loss of testosterone not only causes a decrease in muscle mass in older men, but also is seen an increase of mortality in older men. [123]

In Summary

What have we learned in this chapter?

- The effects of aging in both men and women can be slowed down and even reversed by the beneficial use of BHRT.
- In aging women, hormone replacement is the first line and most effective treatment for menopausal symptoms and improvement of low quality of life due to estrogen deficiency.
- When supplemental testosterone is administered to aging men, it restores their testosterone to youthful levels and increases the production of long protein chains in muscles, total body cell mass, and muscle strength.

Journal thoughts and questions:

_____

_____

_____

_____

_____

_____

_____

_____

_____

_____

_____

_____

_____

_____

_____

_____

_____

_____

_____

CHAPTER 19

Arthritis

Does Bio-identical Testosterone Treat Arthritis?

Arthritis is an inflammatory process that includes red, swollen, and painful joints. Bio-identical testosterone is a natural anti-inflammatory. Once your hormones are balanced at a level of a much younger person, most patients are able to reduce or eliminate the need for arthritis medicines.

Rheumatoid Arthritis

There are many kinds of arthritis. Rheumatoid arthritis is an autoimmune disease that results in a chronic, inflammatory disorder that affects many tissues and organs, but principally attacks flexible joints. Those who suffer from rheumatoid arthritis will feel it progressing gradually over the course of several months or years.

Rheumatoid arthritis is an autoimmune disease that results in a chronic, inflammatory disorder that affects many tissues and organs, but principally attacks flexible joints.

Autoimmune disease is a condition that occurs when the immune system that normally protects us from infection mistakenly attacks and destroys healthy body tissue. There are more than eighty different types of autoimmune disorders. It can be a disabling and painful condition, which can lead to loss of functioning and mobility if not treated.

About 0.6 percent of the United States adult population has rheumatoid arthritis. Women suffer from this disease two to three times as often as men. [124] RA's onset most frequently occurs during middle age, but people of any age can be affected. [125] Rheumatoid arthritis primarily affects joints, however it also affects other organs in fifteen to twenty-five percent of individuals. [126]

What Are the Symptoms of Rheumatoid Arthritis?

Arthritis of the joints is an inflammation of the soft tissue found between the joint capsule and the joint cavity. Joints become swollen, tender and warm, which causes stiffness limiting movement particularly early in the morning on waking or following prolonged inactivity. Most commonly small joints of the hands, feet and cervical spine are affected, but larger joints like the shoulder and knee can also be involved. [127] Eventually there is erosion of the joint surface causing deformity and loss of function.

[128] Rheumatoid arthritis patients are at higher risk of atherosclerosis, heart attack and stroke. [129]

Other body systems can be affected with rheumatoid arthritis such as the liver, anemia, low white blood cell count, increased platelet count that can cause clotting problems, inflammation of nerves, carpal tunnel syndrome and compressing the spinal cord. Other symptoms of rheumatoid arthritis may include low-grade fever, tiredness, morning stiffness, loss of appetite and loss of weight. Local osteoporosis occurs in RA around inflamed joints. The kidneys may be effected causing the deposition of a protein, amyloid, in the kidneys in RA patients. [130]

Smoking places one at a three-times greater risk of rheumatoid arthritis than normal. Men who are heavy smokers may be at even a greater risk. This should be a serious consideration if RA is in the family history. [131] Vitamin D deficiency is common in those with rheumatoid arthritis and may be a cause. [132] Some trials have found a decreased risk for RA with vitamin D supplementation while others have not.

How Can BHRT Help?

Bio-identical Hormone Replacement Therapy using estradiol transdermally causes a significant increase in bone density in postmenopausal women with rheumatoid arthritis. This method of treatment also increases well-being, reduced inflammation in the joints and increased lumbar spine bone density over a one-year period in postmenopausal women with rheumatoid arthritis.[133]

> *Bio-identical Hormone Replacement Therapy using estradiol transdermally causes a significant increase in bone density in postmenopausal women with rheumatoid arthritis.*

Male patients with rheumatoid arthritis usually have low testosterone. IgM rheumatoid factor is a marker for rheumatoid arthritis. Men who have elevated IgM rheumatoid factor have a marked increase risk for rheumatoid arthritis. *Testosterone treatment in men will significantly lower the IgM rheumatoid factor.* Treating men with RA with testosterone also reduces the number of affected joints and in the daily intake of nonsteroidal anti-inflammatory drugs. Testosterone suppresses the inflammation of RA. [134]

> *Testosterone treatment in men will significantly lower the IgM rheumatoid factor.*

Autoimmune and rheumatic diseases such as systemic lupus erythematosus, rheumatoid arthritis, Sjögren's syndrome, autoimmune thyroiditis, and primary biliary cirrhosis, are more common in women. [135] Often abnormalities in the metabolism of estrogen and testosterone are found in these diseases [136] with low concentrations of testosterone in rheumatoid arthritis and Sjögren's syndrome. [137]

There are multiple studies of patients with rheumatoid arthritis and systemic lupus erythematosus demonstrating testosterone therapy provided major improvements in clinical status. [138] Men who have a symptomatic testosterone deficiency often benefit from testosterone replacement by improving quality of life, maintaining lean body mass and preserving bone density. The anti-inflammatory benefit of testosterone may be especially helpful in men with established vascular disease as inflammation determines vascular risk in these men. [139]

Testosterone supplementation also makes bones strong increasing bone mineral density preventing osteoporosis which is so common in patients who are afflicted with arthritis. There are also favorable changes in blood pressure, serum triglycerides, and cholesterol. [140]

In women, estradiol prevents bone loss seen in degenerative arthritis. In a study reported in *Clinical Endocrinology,* women should avoid taking any kind of estrogen by mouth, even estradiol because of potential side effects. However, transdermal or pellet therapy avoids many of these potential side effects. [141]

Other Benefits of BHRT

Hormone replacement therapy prevents long-term degenerative diseases. It has been shown to prevent such diseases as osteoporotic fractures, cardiovascular disease, diabetes mellitus and possibly cognitive impairment if treatment is begun early in the perimenopausal years.

Non-orally (not by mouth) administered estrogens have many advantages. Estradiol used on the skin or under the skin causes no increase in liver enzymes which cause blood clots. Estradiol creams, patches and pellets have cardio-protective effects — they protect the heart and circulation, and are effective in lowering blood pressure.

This is **not** true for oral estrogens such as *Premarin*. Using estradiol in pellet form causes no increase in the risk of developing blood clots in the legs or lungs. In addition, recent indications suggest potential advantages for blood pressure control with non-oral estradiol. [142]

Even though estradiol is obviously beneficial to prevent the degenerative changes in bone by preventing osteoclast (the bone cells that resorb old bone cells) from tearing down bone too quickly. But few know that natural progesterone helps build new bone by stimulating bone cells that lay down new bone cells. This is a similar effect that testosterone has in building new bone. This is why *Bio-identical Hormone Replacement Therapy* may have advantages in preventing degenerative arthritic processes from developing. [143]

So, natural estradiol keeps bone cells from tearing down old bone too rapidly and bio-identical testosterone and bio-identical progesterone help build new bone.

Bio-identical progesterone acts as a hormone that stimulates mineral metabolism. Postmenopausal osteoporosis should be seen as a progesterone deficiency condition as much as a deficiency of estradiol and testosterone. [144]

> *Bio-identical Hormone Replacement Therapy regulates the imbalance in bone remodeling, the process of absorbing and removing old damaged bone cells, and rebuilding new cells in our bones, thereby decreasing bone loss.*

Bio-identical Hormone Replacement Therapy regulates the imbalance in bone remodeling, the process of absorbing and removing old damaged bone cells, and rebuilding new cells in our bones, thereby decreasing bone loss.

Journal thoughts and questions:

_____

_____

_____

_____

_____

_____

_____

_____

_____

_____

_____

_____

_____

_____

_____

_____

_____

_____

CHAPTER 20

Attention Deficit Hyperactivity Disorder

Understanding ADHD

Attention Deficit Hyperactive Disorder is more common in children, but often persists into childhood and even adulthood. The reason it is not as noticeable in many adults is that they have learned to cope and compensate to the symptoms. Much research is being done in this area every year. One thing is for sure: *Attention Deficit Disorder* (ADD) and *Attention Deficit Hyperactive Disorder* (ADHD) are not slowing down in our culture.

Symptoms include difficulty staying focused and paying attention, difficulty controlling behavior, rambling speech, and hyperactivity (over-activity).

This is evident in a study of twins showing that ADHD often runs in families. One or both parents who have ADHD are likely to pass it on to one or more of their children.

It is not known what causes ADHD, but many studies suggest that genes play a large role. It should not be forgotten that hormones control our genes. This is evident in a study of twins showing that ADHD often runs in families. One or both parents who have ADHD are likely to pass it on to one or more of their children. Children with ADHD who carry a particular version of a certain gene have thinner brain tissue in the areas of the brain associated with attention. This difference was not permanent and as children with this gene grow up, the brain often develops to a normal level of thickness. Their ADHD symptoms also improved. But some do not.

It is interesting that anxiety and depression are seen more frequently in patients with ADHD as well as those who have a hormone deficiency. Symptoms in adults are more varied than and not as clear-cut as symptoms seen in children. For an adult to be diagnosed with ADHD, the condition has to have been present as a child and continued throughout adulthood.

The most common type of medication used for treating ADHD is a *"stimulant."* Although it may seem unusual to treat ADHD with a medication considered a stimulant, it actually has a calming effect in patients with ADHD. The most common side effects of such medications are ***decreased appetite and sleep problems.***

ADHD in Adults

Many adults who have the disorder are unaware of it. They may feel that it is impossible to get organized, stick to a job, or remember and keep appointments. Daily tasks such as getting up in the morning, preparing to leave the house for work, arriving at work on time, and being productive on the job can be especially challenging for adults with ADHD.

These adults may have a history of failure at school, problems at work, or difficult or failed relationships. Many have had multiple traffic accidents. Adults with ADHD may seem restless and may try to do several things at once, most of them unsuccessfully. They also tend to prefer "quick fixes," rather than taking the steps needed to achieve greater rewards. [145]

There are very few references to ADHD when considering bio-identical hormones. Most likely the reason is because there are so few studies confirming the benefit of bio-identical hormones in patients who are afflicted with ADHD.

However, Michael E. Platt, M.D., wrote the following:

There are many adults with undiagnosed ADD or ADHD. People who experience sleepiness between three and four in the afternoon or while driving—this is ADD. I use the word "ADD" interchangeably with "hypoglycemia," because when the level of sugar in the brain is low, the person can't focus. People who become workaholics may actually have ADHD and are living on high levels of adrenaline caused by recurrent hypoglycemia.

If you ask a specialist in ADD/ADHD what is causing the problem, they generally say they don't know. I am not aware of any other doctor besides myself who approaches these conditions from a hormonal standpoint. Simply put, I view ADD and ADHD as a matter of too little progesterone, too much insulin, and in the case of ADHD, too much adrenaline. My philosophy is so far removed from the standard of medical practice, which calls for the use of dangerous stimulants to treat the problem, that it can create concerns for traditional practitioners. Yet, as they say, the proof is in the pudding. When I treat symptoms of ADD and ADHD with progesterone and a diet that encourages the lowering of insulin, there are positive results.

There is often a strong family history of associated hormonal problems—a mother with breast cancer, a sister with endometriosis, a brother with bi-polar disorder, children or nephews and nieces who are hyperactive (ADHD). Other commonly associated conditions are type 2 diabetes and also fibromyalgia.

Please keep in mind that adrenaline is not only a hormone but also acts as a neurotransmitter in the brain. Adults with ADHD are often extremely intelligent as well as extremely successful.

Yet utilizing bio-identical hormones, altering the patient's eating habits, and helping them gain insight into their condition often leads to a "miraculous" resolution of these very problems. [146]

Is There Hope? How Can BHRT Help?

It is very common for adults with ADHD to have low hormones. Treating the source of the problem often allows them to discontinue their ADHD medications with their serious side effects.

It is very common for adults with ADHD to have low hormones. Treating the source of the problem often allows them to discontinue their ADHD medications with their serious side effects.

Dwight's Story

Dwight was a forty-three-year-old pharmacist who worked in a compounding pharmacy. Preparing bio-identical hormones for various patients, Dwight had opportunity to listen to many testimonials of the life-changing events of patients using his own products. He eventually came for a consult where he complained about fatigue, poor exercise tolerance, low sex drive and some difficulty maintaining an erection.

Dwight appeared to be healthy. He was not overweight and his blood pressure was good. He was pleasant, but others had begun noticing he was angry and had become short-tempered recently. Dwight's wife, Janice, was nine years younger than her husband and had noticed a drop off of their sex life. *"We used to have a very active sex life."* Janice said, *"We both said the changes in Dwight were just due to his heavy work schedule at the pharmacy."*

Dwight's testosterone was a disappointing 267 ng/dL (normal 800 to 1200 ng/dL). Dwight was disappointed saying, *"But I'm only forty-three. You know, I didn't tell you this, but my family doctor checked my testosterone about six months ago and the result was about the same as yours. But he told me it was OK. I'm glad you confirmed what I thought. Now I know why I'm this way."*

Dwight was treated with bio-identical testosterone pellets. He was given *Revive* to help with erections.

In one month Dwight was so relieved to report, *"My old energy is back. Janice and I are able to enjoy the sex life again we had twenty years ago. The Revive helped but I now hardly ever have to take it. I'm going for a long walk each evening with Janice and still have energy left."*

When Dwight came in for his third treatment at nine months, he said, *"You probably don't remember, but when I first started seeing you, I was on Adderall for ADHD. Now I don't take it any more after being on hormones. This is the first time I've been off that kind of medicine since I was six years old."*

Even though it may seem unusual for an adult to complain of ADHD, it is far more common than one might think. The response Dwight had to *Bio-identical Hormone Replacement Therapy* is often seen by physicians using this therapy.

Journal thoughts and questions:

_____

_____

_____

_____

_____

_____

_____

_____

_____

_____

_____

_____

_____

_____

_____

_____

_____

_____

_____

CHAPTER 21

Breast Cancer

The Fear of Breast Cancer

Perhaps the two scariest words for a woman to hear are *"breast cancer."*
Women dread that annual checkup, often fearing the worst. When the results come back negative and the prognosis is good, they are relieved ... at least for another eleven months. Then the month before their next breast cancer exam, they begin worrying again. It's a vicious cycle.

> *Breast cancer, with its hormonal imbalances, has been directly linked to synthetic estrogens and synthetic progestins.*

Breast cancer, with its hormonal imbalances, has been directly linked to synthetic estrogens and synthetic progestins. In contrast, natural, bio-identical hormones provide necessary balance for the body's well-being without the fear of causing cancer.

The Facts of Breast Cancer

Testosterone begins to decline in men and women as early as the late twenties. But most will begin to develop early symptoms of testosterone decline in the mid-thirties. Most every woman can testify about the stimulatory effect of estradiol on the breast each month. Unchecked by low levels of progesterone and testosterone results in continuous stimulation that can be detrimental to the breast. Testosterone negates these unfavorable effects on postmenopausal breasts. Women who have much lower testosterone as a result of menopause need the protection afforded by testosterone on the breast. [147]

Exposing breast cells to testosterone produces a protective effect. It is known that women who have Polycystic Ovarian Syndrome who have excess testosterone do not have an increased risk of breast cancer. Certainly premenopausal women's self-made testosterone does not increase the risk of breast cancer. [148]

The *Women's Health Initiative* trial in 2002 proved that *Premarin* and *Prempro* caused multiple deadly side effects, including breast cancer, heart attacks, strokes and dementia. But it was actually known that these drugs increased the risk for breast cancer as far back as the 1990s. In 1989 there was an article stating that the combination of *Premarin* and *Provera* (used by most physicians at that time) caused an increase in breast cancer. [149] But it took another thirteen years to convince doctors that they had been fooled by Wyeth Pharmaceuticals. And in those thirteen years, the public suffered greatly.

A study of 98,997 women in France demonstrated that natural micronized progesterone was safer with significantly lower breast cancer risks, compared to synthetic *Provera*. Also women who used the bio-identical hormone-replacement therapy consistently were at lower risk than women who took the hormones occasionally. In other words, women who use hormone replacement were less likely to develop breast cancer. [150]

Women who use hormone replacement were less likely to develop breast cancer.

A nine-year study of postmenopausal women in France produced incredible findings. *There was absolutely no increase in risk of breast cancer in those who used bio-identical transdermal estradiol and bio-identical progesterone!* [151]

A Danish Nurse Cohort studied almost 20,000 women forty-five years old and above who used synthetic estrogen with *Provera*. These women had the highest risk of breast cancer. [152] The short-term effectiveness of *Premarin* and bio-identical estradiol as treatments for relief of hot flashes was comparable. The conclusion was that they both have comparable short-term effects for symptom relief—hot flashes. [153]

The overarching problem with conjugated estrogen is the long-term increased risk of breast cancer, stroke, dementia, and myocardial infarction, which was proven by *The Women's Health Initiative*. This situation leaves us with the very important knowledge that *hormone replacement therapy is an important tool in wellness and prevention.* The type of hormone therapies we choose is what makes the difference and must be carefully considered. [154]

The pharmacological and biological effects of Provera are very different than bio-identical progesterone.

According to virtually every scientific review, *the pharmacological and biological effects of Provera are very different from bio-identical progesterone.*

How can two different compounds be expected to have the same results? Can a tractor be expected to perform like a sports car just because both have four wheels? In many studies comparing synthetic *Provera* with bio-identical progesterone, clearly bio-identical progesterone was safer and more efficacious in every trial. [155]

In well-done studies, synthetic *Provera* has been repeatedly shown to cause negative consequences to breast tissue, whereas bio-identical progesterone has been shown to have a consistently beneficial effect on breast cell stimulation. The often-quoted E3N French and the Danish Nurses studies did not find bio-identical progesterone increased breast cancer risk in women taking various kinds of hormone replacement for more than five years. However, synthetic *Provera* did cause an increase in breast cancer in these women. [156]

Various risks shown to be attributable to *Premarin* and synthetic *Provera* included breast cancer, strokes, dementia and cardiovascular events, [157] but these side effects have never been reported when patients were using bio-identical hormones instead. [158]

Bio-identical estradiol and progesterone have been proven safer to use in women. In addition, when women were prescribed testosterone, which attached to androgen receptors in the breasts, it kept breast cells from being overly stimulated. [159]

Women who have *Polycystic Ovarian Syndrome* have excess testosterone in their bodies. These women experience atrophy, less stimulation, shrinkage of breast tissue and a decreased risk of breast cancer. [160] Women being treated with testosterone should be followed closely by checking their blood levels.

The method of administration is also important. Serum blood levels should not be elevated to abnormal heights in order to have a longer period of time that the testosterone is in circulation. This can happen through the use of injections. Topical testosterone accomplishes a more constant blood level to achieve normal blood levels usually for two or three days. However, *Bio-identical Pellet Hormone Replacement Therapy* accomplishes the same consistent blood level lasting for three to four months with a steady state of delivery. It lasts far longer than simply two or three days. Not only does bio-identical testosterone protect the breast from cancer, but it also improves libido and mood. [161]

Natural estradiol and progesterone have less stimulatory effect on breast tissue than synthetic *Provera* and *Premarin*. [162] When using transdermal estradiol, there is improvement in postmenopausal symptoms with no side effects compared to the use of *Premarin*. [163]

The Postmenopausal Estrogen/Progestin Interventions trial, lasting over three years, confirmed that the use of oral *Premarin* alone or with synthetic *Provera* caused unhealthy changes in cholesterol and more blood clots. However, natural micronized progesterone showed improvement in the lipoprotein profile and lowered blood clots. When synthetic *Provera* is added to the treatment of menopausal women there is a significant loss of the good high-density lipoprotein cholesterol which counters the remarkable benefits of estradiol in menopausal women. But when bio-identical progesterone is given instead of *Provera,* there is a statistically significant endometrial protective effect of estradiol and a positive effect on high-density lipoprotein. [164]

The bottom line? The medical community had been duped for over forty years by the self-interest of the pharmaceutical companies.

It is so unfortunate that the *Women's Health Initiative* trial did not include BHRT in their study, even though bio-identical hormones have surged in usage and have shown consistently positive results. The conclusion they would have reached is that natural hormones are safer and more effective than *Prempro* as used in the WHI. The obvious speculation is that those designing the study, in an effort to give support to a bad hormone produced by Big Pharma, knew that *Prempro* would be shown to be more dangerous as compared to BHRT and that bio-identical estradiol and progesterone would be shown to be protective. The surprise to the entire medical community was just how unsafe these drugs were. ***The bottom line? The medical community had been duped for over forty years by the self-interest of the pharmaceutical companies.***

In Europe *Bio-identical Hormone Replacement Therapy* has been the main type of hormone replacement in menopausal women for years. With it there has been the effective elimination of menopausal symptoms with no long-term negative side effects using BHRT. When the breasts are exposed to at least fourteen days and up to twenty-five days of natural progesterone each month in postmenopausal women, there is a reduction of the stimulation of the breast by estradiol. [165] Bio-identical progesterone proved to be safer and more effective in all trials that involved its usage. [166] *Numerous studies have shown that any estrogen (conjugated estrogen or bio-identical estradiol) combined with synthetic Provera doubles the risk of breast cancer. Can you believe that? The risk DOUBLED!* [167]

Unlike synthetic *Provera*, bio-identical progesterone has been shown to have a consistently limiting effect on breast cell proliferation. [168] The E3N and Danish Nurses studies, which address large populations taking various types of hormone-replacement therapy for more than five years, did not find progesterone to be an increased risk factor for breast cancer – while *Provera* was. When estradiol was used in studies that evaluated its effectiveness in relieving menopausal symptoms, including hot flashes, night sweats, insomnia, mood swings, [169] the results were consistently positive. [170]

Bio-identical progesterone consistently demonstrates a favorable action on the blood vessels and on the brain. However, this has not been shown to be true of synthetic *Provera*. When estradiol is used with bio-identical progesterone there is less or even no risk of breast cancer, as opposed to the use of *Provera*. [171]

There are studies in rats that suggest that the administration of natural estradiol and progesterone may give this protective effect from developing breast cancer secondary to the activation of genes involved in the DNA repair process of breast tissue. [172] The breast tissue in rats that are given estradiol and progesterone (which mimics pregnancy) depresses the growth-promoting cells of breast cancer. [173]

When natural progesterone is added to topical estradiol in treating hormone deficiency in postmenopausal women, there is a reduction in the stimulation in the breast by estradiol. Normal levels of progesterone are important in balancing stimulation and avoiding over stimulation in breast tissue.[174]

In the female, estradiol and progesterone act in concert to establish healthy tissue. In a normal breast, estradiol stimulates the growth of ductal tissue and progesterone, and follows with the development of lobular tissue which provides for secretion. *When estradiol and progesterone are in balance, the result is normal mammary tissue.* Progesterone keeps in check the stimulation of breast tissue by estradiol.

When women have long periods of unopposed estrogen stimulation, not antagonized by progesterone, this may contribute to the development of breast cancer. This may be seen in the perimenopausal years when the ovaries are still producing estradiol but the production of progesterone is diminishing. The balance is lost between estradiol and progesterone. [175] This imbalance can be corrected with the administration of bio-identical estradiol and progesterone. But remember, testosterone also aids in the protection of the breasts from cancer.

Progesterone inhibits the rapid growth of normal breast epithelial cells in women. It also inhibits the rapid growth of breast cancer cells in the laboratory. Not only does progesterone block the over-growth of breast cells, both normal and cancerous, but progesterone actually can cause cancer cells in the breast to die. In the lab, there was a ninety percent blockage of breast cancer cells when exposed to progesterone for seventy-two hours. Forty-eight percent of these cells died and another forty-three percent were in the process of dying after the exposure to progesterone. These results are not seen with all types of breast cancer. [176] When natural progesterone is applied to the breast, there is a significant reduction in the stimulation of the breast by estradiol. [177]

No rational person would say that a woman who is using bio-identical progesterone will never get breast cancer. But the risk factors of having inadequate progesterone certainly increase the odds of breast cancer. It is difficult to justify telling a woman who has had a hysterectomy and still has her ovaries that she does not need progesterone. Most every credible study of natural progesterone in women demonstrates that progesterone is an "anti-estrogen."

Conclusion

The human body is beautiful when all is in balance. That balance occurs in a dramatic fashion between the ages of eighteen and thirty. There is enough testosterone, but not too much. There is a plentiful supply of estradiol to cause the breast to grow each month preparing for possible pregnancy, as well as the inside lining of the uterus preparing for implantation of a fertilized egg. When pregnancy does not occur, the breasts become less swollen and the lining of the uterus sloughs off secondary due to a rapid withdrawal of progesterone.

When the sex hormones are not in balance, the results are again dramatic. Unfortunately, this time it is in a negative way. Perimenopause is a time when testosterone begins its gradual one- to two- percent decline per year, starting at twenty-eight to thirty years old. Progesterone begins to drop off around thirty-five causing sore breasts, fibrocystic breast disease, irregular periods, loss of sleep and anxiety. The ovaries continue to produce estradiol for a while longer not completely stopping until age fifty. However, eight percent of women will be menopausal before age forty.

For those who have had a total hysterectomy where both the uterus and ovaries are removed, they have no more production of the usual sex hormones at all. This causes a total imbalance inside their bodies. And, as many of you can testify, it is a very hard time in life. It is impossible for the human body to function in a beautiful fashion without these hormones.

The great news is that with the replacement of these life-sustaining hormones with the use of bio-identical (not synthetic) hormones, a woman's life can be beautiful again – even in her fifties or sixties or seventies and into her eighties.

Don't let anyone give you the false line that *"The loss of hormones (which occurs at menopause) is just part of life. You'll have to live with these symptoms of hormonal imbalance."* A physician who tells you this is uninformed.

Find someone who will provide you with the protection of bio-identical hormones.

Journal thoughts and questions:

_____

_____

_____

_____

_____

_____

_____

_____

_____

_____

_____

_____

_____

_____

_____

_____

_____

_____

CHAPTER 22

Cardiovascular Disease

Your Heart ... More Critical Than You Know

Testosterone is critical to the proper functioning of the heart. You could save your life or the life of a loved one by knowing and acting upon that knowledge.

Hundreds of reputable studies prove that people with low hormones are more likely to suffer from heart attacks, strokes and blood clots. Bio-identical hormones save lives.

There are more testosterone receptor sites in the heart than any other muscle in the body. Hundreds of reputable studies prove that people with low hormones are more likely to suffer from heart attacks, strokes and blood clots. Bio-identical hormones save lives.

Some of the results of these studies include:

- Women who are menopausal and do not use bio-identical hormone replacement therapy have an increased risk of cardiovascular disease of 1.14. [178]

- Women who have both ovaries removed and do not use bio-identical hormone replacement have an increased risk of cardiovascular disease of 2.62, more than twice the risk of cardiovascular disease than women who are menopausal but still have their ovaries.

- Women who have both ovaries removed before age fifty have an increased risk of cardiovascular disease of 4.55 compared to women who have their ovaries removed after age fifty. [179]

- Women who undergo bilateral oophorectomy and use estradiol hormone replacement therapy have a significant increase in protection against ischemic heart disease. [180] The major benefit of estradiol replacement is seen in women who are now using BHRT and who started treatment within one year or sooner after surgical menopause. There are advantages in beginning bio-identical hormone replacement in the mid-thirties when hormones begin to decline before symptoms begin to appear.

Removal of the ovaries is associated with increased cardiovascular risk and premature death, and an oophorectomy at a young age further increases this risk.

However, hormone replacement therapy that is begun right after surgery or natural menopause will reduce this risk. Estrogen therapy started early after surgical or natural menopause at a young age also appears to reduce this risk.

Not just estradiol, but also testosterone has cardiovascular protective effects. Parental testosterone improves endothelium-dependent and independent vasodilation in postmenopausal women already receiving estrogen. [181] Oral testosterone causes adverse effects on lipids with a reduction in high density lipid levels. This is not true with the use of subcutaneous pellet implants using estradiol and testosterone. There are no significant changes in total serum cholesterol or triglycerides.

How Can BHRT Help Cardiovascular Disease

To understand cardiovascular disease and how bio-identical hormones can retard and perhaps reverse this process of deterioration we must first understand how atherosclerosis (hardening of the arteries) develops. Atherosclerosis, also known as arteriosclerotic vascular disease, is when an arterial wall thickens as a result of the accumulation of calcium and fatty materials such as cholesterol and triglyceride. This reduces the elasticity of the arterial walls and therefore allows less blood to travel through the arteries. This also increases blood pressure.

Atherosclerosis affects the entire arterial tree, but mostly larger, high-pressure vessels such as the heart, kidney, legs, brain, and neck arteries. Too often a patient is told that he/she has a narrowing of an artery in the neck, for example, and that narrowing can be fixed by surgery. That sounds good. *But what they may not realize is that this process of narrowing of the artery in the neck is happening in ALL the arteries in the body from the brain to the feet.*

Numerous studies have demonstrated that estrogen has a protective quality against the development of cardiovascular disease in women. [182]

This process by which atherosclerosis occurs can be significantly inhibited by natural estradiol and progesterone. Epidemiologic studies clearly indicate that women of reproductive age or in the first seven years after menopause have a much reduced incidence of cardiovascular disease compared with age-matched men. [183]

These findings provide evidence that natural estradiol and progesterone are "protective" against the development of cardiovascular disease in women.

A number of studies have shown that in women natural estradiol administration in low doses, or by self-production, is strongly associated with a lower incidence of vascular disease. [184]

The Postmenopausal Estrogen/Progestin Interventions trial, *Gerhard Trial*, and *Estrogen in Prevention of Atherosclerosis* trials have all three demonstrated that *Bio-identical Hormone Replacement Therapy* improves cardiovascular risk factors. Based on the favorable effects on the cardiovascular system, *Bio-identical Hormone Replacement Therapy* may eventually prove to be cardio-neutral or even cardio protective. [185]

Bio-identical Hormone Replacement Therapy improves cardiovascular risk factors

There is ample evidence that estradiol is cardio protective. First, during the reproductive years women have far less cardiovascular disease than men of the same age. Second, at menopause when ovarian dysfunction appears, there is a dramatic increased incidence of heart problems secondary to a decrease in circulating estradiol. Third, when estrogen is replaced with natural estradiol there is marked reduction of cardiovascular risk factors in postmenopausal women. [186]

An article in *Lancet* pointed out that the risk of death from cardiovascular disease was higher for women with early menopauses than for those with late menopauses. For each year's delay in menopause the cardiovascular mortality risk decreased by two percent. [187]

Dr. Rosano demonstrated that estrogen can inhibit the mechanism of constriction (narrowing) of coronary arteries. [188] Progesterone is just as potent as estradiol as an antigrowth factor for the vascular smooth muscle cells which cause atherosclerosis. The risks of cardiovascular disease are seen more often in men and women who:

- Smoke
- Have high blood pressure
- Do not exercise
- Are obese
- Have a diet of too many bad fats
- Have high cholesterol
- Are under excess stress
- Have diabetes
- Have cardiovascular in their family
- Low hormones (especially in men) [189]
- However, of these ten risks of cardiovascular disease, nine can be altered by actions taken by the patient—exercising, get cholesterol down if elevated, if blood pressure is high, see your doctor, eating less fats, weight loss, avoiding stress as much as possible, normalize sex hormones, if blood sugar is high see a doctor to get it down, and not smoking.

Much has been pointed out about the benefits of estradiol and progesterone, especially in women, in the prevention and treatment of coronary artery disease. Even though testosterone is considered by many misinformed physicians only a male hormone, testosterone can be beneficial in protecting and helping to reverse congestive heart failure. The number-one cause of congestive heart failure is the restriction of adequate blood supply to the heart secondary to atherosclerosis. Testosterone supplementation is beneficial to improve physical capacity and reverses insulin resistance in female patients with chronic heart failure. Insulin resistance can lead to diabetes.

Low testosterone is frequently seen in patients with coronary heart failure. [190] And it may be involved in the impairment of skeletal muscle function and exercise tolerance that can occur in coronary heart failure. [191]

Testosterone supplementation in addition to the best medical therapy improves exercise capacity, breathing efficiency, muscle strength, and insulin sensitivity in elderly men with moderately severe coronary heart failure without major side effects. [192]

Insulin resistance, a sign of diabetes, decreased significantly in a group of patients using testosterone treatment, whereas it increased in the control group. High-density lipoprotein (HDL) cholesterol as well as hemoglobin level significantly increased in the testosterone group as compared with the placebo group. Testosterone replacement therapy improves physical capacity and insulin resistance in women with coronary heart failure. [193]

Women who have low physical capacity and insulin resistance with coronary heart failure have a poor prognosis; however, the use of testosterone supplementation in these women has been shown to be beneficial in such women. [194]

Studies show that low-dose testosterone supplementation given in addition to optimal medical therapy improves physical capacity, insulin sensitivity, and large-muscles strength in elderly women with coronary heart failure.

Testosterone in men and estradiol in women protects your heart. Women go through a dramatic decline of estradiol with menopause adding to their chances of heart disease. You could save your own life, or that of a loved one, by knowing and acting upon the knowledge that testosterone and estradiol are critical to the proper functioning of the heart.

Testosterone and Men's Health

Testosterone is very important for men's health.

There are reports that testosterone may be bad for you. This is confusing to many because these reports do not differentiate between synthetic testosterone and bio-identical testosterone. Do not be tricked. Studies demonstrate that the higher the testosterone the lower the chance of one having a stroke from blood-clot-promoting substances in the blood. Some contend that testosterone is not safe and may even cause cardiovascular side effects. However, the type of testosterone used which causes such side effects is testosterone enanthate not bio-identical testosterone.

CHIANTI was a six-year study which demonstrated that one can check the testosterone level in men and predict the likelihood of early death in men. [195] EPIC-Norfolk study was conducted with 11,606 men ranging from forty to seventy-nine years examining the relationship between testosterone over six to ten years. The conclusion was that the higher the concentration of endogenous testosterone the lower the mortality because of cardiovascular disease, as well as all causes. Low testosterone could be a predictive marker for men who have a high risk for cardiovascular disease. In a five-year study of male veterans, it was found that the survival rate decreased as testosterone levels decreased. The lower the testosterone the earlier men die. [196]

In the well-known Rancho Bernardo study in 2008, 794 men were followed for twenty years. Men with total testosterone and bioavailable testosterone in the lowest one-fourth were more likely to die than those with higher levels.[197]

Along with noting the blood levels of testosterone in men and their symptoms it is also necessary to take into account other physical problems he may be experiencing. Low testosterone in men is associated with multiple disease processes including:

- Elevated cholesterol and triglycerides
- Insulin resistance and diabetes
- Obesity
- More likely to cause blood clots
- Lack of exercise
- Smoking
- Excess fat in diet

All of these contribute to several cardiovascular risk factors. [198] As stated in a study from 2010 in the medical journal *Heart*,

"Low testosterone status is therefore associated with mortality and vascular mortality.... This is important because men with manifest coronary artery disease are at a higher risk of cardiovascular mortality and represent a patient population prone to testosterone deficiency."

Those men with angina, chronic heart failure or diabetes may experience particular symptomatic benefit from testosterone replacement therapy. Low endogenous testosterone is related to all-cause mortality—cancers, heart attacks, strokes, diabetes—and especially vascular mortality in coronary disease in men.

Testosterone replacement therapy is helpful in men who have angina, chest pain especially with exertion. Testosterone relieves chest pain by a direct coronary-relaxing effect of testosterone. [199] Sublingual nitroglycerin is commonly used in patients who have chest pain especially when they are exerting themselves. Nitroglycerin is effective for only a short period of time, usually only a few minutes. Testosterone supplementation, especially with pellet hormone replacement, lasts three to four months.

A study by Malkin et al. found that when men were exercised there was a longer time before they began to experience chest pain in patients who had testosterone replacement therapy than those with low testosterone. There were major improvements in mood in the men treated with testosterone. There also were reductions in total cholesterol in the testosterone treated group. The overall level of patient satisfaction was high. The conclusion of the authors was that testosterone therapy offers clinical benefit to this patient group. [200]

The Benefits of BHRT

A very detailed article by Erika T. Schwartz, [201] using 267 medical study references, showed that testosterone replacement therapy has also been proven to reduce insulin resistance, fat in the abdomen, and the chance of having a heart attack. [202] Dr. Schwartz goes ahead to point out that

Based on the extensive scientific data we have reviewed for this article, it is unclear whether any absolute circumstance calls for synthetic versions of hormone-replacement therapy and such use appears unwise. Given the easy commercial availability of bio-identical formulations and the lack of negative data on these hormones, primary care physicians can easily access them for their patients.

Therefore, there is no reason to use synthetic hormones when bio-identical hormones are safer, more efficacious, and readily available. [203]

Men who have coronary artery disease are at a higher risk of premature death. This group of men is far more likely to have low testosterone. Men with angina, chronic heart failure or diabetes may see a great benefit from testosterone replacement therapy. Testosterone hormone replacement therapy is indicated for men who show signs and symptoms of low testosterone. These men who have testosterone levels below what would be seen in a young man often benefit from raising testosterone to 800 ng/dl up to 1200 ng/dl.

Journal thoughts and questions:

_____

_____

_____

_____

_____

_____

_____

_____

_____

_____

_____

_____

_____

_____

_____

_____

_____

_____

_____

CHAPTER 23

Cholesterol

Amber's Story

Amber was fifty-two years old when she was told she had elevated cholesterol levels. Her family doctor immediately placed her on Lescol 40 mg one each evening.

Amber came for bio-identical hormone treatment complaining of hot flashes, night sweats, anxiety, depression, weight gain, tiredness and poor sleep. She said, *"I had a total hysterectomy when I was 43 for endometriosis. I took Prempro for nine years until I heard about the dangers of Premarin from a news story in a women's magazine."*

Her physical exam was unremarkable except for weighing 146 pounds. Amber was only 5'1". She was pleasant and did not appear depressed. Amber said,

I try to cover the stress I feel. I try to smile and put on a good front but I am miserable. I've gained 28 pounds in the last ten years. I used to be 118 and now I weigh 146. My husband and I don't have sex any more. I just don't feel like it. And I don't think he does either. I'm so tired I don't feel like exercising. Inside I know something is missing. A friend of mine told me it might be my hormones.

Her estradiol, progesterone and testosterone were almost non-existent. Interestingly, her cholesterol was still elevated even though she was taking *Lescol*. Her sex hormones were replaced at this office visit. We discussed her need to follow up with her family doctor, suggesting that she might need to make an adjustment in her treatment plan for cholesterol.

Amber returned in four weeks. She was excited about how much better she felt. She explained that replacing her lost hormones had changed her life. This is a very typical story heard many times a day by a doctor practicing bio-identical hormone replacement therapy. It is always exciting to hear the stories over and over through the day.

But Amber also reported about the visit to her family doctor,

She checked my cholesterol and to my surprise and hers as well, my cholesterol was 184. She said that I must be exercising a lot and eating much better to get it to drop that much. I told her no, I started doing BHRT. She didn't know much about it, but didn't seem to believe hormones could have caused such a change.

Amber's story is so typical. Many have been able to decrease their cholesterol medication and some have been able to stop it all together.

What This Chapter Is All About

The goal of this chapter is to determine the best ways to prevent a heart attack or stroke.

Everyone should know their lipid profile. A lipid profile is listing of your total cholesterol, your good cholesterol (HDL), your bad cholesterol (LDL), your very bad cholesterol (VLDL), Lp(a) – which is pronounced *"L p little a"*, and your triglycerides. If you don't know yours, ask your doctor to perform these tests.

It is not commonly known, even by the medical community, that bad cholesterol (LDL) usually increases when women enter into menopause. Good cholesterol (HDL) is stabilized or increased with hormonal balance. Bad cholesterol (LDL) is lowered with natural hormonal balance in most patients. Balancing hormones may prevent the diseases associated with the devastating effects of high cholesterol.

In this chapter we will discuss medications used to reduce cholesterol. A discussion concerning these cholesterol-lowering drugs is not an effort to discourage their use. However, notice what I said at the beginning of this section: *"to determine the BEST ways to prevent a heart attack or stroke."*

The best way to prevent a heart attack or stroke may be something other than beginning with a drug. There are instances when a statin, a cholesterol lowering drug, is necessary – but correcting the cause of the high cholesterol may be more beneficial.

> *There are instances when a statin, a cholesterol lowering drug, is necessary – but correcting the cause of the high cholesterol may be more beneficial.*

What Is Cholesterol?

Let's take a look at the word cholesterol. Notice the last six letters: *"sterol"* — which means cholesterol is a steroid. Cholesterol is produced by all animal cells. We need it. It is essential for us to live. Cholesterol provides for animal cells to not need a cell wall (like plants and bacteria) to protect membrane integrity/cell-viability. This enables our cells to change shape and to move (unlike bacteria and plant cells which are restricted by their cell walls). [204]

Because cholesterol is essential for all animal life, each cell synthesizes cholesterol starting with the intracellular protein enzyme *HMG-CoA reductase*. This enzyme is a good thing—essential for life. But too much of a good thing can be bad. If HMG-CoA reductase produces too much cholesterol, heart attacks and strokes can be a result. However, normal and particularly high levels of fats (including cholesterol) in the blood are strongly associated with hardening of the arteries, *atherosclerosis*. Because the body produces its own cholesterol, the intake of cholesterol in food has little, if any, effect on total body cholesterol or how much cholesterol is in the blood, but it does affect the amount of good cholesterol (HDL) and bad cholesterol (LDL) we have.

The Dangers of Cholesterol

When there are too many LDL molecules they become embedded in the walls of blood vessels because they are so small resulting in atherosclerotic plaque formation, early atherosclerosis (carotid intima-media thickness). [205] These plaques are the main causes of heart attacks, strokes, and other serious medical problems caused by high levels of LDL cholesterol. [206]

HDL particles transport cholesterol back to the liver for excretion or to other tissues that use cholesterol to synthesize hormones. [207] Having high numbers of large HDL particles correlates with better health outcomes. The HDL particles are so large they cannot embed in the walls of the arteries. [208] This means that having small numbers of large HDL particles (good cholesterol) causes cardiovascular disease. [209]

When a physician sees a lab report showing the patient has high cholesterol, the *"knee-jerk"* reaction often is to write a prescription for one of the following drugs: *Lipitor, Zocor, Crestor, Mevacor, Lescol, Livalo, Vytorin* (a combination of *Zocor* and *Zetia*).

> ***When a physician sees a lab report showing the patient has high cholesterol, the "knee-jerk" reaction often is to write a prescription.***

There can be no doubt that as we age there are detrimental changes in the body. The age-associated, progressive changes in the body occur at the same time there is a decrease in hormone levels of testosterone, progesterone and estradiol. The changes seen with aging are important. There is a decline in muscle mass by 20%-40% between the ages of twenty-five and seventy-five. The fat mass doubles and there is a decline in bone mineral density by 0.3% per year after age thirty-five. Low testosterone will lead to more abdominal fat which leads to higher cholesterol and diabetes which causes atherosclerosis, heart attacks and strokes.

The beneficial effects of *Bio-identical Hormone Replacement Therapy* on body composition, to increase muscle mass, reduce the waist line, to reduce fat mass, suggest that an increase in level of natural hormones to those of a young man or woman can prevent some of these age-associated changes. [210]

It is known that at menopause there is often an associated weight gain and an increase in cardiovascular risk factors. However, in women who receive hormone replacement therapy using 17 beta-estradiol, in one study, there was a weight loss of 4.63 pounds in just three months and a decrease of the waist:hip ratio. This was the result of an increase in total energy expenditure. Insulin response to sugar was diminished by 30 percent with hormone therapy. Total cholesterol decreased as well as bad LDL-cholesterol. [211]

Hormone replacement therapy is best achieved by replacing the hormone that is missing (estradiol) rather than by administering an extract of horse urine (conjugated equine estrogens). [212] Indeed, women who are being treated with lipid-lowering agents and *Prempro*, may be in danger of an abdominal aortic aneurysm. [213]

Women who are less than fifty-five years old usually do not have an increase in thickness of the carotid artery, the large artery in the neck that carries blood to the head. However, women who are fifty five or older are far more likely to develop carotid artery intima-media thickness without bio-identical hormone therapy. Women who start the treatment with bio-identical 17 beta-estradiol and progesterone within one year of menopause have a significantly lower total cholesterol than women not receiving these hormones. This gives strong evidence that long-term hormone-replacement therapy with bio-identical estradiol and progesterone, not synthetic hormones, is protective against thickening of intimal of the carotid artery. [214]

How BHRT Can Help Lower Cholesterol

If *Bio-identical Hormone Replacement Therapy* is instituted early in Postmenopause, there is a significant decreased risk of death, heart failure, or myocardial infarction. In women who are started early in menopause and continued for a prolonged duration do not have an increased risk of cardiovascular events such as mortality, stroke, deep vein thrombosis (blood clots in the legs), and pulmonary embolism (blood clots in the lungs). The rate of breast cancer and other cancer is not increased in women treated with bio-identical estradiol. [215]

> *If BHRT is instituted early in postmenopause there is a significant decreased risk of death, heart failure, or myocardial infarction.*

Body composition is better with bio-identical hormone replacement therapy compared to women who do not use BHRT where a significant increase in fat mass and trunk fat is likely in menopausal women.[216] These changes in fat mass may be responsible for the improvement in cholesterol levels in women using BHRT [217] which causes an associated decreased risk in cardiovascular events. Also, healthy postmenopausal women receiving unopposed 17β-estradiol have a significantly less progression of carotid intima media thickness compared with women not on hormone therapy. Using BHRT reduces the risk of breast cancer in women less than fifty years old. Beginning hormone replacement therapy early and with prolonged use does not result in an increased risk of breast cancer or stroke. [218]

Women who have had a total abdominal hysterectomy and are treated with bio-identical estradiol are more likely to see reductions of lipids (a decline in cholesterol, a decreased LDL cholesterol and lowering of triglycerides) especially if given percutaneously (a cream on the skin or a pellet placed under the skin). Any kind of estrogen taken by mouth is more likely to cause blood clots. [219]

Estradiol clearly is protective against the development of cardiovascular disease in women. However, bio-identical progesterone plays a part in protecting the arteries as well. Estradiol shows a seventy-five percent protection and progesterone sixty-four percent. The cardioprotective effect of estradiol and progesterone is supported by the fact that women of reproductive age have a much reduced incidence of cardiovascular disease compared with age-matched men. [220] Also women who have their ovaries removed have an increased incidence and mortality from cardiovascular disease if they do not receive estrogen replacement. [221]

Lowering Men's Cholesterol

Men treated with testosterone have an improvement in lean body mass with an increase in hematocrit, a decline in total cholesterol, and low density lipoprotein cholesterol. [222]

For years uninformed physicians have contended against all reason that testosterone caused cardiovascular disease. Now it is without dispute from a plethora of studies demonstrating that low testosterone rather than high testosterone levels in men is associated with several cardiovascular risk factors including an elevated cholesterol which leads to hardening of the arteries, insulin resistance leading to diabetes, obesity and an elevation of substances in the blood that cause blood clots, a prothrombotic fibrinolytic profile. [223]

Bio-identical Testosterone Replacement Therapy reduces total cholesterol, fat mass, waist circumference and inflammation of arteries which causes atherosclerosis, diabetes, hypertension and abdominal obesity in men. [224] Testosterone also improves the ability of men to function with less shortness of breath, more energy in men with heart failure. [225] Low testosterone is very common in men over sixty years old but many men even in their 40s will have symptoms of testosterone deficiency. [226]

> **Our sex hormones which strongly help to prevent diabetes also can increase HDL and reduce LDL thus reducing the risks of cardiovascular disease.**

All the above information is to demonstrate that our sex hormones which strongly help to prevent diabetes (see the chapter on diabetes) also can increase HDL and reduce LDL thus reducing the risks of cardiovascular disease.

Side Effects of Statin Drugs

The risk of myopathy while taking a statin is increased when one is taking any of a multitude of other drugs. Note the possible side effects of statin drugs such as *Zocor, Crestor, Mevacor, Lescol, Livalo, Vytorin,* or *Zetia*:
Side effects of *Zocor* include:

- Hives
- Difficulty breathing
- Swelling of the face, lips, tongue or throat
- Fever
- Unusual tiredness
- Unexplained muscle pain, tenderness, or weakness
- Swelling
- Confusion
- Memory problems
- Weight gain
- Little or no urinating
- Pain or burning on urination
- Increased thirst
- Increased urination
- Hunger
- Dry mouth
- Fruity breath odor
- Drowsiness
- Dry skin
- Blurred vision
- Weight loss
- Nausea
- Upper stomach pain
- Itching

- Dark urine
- Loss of appetite
- Jaundice (yellowing of the skin or eyes)
- Dark colored urine   Clay-colored stools

This is not an indictment against the use of statins. These medications should be used if other efforts have failed to reduce LDL or to increase HDL or to reduce triglycerides.

It is important to do a risk assessment of your health. Sure, it is important to know your cholesterol level, your HDL and your LDL. However, it is more important to know your testosterone level. Low testosterone is a more accurate marker for early death than cholesterol. Most likely the reason is that testosterone deficiency especially in men and estradiol deficiency in women causes a cascade of changes that lead to cardiovascular disease.

One in three Americans will die from heart disease or stroke, and fully sixty percent will have a major vascular event before they die. The goal of every physician should be the same: to help our patients reduce their risk of cardiovascular diseases and stroke. The overwhelming missing piece to the assessment of the patient who may need to reduce their risk of cardiovascular disease and stroke is the lack of evaluating the patient's blood levels of testosterone, progesterone and estradiol.

Checking sex hormones should be on every blood panel if risk factors for coronary artery disease are suspected. Again, it is more important to know your hormone levels than to know your cholesterol level.

But it is also important to not rely on the so-called "normal" values of most laboratory blood panels. It is not normal to have only ten percent of the hormones one had at their prime.

- If a woman at twenty years old had a progesterone of 15 to 25 ng/ml and now it is .2 ng/ml, this represents less than 1 percent of what she had in her prime. Does this sound healthy?
- If her estradiol was 100 pg/dL (and often up to 800 pg/dL) and now it is 5 pg/dL, this is only 2.5 percent of what she had when she was feeling great.
- If her testosterone is now 4 ng/dL when it was 80 ng/dL when she was at her optimal health, this clearly designates just 5 percent of what she should have to feel complete.

Postmenopausal women have increased incidence of cardiovascular disease caused by plaque buildup from bad cholesterol. Bio-identical estradiol therapy protects the heart. High blood pressure and heart attacks damage heart muscle.

The protection afforded by natural 17β-estradiol is enhanced by progesterone. The facts are self-evident when observing that women in the reproductive age group are protected against cardiovascular disease in comparison with men. [227] Also, at menopause when these life-giving hormones diminish there is a marked increase in cardiovascular disease in women. Plus, the evidence is indisputable that replacing lost natural 17β-estradiol reduces the risk of cardiovascular disease in postmenopausal women. [228]

Correct the hormonal imbalance first and many disease processes will resolve. Telling a patient to stop smoking may do little when he/she has anxiety, depression, and is stressed out. Starting the patient on medication for diabetes may not be the first best treatment. Diagnosing osteoporosis and prescribing a dangerous drug may not be good until the cause of the osteoporosis is resolved. High cholesterol is related to the basic problem beginning in our late twenties and early thirties—loss of health-giving hormones. Correct this and see if many other problems don't resolve before reaching for a drug.

The American Heart Association and American College of Cardiology committee report spends a lot of time talking about changing lifestyles which would lead to lowering of cholesterol. The emphasis of this committee was to encourage changes in "behavior around food" that caused weight gain. But one has to ask, *"What caused this twenty-eight-year-old woman to go from a size four to where she is now a forty-two-year-old who now wears a size sixteen? Did she have such a change in her "behavior around food" that caused the problem?"* Probably not! Think about doing something to help her get back to the way she was when she was 28 years old.

The solution? ***Correct her hormonal imbalance.***

Journal thoughts and questions:

_____
_____
_____
_____
_____
_____
_____
_____
_____
_____
_____
_____
_____
_____
_____
_____
_____
_____
_____

CHAPTER 24

Who Should Not Receive Testosterone Therapy

Exceptions to Bio-identical Hormone Replacement Therapy

BHRT sounds so good – everyone should get it. Right? Not Necessarily.

There are times and cases where people should not receive testosterone therapy. Most of these people will be able to proceed after they have been cleared medically. This chapter outlines when testosterone therapy is not appropriate.

There are times and cases where people should not receive testosterone therapy.

Even though *Bio-identical Hormone Replacement Therapy* is beneficial for improving health, maintaining bone density, sex drive, lowering cholesterol, improving memory, building more muscle mass while lowering body fat, and many other advantages, there are times when BHRT should not be instituted.

Male Breast Cancer

Testosterone replacement may not be right for men with breast cancer. Ninety percent of male breast cancers are estrogen receptor positive. However, there may be a reduced spread of the breast cancer if testosterone is blocked.

Male breast cancer is rare and accounts for only about 1% of all breast cancers. Breast cancer risk in men is increased by elevated levels of estrogen, previous radiation exposure, and a family history of breast cancer. This would indicate that men who have high levels of estrogen should make efforts to reduce these levels in their blood. If the estradiol level is higher than 25 to 45 mg/ml, a man may be able to take DIM I-3-C Complex twice a day, and/or Zinc 50 mg once or twice a day. If this does not reduce the estradiol level, an aromatase inhibitor might be indicated, such as anastrozole 1 mg two or three times a week.

The male breasts may become abnormally enlarged in response to high levels of estrogen. This is called gynecomastia, but is commonly referred to as "man-boobs."

Men who have high levels of estrogens also have an increased risk for development of male breast cancer. Most of these breast cancers in men are estrogen receptor-positive, meaning that they have proteins on the surface of the cells that can receive and transport estrogen through the cell wall and into the interior of the cell. Men that are obese are more likely to have excess estrogen as fat cells produce estrone.

Men with cirrhosis of the liver may also have a higher risk of breast cancer. Some blood pressure medications, medicines to reduce stomach acid, *Valium*, finasteride, and medicines to treat prostate cancer may cause man-boobs to develop.

Male breast cancer is staged just as in women with breast cancer depending on the extent of tumor spread. Surgery is the most common initial treatment for male breast cancer. Chemotherapy, radiation therapy, and hormonal therapy are also administered. The prognosis is dependent on the extent of spread of the tumor.

Prostate Cancer

There is sharp debate whether men should receive supplemental bio-identical testosterone if they have active prostate cancer. Dr. Abraham Morgentaler, associate clinical professor of urology at Harvard Medical School, in his book, *Testosterone for Life* says, *"... the evidence fails to support the long-held concerns that higher testosterone might increase the risk of prostate cancer or that it might cause a hidden, undetected prostate cancer to grow."* [229] This is not to suggest that testosterone causes breast cancer or prostate cancer. Many studies indicate that maintaining testosterone at a healthy level in men may prevent prostate cancer.

Body Builders

Testosterone replacement therapy to achieve supra-physiologic levels to improve one's athletic prowess is inappropriate. Some men wanting to perform well in body-building contests want to achieve blood levels of testosterone of 5000 ng/dl or above. This is inappropriate therapy and a misuse of BHRT.

Penis Enlargement

Testosterone therapy does not cause enlargement of the penis resulting from testosterone deficiency during fetal development. Nor will testosterone therapy correct short stature. Nor is it appropriate to administer doses of testosterone high enough for male birth control, even though supplemental testosterone may cause a decrease in sperm.

Men Who Want to Father a Child

While good levels of testosterone are necessary for normal production of sperm, too much of a good thing is bad. Testosterone replacement therapy may suppress a man's sperm count. If a man has been on testosterone therapy for a while and later wants to become fertile again, normal sperm counts should return after three to six months of not using testosterone supplementation. Also *Clomid* can be used to stimulate a higher sperm count.

Too Many Red Blood Cells

Testosterone stimulates the production of red blood cells in bone marrow. This is a valuable action of testosterone. In men with low testosterone there often is a decreased production of red blood cells causing anemia.

However, it is possible to have an over-production of red blood cells secondary to an increase in testosterone from hormone replacement therapy for men, and very occasionally in women. This condition is called polycythemia—too many red blood cells. This determination is made by measuring a person's hematocrit. Normal hematocrit (Hct) in men is 42 to 54 %. Women's normal hematocrit is 38 to 47 %. Along with the measurement of Hct is hemoglobin. Normal hemoglobin in men is 14.3 to 17.0 g/dL and women's normal is 12.5 to 14.8 g/dL.

In the course of treating men with bio-identical testosterone, the physician should check the patient's blood every three months prior to administering more testosterone. Testosterone replacement is often very beneficial, especially in older men who are anemic. However, if testosterone therapy is too aggressive, a man's hemoglobin and hematocrit may rise too high. In a man if the hematocrit is above 17 g/dL, he should not be treated with more testosterone until he has a therapeutic phlebotomy or donates a unit of blood.

Cushing's Syndrome

Cushing's syndrome is a disorder that occurs when your body is exposed to high levels of the hormone cortisol. It may also occur if you take too much cortisol or other steroid hormones. This condition needs to be treated by an endocrinologist before instituting *Bio-identical Hormone Replacement Therapy*.

Pregnancy

In general, the sex hormones testosterone, progesterone, and estradiol are not used during pregnancy. However, there are anecdotal reports that women who have had frequent miscarriages may benefit from bio-identical progesterone in high doses during the pregnancy.

If a female patient is on BHRT at the time she becomes pregnant, there have been no documented cases of fetal abnormality if she stops the therapy early in the pregnancy.

Young Boys

Boys younger than sixteen, and probably younger than twenty-one, are not candidates for *Bio-identical Hormone Replacement Therapy*. There are various hormonal issues that would need the attention of an endocrinologist familiar with such problems in development in young boys.

During Breast Feeding

Mothers who are breast feeding do not need to use *Bio-identical Hormone Replacement Therapy* until the baby is using other means of feeding. The reason, of course, is the baby would be taking in the hormones administered to the mother.

Active Uterine Cancer or in Treatment

Women with uterine cancer should have these issue resolved before beginning *Bio-identical Hormone Replacement Therapy*.

When PSA is Elevated

A general rule-of-thumb is that no hormonal treatment should be administered to men who have a PSA above 4.0. Actually, the more important lab value to note is the velocity of the change in PSA. In other words, if a man's PSA demonstrates a trend upward from 2.8 ng/ml to 3.4 ng/ml one year later, and again increases to 3.9 ng/ml the next year, this causes a concern. However, a man whose PSA changes from 3.7 ng/ml to 2.9 ng/ml to 4.1 ng/ml to 3.4 ng/ml most likely has a benign issue.

Ovarian Cancer

Perimenopausal women, as their estradiol begins to decline, will have an increase in follicle stimulating hormone. FSH stimulates the ovaries to produce more estradiol in response to the pituitary sensing there is a deficiency of estradiol. There is reason to believe that the constant stimulation of the ovaries every second of the day for the years following the decline of estradiol, usually beginning at age thirty to thirty-five, may be an irritant causing ovarian cancer.

It would be difficult to treat such a patient once ovarian cancer has been identified. However, if she has had her ovaries removed and her oncologic surgeon approves, treatment with bio-identical estradiol may be permissible.

Men with Very Low Testosterone

A man with a testosterone of less than 50 ng/dL may have some other serious unidentified malady. This patient should be evaluated very thoroughly for a multitude of issues, such as occult cancer, before *Bio-identical Testosterone Replacement Therapy.*

Bob was a seventy-one-year-old-retired insurance representative who had smoked for most of his life until he was diagnosed with lung cancer. Bob said,

Doc, I know I have lung cancer and I am having radiation therapy for this now. But, I feel so bad I can hardly get out of bed. My son is having testosterone hormone therapy and he says it helps him a lot. Do you think it might help me?

In this case the reason for his low testosterone level was known. Bob was treated with bio-identical testosterone pellets just as any other man his size and age. He responded nicely. He still had to battle lung cancer and to suffer the side effects of radiation therapy

After just one year of treating Bob, his son returned for his usual three-month hormone insert of testosterone and said, *"Doc, Dad passed away last week. But the family wanted you to know that Dad felt so much better on testosterone and they all wanted me to thank you for what you did for him."*

Active Vaginal Bleeding

Women who have abnormal vaginal bleeding are not to be treated with *Bio-identical Hormone Replacement Therapy* with estradiol until the bleeding problem is resolved. If the patient has a uterine fibroid, or endometrial cancer, or whatever the issue is, this has to be treated first.

Significantly Elevated Blood Pressure

Hormonal balance usually aids in proper control of blood pressure. However, when the patient has been deficient in testosterone for years, the sudden burst of testosterone may cause a very quick increase in blood pressure for a day or two. If the patient has significant blood pressure issues, testosterone should be withheld until there is proper control with medication. If the patient's blood pressure is slightly elevated when bio-identical testosterone is begun, they should receive about half the dosage as would be normally administered. Then the dosage may be gradually increased to normal levels over several months.

Journal thoughts and questions:

_____

_____

_____

_____

_____

_____

_____

_____

_____

_____

_____

_____

_____

_____

_____

_____

_____

CHAPTER 25

Delivery Systems For Hormone Replacement

There Are Options

Hormonal treatments are available in many different delivery systems. In this chapter, we will compare and contrast those options so you will know which is best for you.

Oral Hormones

The problem with oral medications of any kind, especially Prempro, is that the drugs have to pass through the liver when taken by mouth.

Oral medications are taken by mouth. *Premarin* and *Provera* are two examples of oral hormones. When combined together, they form the drug *Prempro*.

There are also bio-identical hormones that can be taken by mouth.

The problem with oral medications of any kind, especially *Prempro*, is that the drugs have to pass through the liver when taken by mouth. This may sound simple, but it is actually very dangerous.

The drug starts out as *Premarin*, a combination of about sixteen different horse estrogens that may be as much as eighty times stronger than the estradiol found in women. This sounds bad, but there is something even more dangerous: the byproducts of *Prempro* as it passes through the liver. The resulting chemicals (drugs) produced from this conversion process in the liver actually cause cancer.

Any kind of estrogen taken by mouth changes clotting factors because of the production of substances that causes the blood to clot more readily. This means the patient is more likely to have blood clots if they take estrogen by mouth. This is why women taking birth control pills have a greater risk of developing thrombophlebitis in the legs and lungs. The exception to oral hormones is progesterone especially if it is taken under the tongue, sublingual, and allowed to dissolve, where it is directly absorbed into the blood stream.

Injections

The most common hormone injected is testosterone. It is not bio-identical testosterone that is injected, but rather a foreign substance. If the dose is not too high, there are relatively few side effects. Unfortunately, these injections do not last long. Men have to repeat this process every seven to ten days. This means a man will feel better for five or six days, but the other four days are a time when the testosterone is either building or declining in the blood.

Most men do not like that roller coaster feeling and would rather opt for something with more consistency.

Testosterone Creams

Men can use a testosterone cream as well as women, but testosterone is not FDA approved for women.

A large majority of men stop using this method of treatment because they do not see the results they were looking for. Creams simply do not relieve most men's symptoms.

Another problem is the user of topical testosterone has to take care to not allow others to come into contact with the area of application as testosterone can be passed to a child or a mate. Testosterone creams do not last long on the skin. This means the patient may have to apply testosterone twice a day to achieve blood levels high enough to relieve symptoms.

Often when a patient who has used testosterone creams has their blood tested a few hours after application, they will find insufficient blood levels to provide benefits of this treatment. Remember, the goal is to try to return the blood levels of testosterone to a level it was before beginning perimenopause or andropause. Testosterone creams are very unlikely to achieve these levels.

Also the body builds a tolerance to skin creams. This requires a higher and higher dose with time to see results.

Estradiol Creams

As bio-identical hormones have been proven to be much safer and more efficacious than synthetic hormones, pharmaceutical companies are now producing topical bio-identical estradiol. This is a marked improvement in oral hormones. Some women experience relief from perimenopausal and menopausal symptoms with estradiol creams.

However, the dose may be adjusted according to how she feels that day. For some, this may be easy – but for others finding the correct dose may be problematic.

Also, the same tolerance can develop with the use of estradiol creams requiring a higher dose periodically. Because estradiol creams do not last all day, many women have to apply the cream twice a day to ward off hot flashes.

Estradiol Patches

Estradiol patches are applied usually every three days. While estradiol may increase the risk of developing cancer of the lining of the uterus, this risk can be decreased considerably by taking progesterone.

Many doctors mix bio-identical estradiol patches with a synthetic "look-alike" progestin, namely *Provera*. This is an effort to counterbalance the stimulation by estradiol of the endometrial lining of the uterus. This makes no sense. The same reason bio-identical estradiol is used is the same reasoning why natural progesterone should be used: it is much safer and effective. If estradiol is used with *Provera*, there is a higher risk of heart attacks, strokes, blood clots in the lungs or legs, breast cancer, and dementia (loss of ability to think, learn, and understand). These consequences seen in the use of *Provera* have not been found in women using bio-identical progesterone.

Examples of estradiol skin patches are *Vivelle-Dot* and *Climera*. There may be problems with the patch staying on for the full three days. Patients report that the patches easily come off in the shower. Also, many women have skin reactions to the adhesive material of the patches.

Estradiol Vaginal Creams and Pills

Vagifem 10 mcg is a pill that is inserted with an applicator into the vagina once a day for one week followed by bi-weekly thereafter. It is designed to relieve symptoms of vaginal dryness, pain and bleeding during intercourse, irritation, soreness, itching in and around the vagina, and painful urination. The product *Estrace* is an example of estradiol used as a vaginal cream.

The interesting question is if a woman has a deficiency of estradiol in her entire body, why not treat the entire body? Having vaginal dryness and irritation are symptoms that a woman needs estradiol throughout her body, not just in the vagina. Systemic (throughout the body) treatment will relieve these symptoms as well as other symptoms of estradiol deficiency.

Pellet Hormone Replacement Therapy

Many doctors are turning to the use of hormone pellets in the treatment of hormone deficiencies in men and women. The treatment is the insertion of a small pellet of estradiol and testosterone, if both are indicated, into a very small puncture site in the upper outer part of the buttocks. This puncture is closed with skin closure strips such as *Steri-Strips*. The patient usually does not have to return for three or four months for another insertion, usually in the opposite hip. The entire procedure is performed in five minutes. An injection of *Lidocaine* is used to alleviate any pain during the procedure.

The advantages of *Bio-identical Pellet Hormone Replacement Therapy* are a constant blood level for a much longer period. Instead of the daily variations requiring frequent dosing changes and inadequate levels achieved for optimal benefits, the patient reaches blood levels of a young adult within a few days and maintains these levels until time for the next insert.

> ***The advantages of Bio-identical Pellet Hormone Replacement Therapy are a constant blood level for a much longer period.***

The two hormones commonly used for hormone insertions are estradiol, varying from 6 mg to 50 mg for women every three to four months. The most common dose is the lowest, 6 mg. Testosterone in women is from 12.5 mg to 100 mg. For some women a dose of 125 mg may be required depending on her weight.

Men require much higher doses of testosterone, usually 1800 mg to 2200 mg, depending on the blood levels before treatment, his symptoms and the size of the man.

For women progesterone sublingual rapid dissolve tablets are used either every night or may be used cyclically twenty-five nights per month allowing for a period.

Blood levels are always checked before each insertion to allow for adjustments in dosing based on the symptoms of the patient and the blood levels desired. ***The important message is that each person is different.*** One woman may need just progesterone and no pellets. Another may require a testosterone pellet and progesterone sublingual tablet. And still another may need estradiol, testosterone and progesterone.

The dosing within each different hormonal deficiency is very much different from one patient to the next and from one treatment to the next. On one visit a woman may need estradiol 6 mg and testosterone 70 mg pellets and oral progesterone 100 mg. The next visit three or four months later, she may require a much different dosage to achieve optimal levels. *Bio-identical Pellet Hormone Replacement Therapy* allows for this personal, adaptive treatment each time.

Conclusion

Administering bio-identical hormones via pellets is the most effective, efficient, and long-lasting treatment available. Most patients are seen by their physicians every three to four months. They are able to maintain hormone levels of a much younger person twenty-four hours a day, seven days a week and avoid many of the side effects associated with unpredictable administrations of creams, patches, and injections.

Journal thoughts and questions:

CHAPTER 26

Depression

Understanding Depression

Antidepressants are a multi-billion dollar business in America. Depression is a dysfunction of the brain. Hormones bathe the brain 24 hours a day with what stimulates the nerve cells to function properly. Replacing lost hormones can give people their lives back and allow them to discontinue anti-depressants with their debilitating side effects.

But pathological depression is different. Depression interferes with daily life and causes pain for you and your family.

Most all of us at one time or another for a short period of time feel sad, blue, unhappy, miserable, or down in the dumps. Usually these feelings are short-lived and pass quickly. But pathological depression is different. Depression interferes with daily life and causes pain for you and your family. During World War II, Prime Minister Winston Churchill of England was plagued with what he called a *"black dog"* that followed him around.

The average age of onset of depression is thirty-two years old.

Many people with depression do not go to a doctor for help. If they do the typical treatments are medications and psychotherapies (counseling). Almost 7 percent of U.S adults experience major depression each year.

Patients with major depression have severe symptoms that interfere with their ability to work, sleep, study, eat, and enjoy life. It is usual for one with major depression to experience several episodes in his/her lifetime.

Signs and symptoms of Depression

Depression is a disorder of the brain perhaps caused by a combination of genetic, biological, environmental, and psychological factors. Brain scans of patients who have depression are different from people without depression especially in parts of the brain involved in mood, thinking, sleep, appetite, and behavior. But these images do not reveal why the depression has occurred.

Scientists are studying certain genes that may make people more prone to depression. Remember, hormones affect our genes. Some genetics research indicates that risk for depression results from the influence of several genes acting together with environmental or other factors.

Depression can result from the influence of genes. Dr. Terry Hertogue has said,

(Hormones) penetrate deeply into the cells, usually acting on the genes in the nucleus, unlocking a portion of the genetic code, accessing the information the cells need to do their jobs (including making hormones). With hormonal deficiencies, the cells simply won't—can't—function as well. Total absence brings total disorder. [230]

Depression is an example of total disorder.

Depression and Hormones

Absence of sex hormones can be a significant reason for depression. Hormones are the fuel that ignites brain function.

Absence of sex hormones can be a significant reason for depression. Hormones are the fuel that ignites brain function. If you are depressed, you probably do not have a *Prozac* deficiency but instead you may have a hormone deficiency.

One hundred and twenty women who had perimenopausal symptoms were treated with hormone pellet implants of estradiol 50 mg and testosterone 120 mg for four years. Progesterone was also given to prevent endometrial hyperplasia. Hot flashes improved in 100 percent of the patients. Depression was resolved in ninety-nine percent and an active libido returned in ninety-two percent of these women. [231]

It is an undisputed fact that many women suffer from the consequences of low testosterone causing depression, changes in mood, loss of the sense of well-being, loss of sexual function, and low libido. Many studies demonstrate that intradermal or transdermal testosterone quickly provides relief from depression brought on by perimenopausal loss of natural testosterone. Women in this age group can still have an active sex life and will not need antianxiety medications and antidepressants. [232]

Audrey's Story

Audrey was forty-seven years old and depressed. She had minor episodes of anxiety but never had significant depression. Audrey explains,

I was married for nineteen years. When I went through "the change," I almost lost my mind. My husband left me and I don't blame him. I felt so depressed I even thought about taking an overdose of Xanax.

You are my last hope. I've seen so many psychiatrists and counselors, even my pastor. No one can help. There are days it's hard to get out of bed. Some days I just stay in bed all day. I go for two or three days and don't eat hardly anything. I've lost a lot of weight, I don't know how much. I lost my job as a teacher over this and had to move in with my dad. My mother committed suicide when I was eighteen.

My sister comes to this clinic. She told me it may be my hormones. Please help me.

Audrey clearly was depressed. She was more depressed than most patients we see. Doctors who treat patients with bio-identical hormones know that it is not uncommon for patients with low hormone levels to experience bouts of depression.

Along with moderate depression, Audrey had multiple symptoms of menopause: hot flashes, poor sleep, headaches, vaginal dryness, tired, sagging of the breast, no libido.

She had twelve different prescription medications in her purse from 7 different doctors including *Percodan, Dilaudid, Xanax, Ambien,* four different SSRIs (antidepressants), *Lithium, Risperdal, Zyprexa* and *Wellbutrin* to help her stop smoking. (She had never smoked until she was 42.)

"Life was good before menopause – but not now."

Audrey was 5'3" and weighed 104 pounds. She was lucid and pleasant. She was not psychotic. She knew that things were not right. *"Life was good before menopause – but not now."*

Audrey had also experienced a mild episode of postpartum depression at age twenty-five after her second child was born. That episode lasted about three months.

Vital signs were normal for the patient. She was clearly underweight. Her sex hormones testosterone, progesterone, and estradiol showed obvious signs of menopause. This was to be expected – her symptoms were telling that same story.

Audrey was treated with bio-identical hormone pellets of estradiol 6 mg, the lowest dose, and testosterone 70 mg because she weighed only 104 pounds. She was given progesterone 100 mg sublingual rapid dissolve tablet to be taken twenty-five days per month at bedtime. For sleep medication, Audrey was asked to gradually stop *Ambien* and begin using melatonin 20 mg at bedtime. She was anxious to stop her *Xanax, Ambien* and *Zoloft,* but she was told to decrease these medications very slowly.

One month later Audrey was a new woman.

She actually was completely free from depression for the first time in seven years.

I use melatonin to help me sleep. I use it instead of Ambien and it works fine. I have to take it earlier in the evening than Ambien, which worked in ten minutes. I hardly ever need my Xanax, but I still carry it with me in my purse. I just feel more comfortable having it nearby. I have cut back on Zoloft to 50 mg a day and I only smoke a half pack a day instead of one pack a day.

Her lab studies showed improvement in every area. Audrey even said she was thinking of trying to get back with her husband.

Antidepressants

The most commonly used antidepressants are called selective serotonin reuptake inhibitors (SSRIs). *Prozac, Zoloft, Lexapro, Paxil,* and *Celexa* are some of the most commonly prescribed SSRIs for depression.

For those doctors who are afraid to prescribe *Prempro* because of the dangers of cancer and stroke, they will prescribe these antidepressant drugs or SSRIs.

The most common side effects with antidepressants that patients complain of are loss of sex drive, an inability to have an orgasm and weight gain.

Depression is often seen in those who have low testosterone. Antidepressants are commonly prescribed for these patients. This is obviously an inappropriate treatment. Testosterone replacement is an effective treatment for depression if hypogonadism is the etiology.

Some physicians may also prescribe a selective serotonin reuptake inhibitor for refractory major depression. Most do not have refractory major depression and do not need an SSRI that carries with it a multitude of side effects. [233]

Patients over fifty years old who have been on SSRIs for five years or more have twice the risk of bone fracture.

Many people experience the side effects of SSRIs.

Dr. Jim was a very prominent dentist who experienced depression after his son took his own life. Jim was placed on *Cymbalta.* He described his response, *"I felt like a zombie on that stuff. I wasn't able to think straight. I was depressed about my son, but this medicine made me feel worse. I had to stop it."*

If *Cymbalta* is not a viable alternative, what is?

When testosterone is added to estrogen therapy in surgically menopausal women, there is an improved sense of well-being and increased energy levels compared to women who received only estrogen. The same response was observed in surgically menopausal women who used a transdermal testosterone patches over a 12-week period. These menopausal women had a significant improvement in 'Psychological General Well Being Index' scores when compared to placebo.

Treatment with testosterone implants (50 mg) in addition to estrogen therapy in postmenopausal women was found to also improve general well-being. Testosterone therapy is used in women who are not yet menopausal but complain of low libido. These women show not just improved libido but also an improved mood and sense of well-being. [234] Three other studies using subcutaneous pellet implants of testosterone reported improve sexual activity, satisfaction, pleasure and orgasm, above that of estrogen therapy alone. [235]

A study in 2011 used compounded bio-identical hormones to provide evidence of the safety of BHRT. In menopausal women using BHRT for three to six months, significant improvements were seen in moderate to severe mood symptoms. These women had a 53 percent decrease in emotional ups and downs, a 58 percent drop in irritability, and a 49 percent reduction in anxiety. This study confirmed that compounded Bio-identical Hormone Replacement Therapy is effective for improving mood symptoms associated with menopause. [236]

It is impossible to justify treating women, who are losing their natural hormones and experiencing depression, with traditional antidepressants. These women develop depression as they are going through perimenopause and menopause ... but they do not suddenly develop an abnormality of the brain. These women are losing their hormones! Why not replace lost hormones instead of giving an antidepressant to try to cover up the obvious?

> *These women are losing their hormones! Why not replace lost hormones instead of giving an antidepressant to try to cover up the obvious?*

Effects of Surgical Menopause

Women who experience surgical menopause have an abrupt drop in estradiol, progesterone and testosterone. They are more likely to have symptoms that can cause a poor sense of well-being, hot flashes, loss of sexual function, and psychological problems. ***Women treated with estradiol alone or estradiol plus testosterone show remarkable improvement in symptoms with no serious side effects.*** Improvement in general well-being can be seen in those using estradiol with or without testosterone. When testosterone is added to estradiol, there is additional improvement in well-being in women who have menopause after surgery.

Some may suggest that women are better off having a hysterectomy even if removing the uterus is done for a benign disease. They imply that women should feel better psychologically and will have improved quality of life and have less depression now that the uterus is gone. [237] *However, it has been recognized by the medical community for years that women who have a hysterectomy with both ovaries removed experience worsening cases of depression.* [238]

Women who have their ovaries removed before menopause or perimenopause have an increased risk of developing anxiety and depression, even if they had no depression before surgery. *This anxiety and depression usually last for years after the ovaries are removed.* [239] These negative effects following both ovaries being removed include premature death, depression, anxiety, cardiovascular disease, loss of reasoning, symptoms of Parkinsonism, dementia, decreased quality of life, loss of sexual function and mental health. *These effects are rarely discussed with women who are considering this surgical procedure.*

Estrogen levels are higher in women who still have their ovaries than in women after removal of their ovaries. This is true even in older women. [240] In the United States more than 1.3 million women will reach menopause each year. [241] Women's transition into menopause represents a dramatic change from the usual abundant supply of hormones that make her a woman. Now she will experience a great deal of variability which brings with it severe vasomotor symptoms such as hot flashes, night sweats, red face, increased risk of osteoporosis, loss of sexual desire and ability to have an orgasm, greater sexual dysfunction, [242] depression, [243] and substantial psychosocial impairment (eg. marriage issues, coping skills, adjusting to new situations). [244]

There are significant antidepressant benefits from estradiol therapy in women in perimenopause and in menopause. This benefit occurs in just four weeks. Longer therapy is even more beneficial. [245]

Case Studies

There is an abundance of evidence that estradiol is beneficial in the treatment of depression. It should be the first line of treatment for perimenopausal women having depression.

There is an abundance of clear evidence that estradiol is beneficial in the treatment of depression. It should be the first line of treatment for perimenopausal women having depression instead of the heavy-laden side effects of most every category of antidepressants. [246]

- Women who experienced depression in the perimenopausal period, usually between the ages of thirty-five and forty-five, were treated with bio-identical 17beta-estradiol for three weeks. They had a significant reduction in sadness, inability to experience pleasure from activities usually found enjoyable, and social isolation.
- Eighty percent of perimenopausal women had a full or partial response in just three weeks from depression using estradiol treatment in a study reported in the *American Journal of Obstetrics and Gynecology* in 2000. *The conclusion of this study was that estradiol replacement is effective in treating depression in women who are losing their hormones.* In just three weeks 80 percent of these women experienced remarkable changes without the side effects associated with the SSRIs.

Even Big Pharma is not going to be able to provide evidence that their antidepressants show a positive response in 80 percent of their patients, no matter how long the patient is being treated – certainly not in three weeks.

It is amazing how quickly patients will respond when we provide what is deficient in their body, instead of giving a drug that is unnatural to the human body. [247]

For years, the diseases diabetes mellitus, hypertension, high cholesterol, osteoporosis, arthritis, fatigue, decreased sex drive, erectile dysfunction, cardiovascular disease, obesity, depression and decreased mental clarity were thought to be a natural process of aging. But now we know that low testosterone is the culprit. [248]

What about the Men?

Decreased sexual desire is primarily affected by the presence of erectile dysfunction and depression. In addition, hypogonadism in men with type 2 diabetes was associated with decreased sexual desire, and more symptoms of depression.

Men with low testosterone not only have a high risk of diabetes but also cardiovascular disease. [249] These men are also more likely to experience sexual dysfunction including erectile dysfunction (ED) and low libido which in turn can lead to depression. [250]

In men, the lower the testosterone the more likely a man is to develop diabetes. He is also more likely to have hypertension, heart disease, to be overweight (high BMI), and to have depression.

Every patient treated with testosterone had a rapid and dramatic recovery from major depression.

A study was conducted of men with mean age of forty years old whose testosterone was mean at 277 ng/dl. This is a very low testosterone when compared to 800 ng/dl to 1200 ng/dl in young men. All these treated men had depression and were not responding to SSRI therapy.

The authors of this study concluded that testosterone replacement therapy may be an effective treatment of depression in men. [251]

Men who are low in testosterone are more likely to be more anxious, less friendly, have a lower sense of well-being, irritable and more tired. Testosterone replacement therapy causes dramatic changes in mood scores. Patients become less depressed, they are less nervous, more alert, and more energetic. [252]

Those who suffer from depression know how debilitating it can be. Therefore treating depression is serious business. When you read a quote that says *"Every patient treated with testosterone had a rapid and dramatic recovery from major depression,"* it makes you stop and seriously consider if testosterone replacement therapy could be the right choice for you.

Journal thoughts and questions:

_____

_____

_____

_____

_____

_____

_____

_____

_____

_____

_____

_____

_____

_____

_____

_____

CHAPTER 27

Diabetes

The Reality of Diabetes

When you have type 2 diabetes – the most common type of diabetes – your body either does not produce enough insulin on its own, or the cells in your body don't use that insulin properly.

Diabetes type 2 is a metabolic disorder that is characterized by high blood sugar in the context of insulin resistance and relative lack of insulin. The classic symptoms are excess thirst, frequent urination, and constant hunger. Type 2 diabetes makes up about ninety percent of cases of diabetes, with the other ten percent due primarily to diabetes type 1 and gestational diabetes. Obesity is thought to be the primary cause of type 2 diabetes.

When you eat food, it gets broken down and turned into a sugar called glucose, which is used for energy within the body. However, in order to use glucose properly, your body needs a hormone called insulin, which helps take that sugar out of your blood and transport it into your muscles, brain, eyes, nerves, bones, etc. to produce energy.

When you have type 2 diabetes – the most common type of diabetes – your body either does not produce enough insulin on its own, or the cells in your body don't use that insulin properly. Instead of using glucose for energy, that sugar stays in your blood, which can lead to a number of serious health problems.

Type 2 diabetes is a serious condition. You may have heard people say they have *"a touch of diabetes"* or *"my sugar is a little high."* These words suggest that type 2 diabetes is not a serious disease. That is not correct.

Type 2 diabetes is associated with many serious health problems. High blood-sugar levels may cause:
- Blindness
- Gum infections in your mouth
- Heart disease
- Kidney disease
- Nerve disease
- Poor blood flow
- Stroke

Between ninety and ninety-five percent of people with diabetes have type 2 diabetes. It is most often associated with old age, obesity, family history, previous history of gestational diabetes, physical inactivity, and certain ethnicities. Eighty percent of people with type 2 diabetes are overweight.

When type 2 diabetes is diagnosed, the pancreas is usually producing enough insulin, but for unknown reasons the body cannot use the insulin effectively, a condition called insulin resistance. After several years, insulin production decreases. The result is that glucose (sugar) builds up in the blood, and the body cannot make efficient use of this main source of fuel.

The symptoms of type 2 diabetes develop gradually. Symptoms may include fatigue, frequent urination, increased thirst and hunger, weight loss, blurred vision, and slow healing of wounds or sores. Some people have no symptoms.

Managing Diabetes

A key to managing type 2 diabetes is controlling blood-sugar levels. The American Diabetes Association suggests:

- For patients diagnosed with type 2 diabetes, healthy blood-sugar levels are 70 to 130 mg/dL (milligrams per deciliter) before meals and less than 180 mg/dL at one to two hours after starting meals
- An A1C goal of 6.5 or less

One way your healthcare provider measures your blood-sugar levels is with a hemoglobin A1C test. It shows your average blood-glucose levels over the last 3 months. It is the best way to learn your overall blood glucose levels during this time.

Another step toward leading a healthy life with type 2 diabetes is learning some new habits. These include:

- Choosing what, how much, and when to eat
- Getting physically active
- Checking your blood glucose
- Going to your doctors' appointments
- Learning all you can about diabetes
- Taking medicine as your doctor prescribes it [253]

Men with type 2 diabetes almost universally have low testosterone. Women with elevated insulin levels have almost a three-hundred-percent increase in breast cancer. Men find that within just one week after testosterone is increased with bio-identical testosterone and estradiol is decreased, there is a marked lowering of blood sugar in the body and increased insulin sensitivity. Hormonal balance often reverses insulin resistance thereby lowering blood sugar to normal levels.

***Hormonal balance often reverses insulin resistance thereby
lowering blood sugar to normal levels.***

Diabetes is a devastating disease that becomes more common as we age and made worse with weight gain and decreased exercise. The *"Metabolic Syndrome"* usually encompasses elevated lipids (cholesterol and triglycerides), low HDL cholesterol, high blood pressure (hypertension), and diabetes or insulin resistance (elevated fasting blood sugar), central obesity (abdominal fat). Metabolic syndrome increases the risk of developing cardiovascular disease, particularly heart failure, and diabetes. [254]

Some studies have shown the prevalence of the metabolic syndrome in the USA to be an estimated 34% of the adult population, [255] and the prevalence increases with age. Bio-identical testosterone therapy produces positive changes by reducing total cholesterol, fat mass, waist circumference and pro-inflammatory cytokines associated with atherosclerosis, diabetes and the metabolic syndrome. [256]

Most diabetics have insulin resistance. They have excess insulin, but the body cannot use the insulin it has. This is called insulin resistance. Women with elevated insulin levels have almost a 300 percent increase in breast cancer. This is why your physician should regularly check your insulin levels and serum testosterone. Even if one is not obese, having low testosterone is a major risk factor for insulin resistance and type 2 diabetes. Also insulin resistance and type 2 diabetes is a strong indication that low testosterone is present. [257]

A major complication of diabetes is nerve damage in the arms and legs. There has been a search for drugs that can protect the nerves from damages caused by diabetes. A study reported in *Neuroscience* in 2007 demonstrated that natural progesterone had neuroprotective effects against diabetic neuropathy.

Chronic treatment for one month with bio-identical progesterone counteracts the impairment of nerve conduction velocity (how quickly a nerve impulse travels through a nerve) and thermal threshold (how long it takes for a patient to feel heat), and restored skin innervation. [258]

Anna, a 53-year-old lady, was seen in the emergency department complaining of swelling in her right big toe. She said,

I have type 2 diabetes and I have trouble controlling my blood sugar. I have three dogs. Four days ago I took a nap and when I woke up one of my dogs was gnawing on my right big toe and I didn't feel anything. When I woke up and saw what happened I put an antibiotic ointment on it and wrapped it up. When it got worse, I saw my family doctor. He gave me some antibiotics, but it keeps getting worse.

Ultimately her toe had to be amputated. If Anna had been on natural progesterone, and had felt the dog chewing on her toe, perhaps she would not have had to have an amputation.

Estradiol is known to inhibit the buildup of plaque in the arteries.

Those with diabetes have a significant risk factor for atherosclerotic peripheral vascular disease (plugged up arteries from plaque buildup). Elevated glucose (sugar) and high insulin levels as is seen in type 2 diabetes stimulates the buildup of the blockage in arteries. Estradiol is known to inhibit the buildup of this blockage. Also natural progesterone inhibits the development of atherosclerotic peripheral vascular disease in patients with diabetes. [259]

Women who have normal levels of estradiol and progesterone, even if they have diabetes, are at lower risk than women who have low levels of natural estradiol and progesterone.

Men with obesity, the metabolic syndrome, and type 2 diabetes have almost universally low testosterone. Conversely, the presence of low testosterone predicts the development of metabolic syndrome and type 2 diabetes. Visceral adiposity (apple shape torso) present in men with low testosterone, the metabolic syndrome, and/or type 2 diabetes causes the production of inflammatory factors. These inflammatory factors cause low-grade inflammation throughout the body, especially in the arteries. These inflammatory markers cause the inside lining of the arteries to narrow down with adverse consequences such as increased risk of cardiovascular disease and erectile dysfunction. [260]

You don't have to be a rocket scientist to know something bad is going to happen.

Think of a car with no headlights and bad brakes. A drunk driver is at the wheel, going too fast on icy roads, with bald tires. You don't have to be a rocket scientist to know something bad is going to happen. With central obesity, metabolic syndrome, type 2 diabetes, hypertension, low HDL, and elevated triglycerides, surely one is looking in the face of a heart attack or stroke.

It's All Inter-Related

Low total testosterone is associated with type 2 diabetes, independent of age, race, and obesity. [261] When one has low testosterone there, is a very good chance type 2 diabetes will be following not far behind. [262]

Because so often type 2 diabetics are obese, which suppresses testosterone levels, obesity is an important factor in the relationship between testosterone and type 2 diabetes. Low testosterone is seen more often in diabetic men than men without diabetes. [263]

In men who have had a bilateral orchiectomy as treatment for prostate cancer the risk of the patient developing diabetes and cardiovascular disease is significantly increased. Not only are obesity, metabolic syndrome, and type 2 diabetes found in men with low testosterone, but also sexual dysfunction is frequently seen, especially erectile dysfunction. [264]

It is easy to see the complex and multidirectional relationships among obesity, metabolic status, low testosterone, and ED in men.

When testosterone is increased with bio-identical testosterone to the levels it should be – and estradiol is decreased, there are improved triglycerides, lowering of blood sugar after eating, and increased insulin sensitivity with substantial improvements in erections and sexual desire – in just one week's time. [265]

One study showed that sixteen percent of men with erectile dysfunction were diabetic and almost one-fourth of the men with diabetes had a testosterone level of less than 300 ng/dl — normal for a young male being 800 to 1200 ng/dl. [266] Decreased sexual desire, depression, and lower luteinizing hormone, the hormone that stimulates the testicles to produce more testosterone, were seen in men with low testosterone and with type 2 diabetes.

Men with type 2 diabetes can have other causes of ED besides low testosterone. These can include:

Poor control of sugar, smoking, alcoholism, use of antidepressants, cardiovascular disease, medications, and medicines for acid in the stomach, antidepressants, recreational drugs, fatigue, systemic illness (eg. liver or kidney failure, COPD, stroke), depression, relationship problems, other sexual dysfunction (fear of humiliation), hypoactive sexual disorder, and sexual aversion disorder. [267]

Weight loss and increased physical activity increased the ability to have erections in men with type 2 diabetes who had ED especially if they increase their testosterone with bio-identical testosterone replacement. [268]

Improved Sexual Performance for Men

Maintaining tighter control of blood sugar may show some improvement in erectile function, but far more benefit is seen with natural testosterone hormone replacement therapy. [269]

Natural testosterone treatment improves the number and strength of nighttime erections, sexual thoughts and sexual desire, number of successful intercourse sessions, scores of erectile function, and overall sexual satisfaction.

Natural testosterone treatment, not synthetic testosterone, improves the number and strength of nighttime erections, sexual thoughts and sexual desire, number of successful intercourse sessions, scores of erectile function, and overall sexual satisfaction in men who had testosterone below 346 ng/dL.

Increasing testosterone in these men to 800 ng/dl to 1200 ng/dl almost always will have dramatic effects in libido and all other aspects of sexual function.

The effects of *Bio-identical Testosterone Replacement Therapy* are greater when *Viagra, Cialis*, or *Levitra* are added to the treatment. Many men with diabetes have benefited from the combination of BHRT with testosterone pellets and daily oral dosing of *Cialis*, showing significant improvement in vaginal penetration, completion of intercourse, and overall treatment satisfaction. [270] *Revive*, a natural male supplement that does not require a prescription, is also very beneficial to add endurance and firmness to erections.

Benefits to the Heart

When men who have low testosterone are treated with natural testosterone, there will be dilation of the coronary arteries supplying more blood to the heart, a decrease in myocardial ischemia (narrowing of the small blood vessels that supply blood and oxygen to the heart due to coronary artery disease) and less chest pain during exercise. [271] *Bio-identical Testosterone Replacement Therapy* will actually improve chronic heart failure—congestive heart failure (a weak heart muscle). [272]

There are more testosterone receptor sites in the heart than any other muscle in the body. This is because the heart is the most important muscle we have, and it is so very much dependent on testosterone to function at its best.

It is common for traditional doctors to give drugs to try to get the heart to beat stronger, to decrease the amount of blood flowing into the heart to take pressure off, or to open up blood vessels after blood passes through the heart, or to give diuretics (fluid pills) to remove some of the fluid the heart has to pump, all in an effort to relieve congestive heart failure, to keep the heart from having to work so hard.

The heart needs testosterone to keep the heart muscle strong enough to do its work.

But none of these treat the real problem—the heart needs testosterone to keep the heart muscle strong enough to do its work.

How Bio-identical Testosterone Replacement Therapy Helps Men with Diabetes

Bio-identical Testosterone Replacement Therapy helps men with type 2 diabetes who are low in testosterone. There will be numerous beneficial effects including:

- Sexual health—less erectile dysfunction, more sexual desire, nighttime erections
- General well-being—less depression
- Body composition—more muscle and less fat which reduces risks for CVD—chances of a heart attack
- Reduction of fat in the abdomen—smaller waist circumference
- Better control of blood sugar—insulin resistance is common in congestive heart failure and will improve with natural testosterone replacement therapy
- Reduction of total cholesterol
- Increase of HDL cholesterol
- Reduction of LDL cholesterol
- Reduction of triglycerides
- Reduction of *Lipoprotein a* (Lp(a)—the strongest positive correlation with premature coronary heart disease than any other component of the lipid profile [273]

None of these clinical trials quoted above reported any adverse effects on blood pressure, cardiovascular events, or mortality. [274] How many of the drugs Big Pharma advertises can say that?

But there is even more evidence demonstrating that it is essential for men to have their health-providing testosterone maintained at a level much higher than seen in aging.

One routine treatment of men who have prostate cancer is to remove the testicles or to give a drug that stops the production of testosterone. The results of such treatments, called Androgen (testosterone) Deprivation Therapy (ADT), gives evidence of what happens to men who have low testosterone.

Various complications occur such as osteoporosis, sexual dysfunction, gynecomastia (man-boobs), and adverse body composition (obesity, loss of muscle mass), metabolic syndrome, elevated blood sugar, type 2 diabetes, decreased quality of life, impotence, decreased sexual desire, and premature death. Some of these complications occur within just three to six months of treatment of ADT. Long-term treatment more than twelve months has even more serious side effects, especially higher prevalence of diabetes, metabolic syndrome, and higher cardiovascular mortality. [275]

Cardiovascular disease, heart attacks and congestive heart failure have become the most common causes of mortality in men with prostate cancer (PCa). In other words, it is common for men with prostate cancer to die of something unrelated to PCa, but secondary to the treatment for PCa. [276] This occurs because removing testosterone from men causes hardening of the arteries, atherosclerosis, leading to cardiovascular disease. These events occur because the body cannot function without hormonal balance. Without testosterone men gain weight, especially around the waist, leading to increased insulin levels which cause an increase in inflammatory cytokines that damage blood vessels. There is a decrease in muscle mass secondary to a decrease of glucose taken into muscle fibers (insulin resistance) which leads to diabetes and soon to follow cardiovascular disease. [277]

Many of the above consequences of men with low testosterone can be prevented with *Bio-identical Testosterone Replacement Therapy* in obese men. [278] Men who have their testosterone removed artificially have a twenty-five percent higher risk of coronary artery disease. [279]

What About Women?

Although low levels of testosterone are seen in men who develop type 2 diabetes, the exact opposite is seen in women. High levels of testosterone in women may cause the development of type 2 diabetes.

But notice, normal levels of testosterone for a young female are found in women who do not have diabetes. Only ***abnormally high levels of testosterone*** are related to diabetes in women. This is frequently seen in women with Polycystic Ovarian Syndrome, a condition of women that produces masculinization and infertility.

Diabetic men have significantly lower levels of testosterone. Women with type 2 diabetes had much higher levels of testosterone and estradiol compared with those with normal blood sugar. [280] This suggests that diabetic women who need hormone replacement should be monitored more closely by regularly checking the patient's blood sugar, testosterone, estradiol and progesterone levels. [281]

> *It is easy to see that hormonal balance is most important—not too much, not too little of each of the health-providing sex hormones.*

In postmenopausal women, treatment with *Premarin* and with *Provera*, not a natural progesterone, causes an increase in blood sugar because of problems with insulin delivery and an increase in insulin resistance. Treatment with natural transdermal estradiol causes no such changes. [282] It is easy to see that hormonal balance is most important—not too much, not too little of each of the health-providing sex hormones. [283]

It may seem strange … but older women had much lower values of estradiol compared with men. Because men have higher levels of testosterone than women, older men have four times higher levels of estradiol. This is because testosterone can convert to estradiol, as we discussed earlier. But remember, high levels of estradiol in men is not a good thing. Men who have levels of estradiol much above 45 pg/ml need to take a low dose of an aromatase blocker. [284] Elevated systolic and diastolic blood pressure may also contribute to diabetes in men. The higher the blood pressure the more likely one is to eventually develop diabetes. [285] Because our sex hormones are so helpful in improving our circulation by dilating blood vessels, *Bio-identical Hormone Replacement Therapy* may be beneficial in the overall scheme of good health.

Healthy levels of testosterone are not just for the prevention of diabetes. But low testosterone is seen in mortality (early death) due to all causes, including cardiovascular disease, and cancer. The higher the testosterone the less the chances one has of cardiovascular disease and cancer. And there is a lower chance of diabetes seen in patients with higher testosterone. Higher levels of testosterone, within the limits of a young man, are associated with increased (LDL) high-density lipoprotein cholesterol concentrations and lower blood pressure, triglyceride, and glucose concentrations. The higher the level of testosterone, the lower the body mass index, waist-hip ratio, and prevalence of type 2 diabetes.

It has been known since 1994, when it was reported in a study, that the higher the testosterone a patient has (within the limits of a normal young male), the less coronary artery disease men will have. [286] Since then other reports have shown the same results in the carotid artery in the neck [287] and in the aorta (the large artery coming out of the heart). [288] It is so difficult to imagine why every cardiologist, cardiovascular surgeon, heart transplant surgeon and family doctor are not checking the testosterone in every male patient regularly. Cholesterol and blood sugar are checked at least annually, but a more important number to know that determines mortality (how long one is going to live) is the patient's testosterone level.

Because suppressing a man's testosterone seems to cause regression of prostate cancer, albeit temporary, concerns were raised that high testosterone might be a risk factor for prostate cancer. [289] However, other studies have not shown testosterone to be a problem for men with prostate cancer. [290] And these studies confirm that providing natural testosterone replacement therapy does not cause worsening of prostate cancer even in one who has this disease. Men are far more likely to die from the complications of withdrawing testosterone in men with prostate cancer than the disease itself. Men are dying far more quickly from heart attacks, strokes, blood clots, and diabetic complications than from the treatment for prostate cancer. [291]

Thirty-one percent of all adult men in U.S. are obese and 2.8 percent are morbidly obese. [292] Knowing the devastating diseases associated with obesity, these observations have profound pathophysiological, clinical, epidemiological, and public health implications. [293]

Normal testosterone for a young male is about 800 ng/dl to 1200 ng/dl. Most studies that report men are not classified as having low testosterone until he drops down to below 250 ng/dl—one-third to one-fourth of normal for a young man. Even in men who are not obese, 26 percent will have levels below what is called low testosterone, which is ridiculous to say 250 ng/dl is normal. Fifty percent of obese diabetic men are below 250 ng/dl.

By age thirty, men begin a gradual decline in testosterone until many by age 70 will have only ten percent of what they had as a young man. Obese diabetic men are far more likely to have low testosterone. Men with low testosterone are far more likely to have type 2 diabetes and obesity.

Bio-identical Hormone Replacement Therapy with testosterone is essential to save the lives of men with cardiovascular disease and diabetes.

Bio-identical Hormone Replacement Therapy with testosterone is essential to save the lives of men with cardiovascular disease and diabetes. But it is equally important to protect men from becoming obese with declining testosterone and developing coronary artery disease. [294]

Journal thoughts and questions:

_____

_____

_____

_____

_____

_____

_____

_____

_____

_____

_____

_____

_____

_____

_____

_____

_____

_____

CHAPTER 28

Erectile Dysfunction

Edith and Jerry's Story

Edith had been receiving pellet hormone therapy for six months with great results. Now sixty-one years old, she came into the consultation with her sixty-three-year-old husband, Jerry. *"I have felt so good since starting hormone treatments and I want Jerry to feel as good as I do. He doesn't seem to be the same warm and loving man I married thirty-nine years ago. Actually, what I want is to have sex more than once a month."*

Edith was blunt – but she expressed what numerous other women have experienced: a renewed sex life. She had problems after menopause with vaginal dryness causing pain on intercourse. This was not much of a problem, however, because she had no libido. To further complicate the problem, Jerry had dropped off a lot in his sexual interest as well.

This couple is no different from thousands of others. Listen to Edith's their story:

The problem came when I regained my sexual interest but Jerry did not. Several times I even pleasured myself. I now have vaginal moisture like I had when I was eighteen. I also have more sexual thoughts like I did then as well. I enjoyed sex before and Jerry did too, but now he just gives up when can't perform.

Jerry's testosterone was only 224 ng/dL, below most men his age, and far below where he probably was thirty-nine years earlier when he married Edith. Jerry had most all of the typical low testosterone symptoms. He reported,

I knew something wasn't right but I didn't know what to do. I blamed it on being so busy. My company is going gangbusters and I'm working long hours to keep it going. I feel so stressed out and sometimes I have trouble concentrating. I feel overwhelmed and have doubts about myself. Edith has changed so much in the past six months. I feel so embarrassed but I don't even think about sex much and more. When Edith and I are together I am afraid I can't keep it hard long enough to put it in. I wish I had her energy. Can you give me what you gave her? [295]

Edith was due for her three month insert of estradiol and testosterone. Jerry began his first treatment receiving only testosterone pellets. [296] Jerry was also started on *Revive TCM*, a supplement to help his erections. He was encouraged to begin a regular exercise program and to follow a low glycemic index diet. Jerry had gained forty-five pounds over the previous ten years, mostly around the waist.

One month later Jerry and Edith returned for their follow-up appointment. There were smiles everywhere. Jerry said,

I really feel like I did when I was thirty! Really. I have energy and can concentrate at work. I have my confidence back at work and at home. [297] *I've already lost eight pounds and I'm down three inches in my waist. I stop off at the gym three days a week on the*

way home from work. [298] *I noticed on the fifth morning after the testosterone treatment I woke up with an erection. I hadn't seen that happen in four years. I think about sex more than before. Used to I wouldn't think about sex even once a week, now I think about sex two or three times a day. And Edith and I are like we're on our second honeymoon, but this one is even better. We have sex almost every day and on weekends more than that.* [299]

The Reality of Sexual Dysfunction

A major health issue men face in aging is erectile dysfunction. Hormonal decline influences many areas of changes seen in the aging process, but few as obvious and damaging to men's feeling of self-confidence as erectile dysfunction. This is seen by the widespread use of PDE5 inhibitors, *Viagra, Cialis* and *Levitra.*

It is important to know that erectile dysfunction is an outward sign of something going wrong inside.

It may be difficult for women to understand the distress a man has when he is not able to perform in bed. This is one of the most important areas in a man's life. He finds much of his identity in how he performs sexually. And when he loses that ability, it can be devastating. It is important to know that erectile dysfunction is an outward sign of something going wrong inside.

The Root Cause of Erectile Dysfunction

The root cause of erectile dysfunction is a decline of testosterone. For years the study of hormones has been reserved for the area of endocrinology. However, more physicians and the lay public have become more conscious of the effects hormones have on wellness and disease prevention. The first physician the patient usually contacts is his or her family doctor. The family physician is becoming more aware of the role hormones play in keeping us healthy (disease prevention). [300]

The overwhelming observation that needs to be made is that PDE5 inhibitors do not influence the cause of erectile dysfunction. Taking cough medicine for pneumonia does not cure pneumonia. *The root cause of erectile dysfunction is a decline of testosterone.* Men do not develop a deficiency of *Viagra* as they grow older. They develop a testosterone deficiency. Does it not make sense to replace low testosterone instead of using *Viagra* so you do not need *Viagra* any longer?

PDE5 inhibitors do not influence the cause of erectile dysfunction. Taking cough medicine for pneumonia does not cure pneumonia.

The Effects of Low Testosterone in Men

Testosterone deficiency not only causes erectile dysfunction (ED) but men will also experience:
- Decreased body hair
- Reduction in muscle mass
- Decreased strength

- Increase in fat mass
- Decreased hematocrit (anemia)
- Decreased libido
- Infertility
- Osteoporosis
- Depression
- Orchitis—often mumps
- Mood changes [301]

Low testosterone may be seen in men who have had trauma to the pelvis or to the testicles, removal of the testicles usually due to cancer or torsion (twisting of the cords to the testicles), or a genetic abnormality. But most often low testosterone is due to aging. [302]

When a patient tells the physician that ...

- He is fifty years old
- Tired
- Has difficulty building muscle even though he exercises regularly
- Has gained weight
- Is somewhat depressed
- Has erectile dysfunction
- Has low sex drive

... the doctor knows that this guy has a very high probability of having low testosterone.

In one primary care office, the risk of men forty-five years or older having low testosterone was almost thirty-nine percent.[303] The increased risks noted above are for men who have a testosterone below 300 ng/dL. But young men of eighteen to thirty years old have testosterone levels of 800 ng/dL to 1200 ng/dL. Many men who use *Viagra* are able to get erections – but have no increase in energy or sexual desire. Many on *Viagra* do not get much benefit because men with low testosterone are less likely to respond to a PDE4 inhibitor.

> ### *Many on Viagra do not get much benefit because men with low testosterone are less likely to respond to a PDE4 inhibitor.*

With the loss of testosterone the nervous system, muscles and vascular system of the penis weaken with less sensitivity, less power and less pleasurable ejaculations. Having and maintaining an erection is more difficult. The penis becomes flaccid and flabby, instead of strong and firm. This does not have to happen, no matter what the age. When low testosterone is replaced to the level of youth, these fat cells return to near 100 percent of the youthful state. [304]

A seventy-year-old man can have a penis as large and functional as a twenty-year-old. Testosterone is not only critical for proper functioning of the penis, but also essential for the brain to respond to sexual thoughts and stimulation, sexual fantasies and desire. It has been said that a young man thinks about sex every eighteen seconds. And an old man has forgotten what it's like to think about sex. Bio-identical testosterone replacement therapy will wake up those centers in the brain and provide the ability to respond when the thoughts occur.

What BHRT Treatment Will Do

Treatment with bio-identical testosterone improves sexual function in men who have low testosterone. Treated men have more frequent erections, more nighttime erections and these erections last longer. Men treated with natural testosterone have more frequent ejaculations and longer and stronger orgasms. [305]

It is easy to think of each of the sex hormones (testosterone, estradiol and progesterone) as an independent acting hormone. This is not true. Women have testosterone, progesterone and estradiol just like men do, but the proportions are very different. Men may have twenty times more testosterone than women. Women will have much more estradiol and progesterone than men. It is important that there is a balance between the three in both men and women. [306]

If a man's estradiol lowers too much, he may experience erectile dysfunction, irritability and loss of libido. [307] Excess estradiol contributes to the development of insulin sensitivity, hypertension, type 2 diabetes, elevated cholesterol and triglycerides, abdominal obesity and low HDL cholesterol. [308]

Bio-identical hormones are manufactured to be molecularly identical to hormones found in the human body. This is certainly good – but when a man is treated with bio-identical testosterone, it is possible for his estradiol level to increase beyond normal. This is somewhat unusual. The treating doctor must always check the patient's estradiol level. If the estradiol level is too high, he should be placed on zinc 50 mg and DIM. If this does not cause a decrease in estradiol, the patient may be given a prescription for an aromatase inhibitor to be taken for a few days. The most commonly used aromatase inhibitors are *Arimidex* or *Femara*.

Some physicians may be hesitant to treat men over fifty-years-old with bio-identical testosterone because of a misperception that testosterone causes prostate cancer. For more than sixty years, doctors were told that testosterone caused a significant risk factor for prostate enlargement. The assumption was that high testosterone levels served as fuel for prostate cancer. Blocking testosterone in men, or actually giving men estrogen, is still the standard of care for prostate cancer therapy even today. [309]

The idea that higher testosterone causes growth of prostate cancer originated from the publication in 1941 of two papers based on one patient. After more than seventy-three years and many hundreds of studies discounting this connection between prostate cancer and higher testosterone levels, there is still a reluctance to treat men with bio-identical testosterone because of fear of causing prostate cancer or fueling prostate cancer already present at a sub-clinical or microscopic level.

Treating men with bio-identical testosterone has little or no effect on prostate cancer risk.

There has never been a well-designed study that has shown a direct correlation between total testosterone levels and prostate cancer. After almost seventy-five years, it should be clear that treating men with bio-identical testosterone has little or no effect on prostate cancer risk. The theory that testosterone causes prostate cancer is beyond reason when we know that men are far more likely to develop prostate cancer when their testosterone levels are at their lowest, not when they are elevated. [310]

Erectile dysfunction may also be seen in men who are anemic—low hemoglobin and hematocrit (low red blood cells). Testosterone stimulates the production of red blood cells in bone marrow and the spleen. In low testosterone conditions RBCs are not manufactured in sufficient numbers to maintain good health. This is important when remembering that the penis fills with blood causing an erection. With low blood counts erectile dysfunction may result. [311]

Wives' Responses to BHRT

It is interesting to note the responses wives have after their husbands receive testosterone replacement therapy. It is clear that testosterone is an important factor determining sexual behavior in men. The sexual behavior of men affects relationships just as it does in women. The bottom line: when people feel good about themselves, there is better sexual functioning.

When testosterone levels were low, men reported that they had a decline in mood. They felt 'flat,' they didn't care, were less affectionate and generally 'down.' Some wives commented that when their husband's testosterone was low, he was temperamental and less tolerant. As testosterone fell in both married and single men, there was a decline in the ability to concentrate and ability to think clearly and remember. These men commented that when their testosterone was low, they reported feeling fatigued and drained. They tired easily and found it difficult to complete tasks. It is interesting that the partners of these men reported the same effects about their husbands. [312] But when these men had Bio-Identical Testosterone Replacement Therapy they reported that they felt more confident, more talkative, could concentrate better. Many said they felt more macho and aggressive.

Testosterone therapy with pellet implants affects the ability to have intercourse and libido more than just having an erection. Testosterone replacement is safe and almost always successful by all methods, but pellet implants are the most effective in maintaining sexual function and have fewer side effects. [313] As we have seen, maintaining an erection is more difficult, if not impossible and having nighttime erections is rare, when testosterone is low. BHRT will change that.

A Physician's Responsibility

When a physician is consulting with a male patient, it is important to assess his sense of well-being and the sense of maintaining his masculine self-concept. Physicians not only need to be good "diagnosers," they also need to be good listeners. Listen to what your patient is telling you. When they describe the symptoms they are experiencing, they are telling you what is wrong. Their words will point you to the correct diagnosis.

Relationships are important and replacing low testosterone in men with bio-identical (not synthetic injections) testosterone often rekindles such attractions. Sexual counseling should be a part of an overall evaluation of each adult patient.

Journal thoughts and questions:

_____

_____

_____

_____

_____

_____

_____

_____

_____

_____

_____

_____

_____

_____

_____

_____

_____

CHAPTER 29

Fibromyalgia And Chronic Fatigue Syndrome

Meet Danielle

Danielle was depressed.

Now thirty-nine, she had a total hysterectomy five years earlier. She was experiencing all of the side effects from it. She said,

I had to have a hysterectomy when I was thirty-four because of endometriosis. The surgeon told me he was going to also remove my ovaries because without a uterus, I had no need of the ovaries. He said if he didn't remove the ovaries, there was a chance I might get ovarian cancer later on. So I consented.

Later, I read in a book about menopause that I should not have consented to this because the ovaries still make good hormones for a long time. But by that point, it was too late. Way too late.

Danielle had seen seven different doctors since her surgery, complaining of being so tired she could hardly get out of bed in the morning. Seven! At least she was persistent! She said,

I am as tired when I get up as when I went to bed the night before, which is usually six or seven in the evening. One doctor told me she thought I had Mono and I should stay in bed for six weeks. Another one told me I was depressed. One doctor told me he thought I was just imagining the pain. And another one told me I should go back to work and forget it.

I can't do that. I used to work at General Dollar as an assistant manager but asked to be laid off. I couldn't handle the stress and had so much pain. I have headaches all the time and every muscle in my body aches. I went on disability. I take six different medicines a day, most of them three or four times a day but nothing helps.

Danielle went on to say she had become forgetful, was not able to concentrate and became easily confused. Her family told her that she was more irritable. At times she has had a sore throat and fever of 100 to 101. Her family doctor noticed sore lymph nodes in her neck and gave her four different antibiotics over six months ... but nothing helped. She had the typical symptoms of menopause—hot flushes, night sweats, vaginal dryness, mood swings, and no libido at all.

Most of the doctors told her they could not find anything wrong physically, but they suspected fibromyalgia. Two of the seven doctors told her she had chronic fatigue syndrome. Every one of the seven doctors suggested antidepressants.

I took four different kinds of antidepressants. One would help for a month or so. But then they didn't help at all. And they made me gain weight. I had no sex drive at all. I didn't know if it was from the surgery I had or the medicines. After three years of going through all this my husband left me.

This history is so typical of patients whose ovaries have been removed.

Danielle wanted to feel good ... but didn't have the energy.

She described various stressful situations where she reacted in an irrational way over minor things. The morning of the first visit, her son forgot his lunch. When she saw it on the kitchen counter she became almost hysterical. Danielle said, *"I can't handle stress anymore."*

Her medication lists included two antidepressants, *Paxil* 10 at bedtime and *Zoloft* 50 mg twice a day. These two medications were prescribed by two different doctors. She was using *Ambien* 10 at bedtime for sleep. She was taking a diet capsule every morning: phentermine 37.5 mg. For pain she took four pills a day of hydrocodone 10 mg. Also *Xanax* 1 mg was used three times a day as needed for anxiety. She used *Reglan* for an irritable bowel four times a day.

She had never had her hormones checked except her thyroid, which was borderline low. Two years ago her TSH was high, indicating the thyroid may be low. Her T3 and T4 were marginally low. Danielle completed a survey, checking off symptoms such as fatigue, sleep problems, comprehension problems ... all of which were suggestive of chronic fatigue and fibromyalgia.

> ### She completed a survey, checking off symptoms such as fatigue, sleep problems, comprehension problems ... all of which were suggestive of chronic fatigue and fibromyalgia.

At her initial examination, Danielle looked exhausted. More "tired" than depressed. She looked older than thirty-nine. She said, *"Sometimes I think I look older than my mother."*

She weighed 185 pounds – she had gained thirty-seven pounds in the five years since her surgery. That was one of the side effects of being on antidepressants for four-and-a-half years. She was 5' 4" tall. Her blood pressure was low at 92/56. Her muscle strength was poor. Her temperature was recorded at 99.8. She had pain on pressure at 15 of the 18 tender points, indicative of fibromyalgia. She did not have pain in the joints, but near the joints on pressure.

She commented, *"When my doctor pressed on the trigger points, I hadn't realized I was sore there before that time."*

Her testosterone was low at 12.1 ng/dl (normal 60 to 80 ng/dl), estradiol of 14.6 pg/ml (normal 100 pg/ml or higher), follicular stimulating hormone 53 mIU/mL (normal 1 to 4 mIU/mL) and progesterone was only 1.7 ng/ml (normal 15 to 25 mg/ml). Her fasting blood sugar was slightly elevated as well as her C-reactive protein, evidence of inflammation in her body. Her TSH was higher than it was two years earlier at 5.4 mIU/L, suggesting hypothyroidism. Danielle obviously had fibromyalgia and/or chronic fatigue syndrome. A sleep study was performed on the patient showing abnormal alpha waves, which is commonly seen in fibromyalgia.

All of her sex hormones were low, so Danielle was treated with bio-identical estradiol pellets, progesterone oral sublingual tablets and bio-identical testosterone pellets. She was given a prescription for oral *Armour Thyroid* 15 mg each morning before eating.

As with most who are on antidepressants, like Danielle, she wanted to find a way to stop her SSRIs, but was counseled to not discontinue these quickly. As she was on such high doses, stopping suddenly would cause withdrawal symptoms. She was using the diet medication to lose weight, but also to help her get going in the morning. She said she would try to cut back on this also.

A New Person

She returned in one month. All of her sex hormones were within the higher range of a normal woman in her twenties. Her thyroid studies were now improved. She had lost three pounds in the previous month and had no fever. Her blood pressure was 102/ 66.

Danielle was able to discontinue the morning dose of *Zoloft* and broke her *Ambien* in half to 5 mg at bedtime. She was now taking her *Fastin* diet medication only every other day. She now needed *Xanax* 1 mg only occasionally.

On exam she was still was not chipper – but far from the depressed patient she was thirty days before. She said,

I don't have hot flashes or night sweats now. None. Those stopped in seven days. My husband has moved back in and now we have a great relationship. I have my vaginal moisture back and my husband and I make love three or four times a week. He is thrilled to death. I spoke to my boss at General Dollar about coming back to work three days a week. He was happy about that.

Danielle wants to get off her antidepressants completely. *"They make me feel awful."* She will stop her *Fastin* in the next few days and wants to start walking outside a little. She rarely takes her *Lortab* now.

As a physician, I want you to know how encouraging Danielle's story is to me. I've heard stories like that hundreds of times now – and I hope your story will be equally as encouraging.

The Other Side of the Equation

Unfortunately, not everyone has heard about Bio-identical Hormone Replacement Therapy. They are being treated by "traditional" doctors – and seem caught in the same traps that Danielle had been in.

> ### Some of the most disheartening words that patients hear from their doctors are, "There's nothing wrong with you. All your tests are normal."

Some of the most disheartening words that patients hear from their doctors are, *"There's nothing wrong with you. All your tests are normal."* Or, *"There's nothing we can do to help you. You have a condition that has no treatment."*

If you hurt all over and feel worn out, you may have fibromyalgia or chronic fatigue syndrome. Both are serious chronic illnesses that have specific criteria for diagnosis, but may be overlooked because blood tests are typically normal. Also, the distinction between fibromyalgia and chronic fatigue syndrome is rather fuzzy, with up to seventy percent of patients meeting the diagnosis for both. [314]

The most common group to experience fibromyalgia is women in the perimenopausal and menopausal transition. *Bio-identical Hormone Replacement Therapy* stabilizes this group who too often have been placed on antidepressants to treat a hormone deficiency problem. It is extremely frustrating to be diagnosed with depression when dealing with issues like the inability to sleep, aching all over, and pain in muscles and tendons.

Patients with fibromyalgia do not usually have an antidepressant deficiency. They usually have a hormone deficiency.

Patients with fibromyalgia do not usually have an antidepressant deficiency. They usually have a hormone deficiency. A physician has to consider why this patient now has fibromyalgia or chronic fatigue syndrome when two years ago she was active, working, being a productive wife and mother. And now, two years later, she has difficulty even caring for herself, much less others. If a physician is observant and asks, *"What is different in your life now?"* she might reply, *"I am going through the change. Can you check my hormone levels?"*

On the Path to Wellness

Estradiol serves to regulate the influence serotonin has on the brain improving a patient's pain and mood perceptions. Estradiol can also increase dopamine, which is a chemical that transmits signals from one neuron to another that helps control the brain's reward and pleasure centers and emotional responses. Dopamine, under the influence of estradiol, enables us not only to see pleasure, but to take action to seek what makes us feel good and to enhance thinking about memorable experiences, joy, and excitement. Without estradiol, there are less pleasurable experiences.

Fibromyalgia can be difficult to diagnose. In fact, for many people it can take years. But getting that diagnosis can start a patient on the path to treatment. If the patient understands how fibromyalgia is diagnosed, she may be able to reach the point of being treated sooner. *This begins by finding a physician who is familiar with perimenopause and menopause and how Bio-identical Hormone Replacement Therapy is used to treat fibromyalgia and chronic fatigue syndrome.*

Fibromyalgia is a unique syndrome with pain in various areas of the body, but especially the muscles and tendons. Usually these painful areas are paired, the same pain will be in the same spot on the opposite side of the body also. *Along with fibromyalgia, chronic fatigue syndrome is often diagnosed as many of the symptoms are similar or identical.* Doctors may rule out rheumatoid arthritis, lupus, multiple sclerosis, Lyme disease, and mononucleosis. Often fibromyalgia and chronic fatigue syndrome are diagnoses of exclusion—after all other possibilities are excluded.

Fibromyalgia sometimes occurs with other chronic conditions such as irritable bowel syndrome, chronic fatigue syndrome, migraine headaches, restless leg syndrome, temporomandibular joint disease (TMJ) – pain in the jaws, and myofascial pain syndrome – trigger point pain areas similar to fibromyalgia. Many patients with chronic fatigue syndrome or fibromyalgia have depressive symptoms. More than fifty percent of patients with depression have had these symptoms for a lifetime. [315]

Fibromyalgia is an extraordinarily complex disorder, but a physician should always be mindful that this syndrome often begins with hormonal changes and may be treated very successfully with bio-identical hormones after a careful investigation of the patient's serum hormone levels. [316]

Routine lab tests do not detect the widespread pain of fibromyalgia. Instead, the diagnosis is made by a physical exam of pressure points that takes about five minutes. When light pressure is applied to the surface of the muscles throughout the body, patients with fibromyalgia find this painful, especially at the specific tender point areas used for diagnosis.

To meet the fibromyalgia criteria for diagnosis, patients must have:

1.   **Widespread pain in all four quadrants of the body for a minimum of three months**

2.   **At least 11 of the 18 specified tender points**

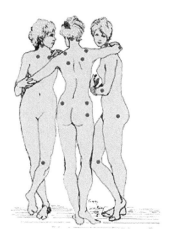

The eighteen sites used for the fibromyalgia diagnosis cluster around the neck, shoulder, chest, hip, knee, and elbow regions. The finger pressure that your doctor must apply to these areas during an exam is just enough to cause the nail bed to blanch or become white. [317]

The physical exam will very often show "tender points" or trigger points. There are eighteen potential tender points that may be pointed out by the patient, but often the patient doesn't even know she has a sore spot until the observant practitioner presses on it. The typical symmetrical tender points are at the inside margins of each shoulder blade, just below the clavicles, the elbows, the inside of the knees, the posterior superior pelvic bone, the insertion of the femur into the pelvis, at the base of the skull and the anterior neck.

When a physician presses on a trigger point (or tender point) of one without fibromyalgia the patient only feels pressure as opposed to pain sensed by the afflicted patient. There is no tenderness in the joint itself but near the joint. A diagnosis of fibromyalgia is strongly suspected if the patient has at least eleven of these trigger points identified. Often these trigger points are where muscles and tendons attach. The pain of fibromyalgia is often severe enough that one cannot work or has to take more time off than is acceptable. The real difficulty here is that, from the outside, the patient looks completely healthy. This leads to the impression that she is inventing her pain ... in other words, it is purely in her mind.
[318]

How BHRT Helps Fibromyalgia and Chronic Fatigue Syndrome

Fibromyalgia is ten times more common in women than men.

It is not surprising that estrogen plays an important role, as most of these women are perimenopausal or menopausal. If the physician checks the patient's blood, her estradiol level usually will be lower than healthy women of the same age. Many physicians using *Bio-identical Hormone Replacement Therapy* have found great success in treating patients who have fibromyalgia or chronic fatigue syndrome with BHRT.

Patients with fibromyalgia show alpha waves usually seen when one is awake or REM sleep (rapid eye movement seen in deep sleep). These alpha waves begin slipping into non-REM or deep sleep which progresses into stage three and four sleep, which is a necessary part of restorative sleep. [319]

This abnormality in sleep pattern is under the influence of serotonin, a neurotransmitter. Estradiol is particularly important in this process. [320]

Serotonin acting as a neurotransmitter (a chemical that transmits signals from one nerve cell to another) is essential for restful sleep. In patients with fibromyalgia there are changes in the diurnal rhythm of sleep—patterns of activity that follow day-night cycles, also known as circadian rhythm. [321] Sex hormones may be affected by these alterations in fibromyalgia as there is such a preponderance of women affected by this illness. [322]

The significance of hypothyroidism (low thyroid hormone) in identifying and treating fibromyalgia and chronic fatigue syndrome is pointed out in an article by Erika T. Schwartz, MD. Often the symptoms are similar to those listed above when referring to fibromyalgia—fatigue, weakness, weight gain, cold intolerance, muscle aches, headaches, decreased libido, depression, hair loss, and dry skin. The patient may have edema, dry skin, pale color of the skin, hair loss, loss of the outer one-third of the eyebrows, and cold hands and feet. The patient with hypothyroidism might also have high blood pressure, hardening of the arteries, high cholesterol, irregular menstrual periods, infertility, PMS, chronic fatigue syndrome, fibromyalgia, fibrocystic breasts, polycystic ovary syndrome, depression, diabetes, and insulin resistance. There is a twofold to threefold increase in the incidence of thyroid dysfunction as we age. [323]

When looking at the possibility of fibromyalgia knowing that the large majority of these patients are women in the perimenopausal stage of life, the consideration should be replacing lost sex hormones — estradiol, progesterone and testosterone. But often other unsuccessful options are chosen that do not address the root cause — hormone deficiency.

Some may doubt the benefits of estradiol in this age group of women, [324] but in the case of patients with fibromyalgia, the risk of using an antidepressant may not be worth the side effects. This reasoning seems to be so powerful when one remembers that very likely the loss of estradiol, progesterone and testosterone is the initial insult to the body causing fibromyalgia.

Declining testosterone for men and women can be an underlying cause of chronic fatigue syndrome.

For women, progesterone and especially estrogen might also be low. Chronic fatigue develops after a long period of stress and hyperactivity.

A physician must search for the etiology of the patient's fatigue including anemia, cancer, vitamin deficiency, thyroid deficiency, multiple sclerosis. A multitude of potentially incapacitating hormonal deficiencies are often found. Small doses of the hormones the patient lacks can bring a veritable resurrection. About fifty-to-ninety percent of cases of chronic fatigue will improve considerably with proper hormone treatment, even where no other treatment has worked.

Journal thoughts and questions:

_____

_____

_____

_____

_____

_____

_____

_____

_____

_____

_____

_____

_____

_____

_____

_____

_____

CHAPTER 30

High Blood Pressure

Understanding the Dangers of Hypertension

One of the major misconceptions about high blood pressure, or hypertension, is that it is not serious.

The higher the blood pressure the earlier in life that person will die.

You may hear someone say, *"My blood pressure is a little up. My doctor said I need to watch it."* It's a lot more serious than that! A general rule is: *the higher the blood pressure, the earlier in life that person will die.*

One very common cause of high blood pressure is a narrowing of the arteries. Testosterone in men and estradiol in women relax these muscles, widening the arteries. Balancing your hormones may very well lower your blood pressure.

It is very common for high blood pressure to occur as we age. How do we deal with that?

Treating High Blood Pressure

Many people take blood pressure medications to open up their blood vessels.

It is important to know that testosterone acts as a potent calcium channel blocker, and therefore lowers blood pressure. Men with low testosterone frequently develop angina, or chest pain due to poor circulation to the heart. These men may especially benefit from supplemental testosterone to dilate these narrow blood vessels. [325]

High blood pressure is intimately related to low testosterone, cardiovascular disease, how the inside lining of the arteries functions, type 2 diabetes, lipid profiles (cholesterol and triglycerides), inflammation inside the arteries, and constriction of the arteries. [326]

Hormones Are Important for Health and Survival

Men must have high levels of testosterone in order to be healthy. Low levels of testosterone have been found in men who die at an earlier age because of an increase in cardiovascular disease.[327] The same was found in the six-year *CHIANTI* study. [328]

Low levels of testosterone have been found in men who die at an earlier age because of an increase in cardiovascular disease.

When there is an imbalance between the blood vessels opening up and narrowing down, hypertension can result. [329] When the endothelium is functioning normally, there is a balance in coagulation. The blood does not clot too much or too little. The immune system fights infection. There is just the right amount of blood volume and electrolytes. And the blood pressure is normal.

Hormones influence every cell in the body, including the endothelium of blood vessels. Hormonal imbalance causes endothelial dysfunction. This is seen in diabetes, hypertension, high cholesterol, angina, cigarette smoking, heart disease, atherosclerosis, dementia, just to name a few. [330]

As many as one-half the women with chest pain have endothelial dysfunction—spasm of the arteries around the heart. [331]

The production of nitric oxide is stimulated by testosterone. Low production of nitric oxide is the hallmark of endothelial dysfunction resulting in high blood pressure. [332] The inability of arteries to dilate due to lack of nitric oxide (which may result from low testosterone) is the key dysfunction contributing to atherosclerosis, angina, blood clots, and poor circulation.

Hypertension can be improved significantly by exercise, smoking cessation, weight loss in overweight or obese persons, and improved diet. Big Pharma wants to treat hypertension and hypercholesterolemia with a long list of drugs such as statins, renin angiotensin system inhibitors, new third-generation β-blockers and 5-phosphodiesterase inhibitors. [333]

Drugs such as these may eventually be necessary in some patients, but using natural testosterone, progesterone and estradiol would be the first step to bringing back balance to the circulatory system. Testosterone has been shown to benefit the inside of arteries by providing for dilation therefore lowering blood pressure. [334] As testosterone dilates blood vessels, there is less pressure on the heart. Reducing pressure on the heart aided by testosterone prevents early mortality in men. [335]

> ### *Using natural testosterone, progesterone and estradiol would be the first step to bringing back balance to the circulatory system.*

The relationship between testosterone deficiency, hypertension, blood clots, endothelial dysfunction, diabetes, high cholesterol and vascular disease is very complex. ***However, we know that the sex hormones help to regulate and improve each of the above conditions.*** [336]

How early we die is intrinsically related to the level of testosterone one has as surely as a well-functioning car is related to the motor, transmission and tires. The cause of death may not be noted as "hypertension," but high blood pressure is related to the function of the heart. An enlarged heart occurs as pressure is placed on the heart because the arteries do not open well. Hardening of the arteries occurs because of high cholesterol and triglycerides. High lipids may occur because of a poor diet, obesity, or diabetes.

Diabetics are known to have low testosterone in high percentages.

Testosterone is inversely related to mortality—the lower the testosterone the higher the rate of death because of cardiovascular disease. The survival rate improves when testosterone is brought up to normal levels. [337] The same is true in dialysis patients. [338] And low testosterone is a cause of early mortality in patients with respiratory diseases. [339]

The lower the testosterone the higher the rate of death because of cardiovascular disease.

Multiple studies have demonstrated that testosterone dilates arteries thereby lowering blood pressure. Testosterone opens blood vessels by relaxing the smooth muscles in the arteries as a calcium channel blocker blood pressure medicine would. [340]

Testosterone opens the coronary arteries producing increased flow. [341] This action by testosterone alone is extremely valuable in patients who have angina. There are medicines that dilate these blood vessels, some of them acting for only seconds. Bio-identical testosterone, especially in pellet form, dilates coronary arteries for months.

Bio-identical testosterone, especially in pellet form, dilates coronary arteries for months.

As testosterone levels decline with age, men who have hypertension have lower testosterone levels. [342]

Men who are being treated for prostate cancer by artificially lowering their testosterone had an elevated blood pressure. [343]

The metabolic syndrome is a combination of hypertension, elevated lipids, central obesity, diabetes, and low HDL. All of these contribute to cardiovascular disease.

It is impossible to separate the disease of hypertension from each component—they are all interconnected. They are all interrelated as much as summer time is related to warm days, vacations and sunburns. When high blood pressure is present, a physician should look for type 2 diabetes. If hypertension and diabetes are present, most likely high cholesterol and triglycerides will be present. If hypertension or type 2 diabetes or high cholesterol or triglycerides is present, the physician should look for low testosterone in men or low estradiol in women.

These disease processes are very commonly seen in obesity. If a patient has any or all of the above pathologies, surely this patient must have his testosterone checked. Treating this patient with *Bio-identical Testosterone Replacement Therapy* may help with weight loss, an exercise program, lowering of cholesterol, elevating HDL cholesterol, lowering blood sugar and lowering blood pressure. [344]

Meet Roger

Roger was a diabetic at forty-six years old. Like many with diabetes, he was forty-two pounds over-weight and had high blood pressure. He was taking *Zestril* 20 mg twice a day and for his cholesterol *Crestor* 40 mg a day. He was taking metformin (*Glucophage*) 1000 mg twice a day and *Lantus Insulin* 30 units a day.

Roger explained,

I just wanted to feel better. I know I'm way overweight – but I don't even feel like exercising on by days off because I am so tired. My wife tries to help me eat right, but I cheat sometimes. Mentioning my wife, we haven't had real sex for three-and-a-half years. I just can't keep it hard, not even on Viagra, or Cialis, or Levitra. I've tried them all, even taking two at a time doesn't help. I'm worried about having a heart attack. My dad died at forty-nine from a massive heart attack and my mother died of a stroke when she was fifty-seven.

Roger was a great guy ... but he was miserable.

His blood pressure was still elevated at 142/90 even on *Zestril*. He weighed 204 pounds at 5'8". Even on insulin and metformin, his blood sugar non-fasting was 186 mg/dL. He had taken his 30 units of *Lantus Insulin* 3 hours before his blood was drawn. His cholesterol was 248 mg/dL (normal less than 200 mg/dL) and his triglycerides were 385 mg/dL (normal less than 150 mg/dL).

His blood work for sex hormones told the story.

His testosterone was 204 ng/dL. When he was twenty-five years old, he probably had a testosterone level of 900 to 1200 ng/dL. Having such a low testosterone would cause his fatigue, erectile dysfunction and weight gain, but to make things worse, his estradiol was 86 pg/ml (normal 35 pg/ml) causing his ED to be even less responsive to *Viagra*.

Roger was sincere. He knew he was in trouble. *"I've had four different doctors. But all they do is give me more pills and I never get any better."*

Roger's main problem was low testosterone leading to multiple symptoms. He was treated with 2000 mg of bio-identical testosterone. He was given a prescription for an aromatase inhibitor to be taken three times a week to lower his estradiol. Roger was to take *Revive* once a day for his erectile dysfunction, coenzyme Q10 100 mg twice a day and omega-3 fish oil twice a day to protect against further atherosclerosis. He was encouraged to begin an exercise program daily. Finally, a dietitian reviewed with him a low glycemic diet.

In one month, Roger's blood work showed this testosterone was 976 ng/dL and his estradiol was down to 44 pg/ml. He said,

I check my sugar two or three times a day. I haven't had to take any insulin in three weeks, and I take my metformin 1000 mg just a half a tablet a day. If I can lose a little more weight I believe I can get off of it completely. My doctor checked my cholesterol. He asked me what I've been doing. He couldn't believe it was down to 189. Oh, and my sex life, my wife says I'm like a twenty year old.

Roger was able to stop his metformin and Lantus over the course of the next year. He still took *Zestril*, but cut back to 5 mg a day to protect his kidneys. (Lisinopril being an ACE Inhibitor should be used in all diabetics to protect the kidneys.) He no longer needed *Crestor*, perhaps because he was walking five miles every day and his weight was down to 163 pounds.

Roger's experience is not unusual. Each discussion concerning diabetes, cholesterol, erectile dysfunction, hypertension, or the cardiovascular systems is replete with studies confirming what every doctor experiences daily when replacing diminished hormones with bio-identical hormones.

Four Studies: Conclusive Evidence

- A study by Dr. Marin [345] showed that testosterone therapy for obese men reduced diastolic blood pressure significantly.
- Another study [346] showed the same result in which both resting systolic and diastolic blood pressure were significantly lowered during treatment with testosterone being used for almost ten years.

- Another study [347] demonstrated significant lowering of diastolic blood pressure in men with hypertension and osteoporosis when their low testosterone was replaced.
- Another showed testosterone therapy in obese men lowered blood pressure. [348]

Men with low testosterone who have high blood pressure and cardiovascular disease can benefit significantly from testosterone replacement therapy.

These studies and hundreds more provide ample evidence that men with low testosterone who have high blood pressure and cardiovascular disease can benefit significantly from testosterone replacement therapy. [349]

Journal thoughts and questions:

_____

_____

_____

_____

_____

_____

_____

_____

_____

_____

_____

_____

_____

_____

_____

_____

_____

CHAPTER 31

Homocysteine

The Amino Acid You've Probably Never Heard Of

Homocysteine. Ever heard of it? Most people haven't.

It may sound innocuous, but it isn't. Everyone should know their blood levels of this amino acid. Homocysteine promotes vascular disease.

Elevated homocysteine in the blood is an indication that a person may be at high risk for a heart attack or stroke.

Elevated homocysteine in the blood is an indication that a person may be at high risk for a heart attack or stroke. Levels rise with menopause and andropause. ***Lifestyle changes and BHRT lower homocysteine levels.***

The Effects of High Homocysteine Levels

When a woman is young, her homocysteine levels are usually low. These levels rise in menopause, which promotes "free radicals." Free radicals are molecules that lack an electron. Therefore, this makes the molecule unstable. It will eventually "take" an electron from a normal cell, which causes the death of that cell. This process of oxidative stress is what causes vascular disease. This causes inflammation throughout the body.

Hormones promote proper protein function by stimulating DNA to produce proteins which are the building blocks for the human body.

Elevated homocysteine levels damage arteries throughout the body. If one has narrowing of an artery in the neck, for example, there is an excellent chance the same condition will be present in various other areas of the body. Atherosclerosis does not select just one certain artery to damage ... but causes havoc throughout the whole body. Internal inflammation from free radicals results from the body's inability to detoxify itself. This condition is seen especially as we age, menopause in women and andropause in men.

High homocysteine causes a decrease in the production of nitric oxide, which leads to high blood pressure, which may lead to cardiovascular disease. Also, a decreased production of nitric oxide may lead to erectile dysfunction. Therefore, erectile dysfunction may be an early indication of cardiovascular disease.

An elevation of cholesterol and triglycerides may be a consequence of elevated homocysteine, again a precursor to cardiovascular and peripheral vascular disease. Peripheral vascular disease may cause leg pain, restless leg syndrome, pain in the legs when walking, cramping, and burning feet when the feet are actually cold and blue.

High levels of homocysteine also contribute to strokes, heart attacks and angina.

Heart disease is the number-one killer of women in the United States. Nine million women each year die from heart disease worldwide. Over five hundred American women die daily from heart disease.

Women under age 55 continue to have an increased incidence of death in American. Homocysteine levels also affect the risk for developing cancer, diabetes, thyroid disorders, and Alzheimer's disease.

According to an article in the *New England Journal of Medicine* in 1997, our homocysteine level should be below 9 μmol/L with optimal levels as low as 6 μmol/L.

- Patients who have levels above 9 μmol/L *are more likely to die prematurely.*
- Homocysteine levels above 9 μmol/L with hypertension (high blood pressure) *are as much as twenty-five times more likely to suffer a heart attack or a stroke*.

How to Lower Homocysteine Levels

Lowering homocysteine may be aided by reversing harmful life-style choices. Among those are:

- **Stop smoking.** You know it's bad for you.
- **Lose weight.** I know you've tried. Get some help. Find a group to which you can be accountable for diet and weight loss.
- **Start exercising.** Even if it is just walking around the block, get started. Join a health club. Find something you enjoy doing – and stick with it.
- **Lower your blood pressure** – even with medication if necessary.
- **Lower your exposure to stress.** There are many helpful books on stress reduction, many from a faith-based perspective. Find some help there.
- **Supplement your diet with vitamins.** B12, B6 and folate are beneficial in lowering homocysteine.
- **Additionally, *Bio-identical Hormone Replacement Therapy* may lower homocysteine and cholesterol.** This is especially true when lost estradiol is replaced.

Women lose estradiol very rapidly with menopause and should be supplemented with a goal of serum blood levels of 60 pg/dL.

Men need some estradiol also. A good goal of estradiol in men is 25 to 35 pg/dL. The best way for men to have healthy levels of estradiol at an optimal level is not to have supplemental estradiol but to have bio-identical testosterone replacement as testosterone naturally converts to estradiol.

Think about the factors that cause heart disease. Among them are high blood pressure, high LDL cholesterol, and smoking. Lack of physical activity, obesity, and excessive alcohol consumption may be on the list. But few think about homocysteine as an independent factor for heart disease.

Eating healthy food, regular exercise, keeping your blood pressure below 130/90, vitamin supplementation, maintaining a healthy weight and balancing your hormones to a youthful state will decrease your chances of having a heart disease.

It is known that those with higher intake of folate, vitamin B12 and vitamin B6 have lower homocysteine levels. When comparing coronary artery blockages in 750 patients under sixty years old with 800 healthy patients, homocysteine was considered as great a risk as smoking or high cholesterol. [350] Healthy homocysteine values are between 5 μmol/L and up to 15 μmol/L and optimal levels are 6 μmol/L or less. Patients who take folate, vitamin B12 and vitamin B6 have a 66 percent less risk of heart disease. Dozens of studies have reported the advantage of maintaining low homocysteine. [351]

> ***Dozens of studies have reported the advantage of maintaining low homocysteine.***

Preventing the number-one cause of heart disease requires an overall healthy balance.

Journal thoughts and questions:

_____

_____

_____

_____

_____

_____

_____

_____

_____

_____

_____

_____

_____

_____

_____

_____

_____

_____

_____

CHAPTER 32

Hot Flushes And Night Sweats

Is It Hot In Here?

"Is it hot in here?" What husband of a menopausal wife has not heard those words? And what menopausal woman has not dreaded their onslaught?

Hot flashes (or flushes) can be very embarrassing. They come at unexpected times. Women entering into perimenopause may have a hot flash once a week – but later will have profuse sweating every hour.

Large-scale studies have been conducted in Europe where *Bio-identical Hormone Replacement Therapy* is the main type of hormone supplementation in menopausal women. These studies repeatedly demonstrated effective elimination of menopausal symptoms and a lack of long-term negative side effects with the use of bio-identical preparations. [352]

It is crucial to understand that even though the elimination of menopausal symptoms may be an important goal, there is something far more important: maintaining good health.

> ***Menopausal symptoms are an outward sign that something is wrong inside.***

Menopausal symptoms are an outward sign (breaking out in a sweat for no apparent reason) that something is wrong inside. This is a sign that your estradiol is dropping. *"So, what's the big deal? My doctor told me it would pass and I'd be fine."*

But you know it isn't!

What Does Estradiol Do for Me?

The big deal is that ***estradiol provides many essential benefits to help you maintain good health***:

- Estradiol prevents bone loss and bone breakdown
- Estradiol prevents weakness in muscles
- Estradiol prevents loss of muscle mass
- Pubic hair thins without estradiol
- Estradiol provides for body hair especially in the scalp—without estradiol women may have thinning of scalp hair
- Estradiol assures adequate size of the clitoris. The lips of the vagina may be thin and lax when estradiol is low
- Estradiol provides for vaginal moisture especially with sexual stimulation

- Estradiol helps prevent the breasts from being smaller
- Estradiol helps prevent sagging of the breasts
- Estradiol provides sensitivity of the nipples especially with sex
- Estradiol increases a positive mood helping to prevent a flat mood
- Estradiol aids in memory. Without estradiol, you may have trouble passing some simple memory tests
- Estradiol stimulates sexual interest
- Estradiol provides for sexual fantasies
- Estradiol aids in sensitivity to sexual stimulation of the breasts or clitoris
- Estradiol provides for more intense orgasms. You require less effort to obtain an orgasm. They last longer and come more often
- Estradiol assures a woman will be happy with her body
- Women with adequate estradiol will usually masturbate more often
- Estradiol provides for more desire for sex
- Estradiol stimulates growth of uterine lining
- Estradiol acts as a natural calcium blocker which opens up arteries
- Estradiol protects against macular degeneration
- Estradiol aids in the formation of serotonin which decreases depression, irritability, anxiety and pain sensitivity
- Estradiol maintains collagen in the skin
- Estradiol lowers lipoprotein A
- Estradiol lowers LDL
- Estradiol increases HDL
- Estradiol decreases plaque in the arteries
- Estradiol increases metabolic rate
- Estradiol decreases chances of colon cancer
- Estradiol increases insulin sensitivity
- Estradiol helps to maintain memory
- Estradiol helps to maintain water content in the skin—fewer wrinkles
- Estradiol reduces homocysteine
- Estradiol decreases risk for cataracts
- Estradiol decreases platelet stickiness
- Estradiol decreases total cholesterol
- Estradiol helps absorption of calcium, magnesium, zinc
- Estradiol improves sleep
- Estradiol improves endorphins
- Estradiol acts as an antioxidant
- Estradiol decreases triglycerides
- Estradiol increases growth hormones
- Estradiol helps maintain potassium
- Estradiol reduces palpitations
- Estradiol thickens the vaginal wall
- There is less urinary leakage when estradiol is present
- Estradiol helps prevent urinary tract infections

What about Progesterone?

And don't forget about progesterone:

- Progesterone protects a woman's breasts and maintains the endometrial lining of the universe
- Progesterone acts as an anti-inflammatory
- Progesterone in women inhibits breast tissue overgrowth
- Progesterone lowers cholesterol and increases HDL cholesterol
- Progesterone decreases coronary artery spasm
- Progesterone helps to maintain sex drive
- Progesterone acts as an antidepressant
- Progesterone thins blood, prevents blood clots
- Progesterone makes bones stronger
- Progesterone mobilizes fluid/decreases swelling
- Progesterone in women reduces breast tenderness
- Progesterone increases metabolism/weight loss
- Progesterone reduces craving for carbohydrates and sweets
- Progesterone increases the breakdown of fat into energy
- Progesterone decreases PMS symptoms and menstrual flow
- Progesterone acts as a natural diuretic
- Progesterone enhances the action of thyroid hormone
- Progesterone protects against fibrocystic breast disease
- Progesterone promotes proper cell oxygen levels
- Progesterone converts to other sex hormones
- Progesterone normalizes zinc and copper levels
- Progesterone helps maintain sex drive (libido)
- Progesterone helps keep blood levels normal
- Progesterone maintains the lining of the uterus

OK, What About Testosterone?

Testosterone has benefits for both men and women. It really is the male *and* female hormone:

- Testosterone stimulates an increase in the sex drive in men and women
- Testosterone helps prevent headaches
- Testosterone helps prevent hot flashes in men and women
- Testosterone helps to restore sexual dreams in men and women
- Testosterone stimulates sexual fantasies in men and women
- Testosterone stimulates sexual thoughts in men and women
- Testosterone increases clitoral sensitivity in women
- Testosterone increases the immune system in men and women
- Testosterone increases muscle strength in men and women
- Testosterone decreases the amount of fat and increases muscle development in men and women
- Testosterone improves bone development and decreases bone loss in men and women
- Testosterone improves the sense of well-being in men and women

- Testosterone causes hair growth on the scalp and body
- Testosterone reduces the incidence of erectile dysfunction in men
- There is lower incidence of diabetes with elevated testosterone
- Testosterone lowers total cholesterol as well as LDL (bad cholesterol)
- In men testosterone protects the heart from heart attacks
- Testosterone adds vigor and vitality in men and women
- Testosterone stimulates sexual responsiveness in men and women
- There is increased pleasure with sex secondary to testosterone in men and women
- Testosterone increases sexual arousal in men and women
- There is less depression when testosterone is elevated in men and women
- There is improved cognition and lower rate of dementia with testosterone in men and women
- There is less breast cancer in women who have adequate levels of testosterone
- Testosterone opens up arteries in men and women
- Testosterone dilates coronary arteries around the heart in men and women
- Testosterone lowers blood pressure in men
- Testosterone improves prostate health in men
- Testosterone lowers blood sugar levels
- Testosterone lowers the risk of blood clots
- Testosterone lowers healing time in men and women
- Testosterone increases ejaculation in men
- Testosterone lowers anxiety [353]
- As you read those three lists, it should be understood that this represents only a small portion of the essential beneficial effects of hormones in maintaining our health mentally, physically, and sexually.

The significance of this list is immense when the large majority of patients who see their doctor for symptoms of andropause or menopause are told, *"Here is an antidepressant. This will help you get through this phase of your life."* Or maybe they give you a sleeping pill or something for anxiety or for the symptoms of hormonal loss. Perhaps it is *Viagra*, a headache medicine, something to reduce the loss of bone mass, a cholesterol-lowering medicine, a pill for angina (chest pain), a blood pressure pill, or a weight-loss pill. Whatever it is, it is simply dealing with the symptoms and not the cause.

You may take these drugs and believe *"It's all going to be okay now. I can have an erection, my chest pain is better, and I've lost eight pounds on this diet pill."*

There's only one problem: the root causes of these symptoms are still there!

Those three long lists of the benefits of the three sex hormones – estradiol, progesterone, and testosterone - demonstrate that when sex hormones are lost, the effects are drastic. Life changes … and you don't get over it by taking an antidepressant or nerve pill.

Journal thoughts and questions:

_____

_____

_____

_____

_____

_____

_____

_____

_____

_____

_____

_____

_____

_____

_____

_____

_____

CHAPTER 33

Hypoactive Sexual Desire Disorder

Do You Understand What's Wrong?

Many women have a condition of which they are not aware. They know something is wrong. They just can't get their head around it.

Their husbands know something is missing, too. What is it?

Sexual desire.

Doctors come up with all kinds of explanations why a woman reaches a point where she has no desire for sex. A few short years ago, she was sexually active and received much pleasure from it. But now? All that traditional medicine can offer are the hollow words, *"It's just your age ... Every woman is like this ... You're depressed ... You're under a lot of stress."*

That message resonates death. It is not comforting. It does not give hope. And most of all, it's untrue.

So What's The Truth?

Hypoactive Sexual Desire Disorder (HSDD) is defined as *persistent deficiency or absence of sexual thoughts, fantasies, and/or receptivity to sexual activity that causes personal distress.* [354]

Women with HSDD experience large and statistically significant declines in health status, particularly in mental health, social functioning, vitality, and emotional role fulfillment. Women with HSDD experience greater health burdens, including more multiple medical conditions, and are nearly twice as likely to report fatigue, depression, memory problems, back pain, and lower quality of life. [355]

HSDD is highly prevalent and is a great burden on health and quality of life.

There is now compelling epidemiologic data indicating that hypoactive sexual desire disorder is highly prevalent and is a great burden on health and quality of life. Large-scale surveys have demonstrated that sexual satisfaction in women is associated with general well-being. [356]

Listen to Julie's Story

One forty-two-year-old, Julie, had seen her personal physician for pelvic pain over the past three years. She complained that she rejected sexual relationships. This very nice woman was crying as she told her story. She said, *"I used to like sex, but now I rarely even think about it. It is so uncomfortable that I actually have nausea when my husband comes near me. This has affected our relationship to the point we are considering divorce."*

At the examination, she was anxious and clearly depressed. Vaginal dryness was evident with thinning of the vaginal mucosa. The uterus was small and a fibroid was felt, but the ovaries could not be felt. The vaginal exam was moderately uncomfortable.

Her lab values demonstrated marked loss of hormones. Her thyroid was normal. All other blood work was within normal limits.

This hormonal picture clearly demonstrates the problem. She was menopausal – and had been for some time. This is not unusual. Eight percent of women will go through menopause before age forty, even those who have not had a hysterectomy. Up to twenty-five percent of women will have a hysterectomy in the United States. So, it is easy to see that there are a large number of women suffering from hormonal issues that go undiagnosed or ignored unless their hormones are checked.

Julie was treated with testosterone and estradiol *Pellet Bio-identical Hormone Replacement Therapy* and oral rapid dissolve progesterone sublingual. In one month her testosterone, estradiol, FSH and progesterone rebounded to normal levels.

At the office visit she was crying again ... but this time they were tears of joy as she said, *"I have no pain and sex is almost a daily experience now. I actually look forward to time together with my husband. Thank you. This saved my marriage."*

Treatment for Hypoactive Sexual Desire Disorder

There is currently no FDA-approved pharmacologic treatment for hypoactive sexual desire disorder.

There is currently no FDA-approved pharmacologic treatment for hypoactive sexual desire disorder. In other words, the FDA says they have no solution for this condition. Many clinicians, however, prescribe testosterone and monitor side effects. [357]

It is the androgens, including testosterone, androstenedione, DHEA, and DHEA-S, which are primarily responsible for subtler feelings, such as arousability, sexual desire, and fantasy, as well as frequency of sexual activity, orgasm, and satisfaction and pleasure from the sexual act. [358]

Dehydroepiandrosterone (DHEA) and DHEA-S, converted in peripheral tissues to testosterone, are the most abundant hormones in the body. These hormones decline steadily as a function of age, beginning as early as the late twenties in women. [359]

Why Is HSDD Under-Diagnosed?

If sexual problems are so common to women, why are they so often underdiagnosed and undertreated?

Some of the more significant reasons why physicians fail to recognize and treat hypoactive sexual desire disorder may be:

- Physicians and patients alike are not aware that such a condition exists and is so prevalent

- Care givers including nurse practitioners, physician assistants, counselors, and physicians are not adequately trained in sexual medicine
- Care givers have such a tight schedule there is not enough time to listen and understand the pain these women have
- The reimbursement is so low that a medical office cannot afford to spend the necessary time to diagnose and treat hypoactive sexual desire disorder
- If the FDA says there is no available treatment for this condition, caregivers are not motivated to spend time trying to diagnose a condition they cannot treat
- Many caregivers have difficulty communicating to patients about sexual disorders [360]

The major problem physicians have in diagnosing and treating hypoactive sexual desire disorder is that sexual problems are not a high priority. How these sexual issues significantly affect quality of life of women and their partners is not on the radar for most traditional doctors. Other medical problems take the forefront of a physician's time: such as headaches, blood pressure, diabetes, gastrointestinal issues, and chest pain.

When a patient complains of having headaches, the doctor has a tendency to concentrate only on the headaches. Skull X-rays and a CT scan may be ordered. Perhaps a cervical spine X-ray is ordered because the patient may have arthritis or muscle spasm in the neck causing headaches. Sinus X-rays may be necessary as sinus congestion may be the cause.

But what about hypoactive sexual desire disorder? Both the patient and the doctor may be reluctant to talk about sexual desire.

The medical community can no longer plead ignorance about the significance of hypoactive sexual desire disorder. There is a large collection of data demonstrating the extreme burden hypoactive sexual desire disorder has on patients. Until caregivers begin to recognize HSDD as a legitimate medical issue, women will go untreated and will suffer in their health, quality of life and in their relationships with their sexual partner and others.

Hypoactive sexual desire disorder may be secondary to serious mental and emotional issues or to physical problems with the pelvis and/or vagina causing pain with sexual intercourse. These potential issues must be addressed.

However, it is far more common that these are hormonal issues.

HSDD is more often seen in women in the perimenopausal and menopausal years.

The treatment algorithm used by mainstream medicine for women with hormonal issues is to give younger women some type of birth control. Doctors often have a particular favorite.

There is no blood test or any other type of measurement that would determine if this treatment is appropriate. The doctor cannot measure the patient's norethindrone plus ethinyl estradiol blood level. There is no norethindrone in a human's blood. Nor can ethinyl estradiol be found in a young woman.

So, how would a doctor decide if this is right for the patient? Or how would one determine if the dose needs to be adjusted up or down? Ovral is a combination of norgestrel (actually dextro-norgestrel and levo-norgestrel) plus ethinyl estradiol.

Now that you've got your antenna up and are aware of the dangers of some of these medicines, do these chemicals sound healthy to you? Probably not!

Remember the term "*progestin*"? Norgestrel and norethindrone are progestins. Medroxyprogesterone acetate (*Provera*) is a progestin. *Provera* was the progestin used in the drug *Prempro* which caused breast cancer, cardiovascular disease, stroke, and blood clots.

Do those side effects sound familiar? You would win at *Jeopardy* if you said, "*Alex, I'll take 'Side Effects found in the Women's Health Initiative Study' for two hundred, please.*"

Rebecca's Story

Rebecca is a fifty-two-year-old court recorder. She told the story of being on oral contraceptives for almost thirty years. Six months before, she had thrombophlebitis in her left leg.

My doctor put me on birth control pills to help regulate my periods and to keep me from having any more children. When my periods stopped six years ago she told me to keep taking the same Lo Ovral. I don't know why. But I did what she said. When I had the blood clots in my leg, she told me to stop the birth control pills.

She told me the reason I had the clots was because I sit a lot at work. She told me I could never again take hormones. I am confused. I have been reading about bio-identical hormones. They seem safe. If sitting at work caused the blood clots than why should I stop birth control pills? Could the pills have caused the blood clots instead of my work?

These are all great questions. It is so unfortunate that she was taking artificial hormones for so long.

Most physicians will have the patient get off of oral contraceptives for a month or so each year because of the side effects, especially the risk of blood clots. This patient did not stop her medication for over twenty-nine years per her physician's advice. Rebecca says,

I was placed on Coumadin after the blood clots. I am hoping I can stop this medicine soon. I have easy bruising and have read that this medicine can be dangerous causing bleeding.

Rebecca had read Suzanne Somers' book, *I'm Too Young for This* and Dr. Vliet's book, *The Savvy Woman's Guide to Testosterone*. She asked, "*If the birth control pills caused my blood clots, why can't I take bio-identical hormones?*"

Another great question.

There are very few if any studies that address this question directly. Traditional doctors are going to absolutely forbid Rebecca from ever using hormones of any kind again. But they do not have studies to support this position.

Can Rebecca take bio-identical hormones? It is known that women who have had breast cancer, even estrogen positive breast cell, can be treated with bio-identical hormones with no greater chance of recurrence. The question is the same as why bio-identical hormones are labeled with the same side effects as traditional synthetic drugs when they are not the same. What caused Rebecca's thrombophlebitis? It was oral contraceptives ... not bio-identical hormones.

The chemical structures of birth control pills are not the same as bio-identical hormones.

But the most important factor is that *Lo Ovral* birth control pill is a pill, taken by mouth. Any kind of hormone taken by mouth has to pass through the liver, which changes the chemical structure of the drug dramatically to a compound that can cause blood clots. Bio-identical hormones, either pellets placed under the skin or creams placed on the skin, do not have the problems with "first-pass metabolism" through the liver; thereby, avoiding the clotting problems seen with traditional synthetic hormones.

Oral *Premarin* causes a significant increase of 3.5 times in clotting factors in the blood leading to an increased incidence of thrombophlebitis (blood clots especially in the legs). [361] When bio-identical hormones are used on the skin or under the skin, this avoids first pass metabolism.

> **When bio-identical hormones are used on the skin or under the skin, this avoids first pass metabolism.**

Older women who are entering into perimenopause or menopause who have major symptoms of hormone deficiency, replacing lost hormones may be considered. The major problem is the findings of the *Women's Health Initiative Study* of 2002.

Before this study, doctors regularly prescribed the synthetic conjugated equine estrogen plus the synthetic progestin *Prempro* to women with hot flashes, night sweats, mood swings, anxiety and vaginal dryness. **After the results of the study were announced, the sales of this four-billion dollar drug dropped by about seventy-five percent.**

Unfortunately women are still being given these dangerous hormones. And women are still getting breast cancer and blood clots from these prescriptions with no relief from Hypoactive Sexual Desire Disorder. How sad!

Journal thoughts and questions:

_____

_____

_____

_____

_____

_____

_____

_____

_____

_____

_____

_____

_____

_____

_____

_____

_____

_____

CHAPTER 34

Elevated Lipoprotein A – Lp(A)

What Is It? What Does It Do?

Lipoprotein(a) is a small cholesterol particle. Its physiological function is still unknown. But what we do know is that Lipoprotein A has been identified as a risk factor for coronary heart disease and stroke.

Small cholesterol particles like Lp(a) more easily penetrate the walls of blood vessels causing vascular damage and inflammation leading to narrowing of the arteries and cardiovascular disease.

An example of a large cholesterol particle that is not harmful is HDL cholesterol, high density lipoprotein.

What Are the Dangers of an Elevated Lp(a)?

If your Lp(a) is elevated, there is a seventy percent greater chance of heart disease over the next ten years.

High Lp(a) in blood is a risk factor for coronary heart disease, cerebrovascular disease, atherosclerosis, thrombosis, and stroke. [362] The association between Lp(a) levels and stroke is not as strong as that between Lp(a) and cardiovascular disease. [363]

Lp(a) concentrations may be affected by disease states like kidney failure, but are only slightly affected by diet, exercise, and other environmental factors. Most commonly prescribed lipid-reducing drugs have little or no effect on Lp(a) concentration. Results using statin medications have been mixed in most trials, although a meta-analysis published in 2012 suggests that atorvastatin may be of benefit. [364]

Niacin (nicotinic acid) and aspirin are two relatively safe, easily available and inexpensive drugs known to significantly reduce the levels of Lp(a) in some individuals with high Lp(a).

If your Lipoprotein(a) is less than 14 mg/dL, you are relatively safe. You are borderline if your Lp(a) is between 14 mg/dL and 30 mg/dL. High risk is if your Lp(a) is as high as 31 mg/dL and no more than 50 mg/dL. If your Lp(a) is over 50 mg/dL, you are at a very high risk for coronary heart disease, cerebrovascular disease, atherosclerosis, thrombosis, and stroke. [365]

Elevated lipoprotein(a) causes clots to form. This is beneficial to prevent excess bleeding. But if lipoprotein (a) is too high, there is an increased chance of heart attacks and strokes. This condition is more prominent in menopause, andropause and in diabetics.

Lp(a) concentrations vary over one thousand-fold between individuals. If one person has only .2 mg/dL and another may have 200 mg/dL, who is more likely to have a dangerous elevation of Lipoprotein A?

Your heredity plays a role here. All populations can have a wide range of concentrations of Lp(a). However, people of African descent are more likely to have a two to three-fold elevated Lp(a) compared to Asian, Oceanic, or European populations.

What Can Be Done About an Elevated Lp(a)?

Lipoprotein (a) is genetically determined and inherited.

However, one can lower lipoprotein (a) with *Bio-identical Hormone Replacement Therapy,* especially estradiol. Also coenzyme Q-10 100 mg twice a day and Vitamin C up to 4 grams a day may be beneficial.

Journal thoughts and questions:

_____

_____

_____

_____

_____

_____

_____

_____

_____

_____

_____

_____

_____

_____

_____

_____

_____

_____

_____

CHAPTER 35

Migraine Headaches

Susan's Headaches

Susan was a beautiful, vivacious 5'5" thirty-year-old blond, upwardly mobile in her business of television media sales. Life was great. She had a fiancée whom she later married.

She came to my office suffering from severe migraine headaches:

Last week I read an article in a women's magazine about migraine headaches and how they might be related to hormones. I don't understand how hormones have anything to do with my severe headaches, but it make sense because my headaches start about the same time of my cycle each month.

They always start on one side of my head, usually the left side. They are so bad I have to go to bed and try to keep the light out of the room. It also has to be as quiet as possible. They usually last two days. I cannot work with my headaches and this is causing problems at work and with my fiancée.

Susan said she was having fairly regular periods, but they were very light. She was frequently anxious and maybe depressed.

She was extremely pleasant, but desperate to do something about her migraine headaches. *"I take Imitrex when I have a migraine, but it seems to take so long to work."*

Her blood work confirmed what her problem was. Her estradiol and progesterone were both low. Because she was only thirty years old and knowing that progesterone converts to estradiol, she was placed on oral sublingual progesterone rapid dissolve tablets. We saw Susan three months later.

"I haven't had a migraine since starting on progesterone, and I rarely have to take Xanax any more. I haven't missed a day of work. I wish more doctors knew how to treat migraine headaches with hormones."

What Is a Migraine?

Have you ever wondered why women have more migraine headaches than men?

Nearly thirty million people in the United States suffer from migraines.

You would be right if you said *"Hormones."*

Nearly thirty million people in the United States have migraines. And women have more than three times as many migraines as men.

Migraines are pulsating headaches, often on one side of the head. Physical activity may intensify the pain, but symptoms can vary from person to person and from one attack to the next.

"In patients who have migraines, we're going to treat all of their headaches as potential migraines," says Anne Calhoun, MD, partner and cofounder of the *Carolina Headache Institute*, in Chapel Hill, N.C. [366]

A migraine is a chronic neurological disease characterized by recurrent moderate to severe headaches often in association with a number of autonomic nervous system symptoms.

What Are the Symptoms?

The word migraine derives from the Greek, *"pain on one side of the head."*

Typically the headache affects one-half of the head. It is pulsating in nature, and lasts anywhere from two- to seventy-two hours. Associated symptoms may include nausea, vomiting, and sensitivity to light, sound, or smell. The pain is generally made worse by physical activity. [367]

Up to one-third of people with migraine headaches perceive an *"aura."* The most common auras are visual, such as flickering lights, spots or lines. Auras typically last between five minutes and an hour and often signal that the headache will soon occur. [368] Occasionally an aura can occur with little or no headache following it.

Bright lights and loud noises can trigger a migraine or intensify the pain

Other symptoms can include:
- Depression, irritability, or excitement. Mood changes can be a sign of migraines
- Waking up tired or having trouble falling asleep are common problems for people who suffer from migraines
- Some people with migraines have sinus symptoms: a stuffy nose, clear nasal drainage, or tearing
- Pulsating, throbbing pain on one side of the head
- Migraine sufferers often experience pain right behind one of their eyes
- Neck pain can often signal the early stage of an on-coming migraine
- Frequent urination – if you have to go a lot, it can mean a migraine is coming
- Numbness or tingling – symptoms of sensory aura
- Nausea or vomiting. 73% of migraine sufferers experience nausea and 29% have vomiting [369]
- The migraine sufferer tends to seek refuge in a dark, quiet place. Bright lights and loud noises can trigger a migraine or intensify the pain
- Vertigo or double vision
- After the migraine passes, a person may feel like his or her body has been pummeled. Migraine patients commonly experienced symptoms such as fatigue, trouble concentrating, weakness, dizziness, lightheadedness, and loss of energy during the post-migraine period

What Causes Migraines?

Migraine headaches are frequently disabling, with the largest majority causing disability in women.

A change in progesterone and/or estradiol may cause a migraine. It is common for this to occur after mid-cycle when estradiol begins to drop and progesterone is still elevated. When estradiol declines the arteries may constrict causing the tiny muscles in the arterial walls to become tense. Declining estradiol may cause a decreased flow of blood to the brain due to vasoconstriction. This is what causes the aura of migraine headaches. This same drop in estradiol in the brain causes a decrease in serotonin which causes more vasoconstriction even to the point of possibly causing a stroke.

Migraines are believed to be due to a mixture of environmental and genetic factors. [370]

The exact mechanisms of migraine are not known. It is, however, believed to be a neurovascular disorder. [371] The primary theory is related to increased excitability of the cerebral cortex and abnormal control of pain neurons in the trigeminal nucleus of the brainstem. [372]

The risk of migraines usually decreases during pregnancy.

Is There Help?

Bio-identical hormone replacement with bio-identical estradiol and progesterone may be beneficial to those suffering migraine headaches secondary to declines in these hormones. You may try Coenzyme Q-10 100mg twice a day or up to two capsules twice a day. Many have found some relief by adding magnesium 800 mg twice or three times a day. The side effect of magnesium is diarrhea. Remember to have some milk of magnesium on hand.

Journal thoughts and questions:

_____

_____

_____

_____

_____

_____

_____

_____

_____

_____

_____

_____

_____

_____

_____

_____

_____

_____

_____

CHAPTER 36

Muscle Mass Loss

One of the "Inevitabilities" of Aging

Our muscles grow every day from the time we are born to our mid-thirties. But at some point in our thirties, we begin to lose muscle mass and function, a condition known as sarcopenia.

People who are physically inactive can lose as much as three to five percent of their muscle mass per decade after age thirty.

Even people who are physically active will lose muscle mass as they age. However, those who are relatively inactive can lose as much as three to five percent of their muscle mass per decade after they turn thirty.

It is a factor in the occurrence of frailty and the likelihood of falls and fractures in older adults.

Sarcopenia accelerates around age seventy-five, although it may happen earlier or later. Those who begin losing testosterone more rapidly will experience muscle loss much earlier – perhaps starting in their fifties.

Symptoms of Muscle Mass Loss

In women, an accelerated loss of muscle mass and strength occurs at an earlier age than in men, but life expectancy is higher in women compared with men. Thus, as women tend to live longer, they are more susceptible to age-related health problems and in particular to declines in muscle mass when compared with men. [373]

Men will begin to notice they do not have the muscle definition they once had. They will see a loss of strength ... even to the point where they are asking others to do what they once were able to do easily.

The rate of loss is about ten ounces of muscle per year after age thirty. This is equivalent to a nice sirloin steak per year. This loss of muscle mass almost always converts into fat being deposited around the abdomen. This kind of fat is especially dangerous as these men are more likely to have coronary artery disease.

Causes of Muscle Mass Loss

Although muscle mass loss is most frequently seen in people who live a sedentary lifestyle, it also occurs in people who are very physically active. Inevitably, it affects almost everyone.

The following factors play a role in sarcopenia:

- Loss of production of testosterone by the testicles or ovaries
- Our nerve cells become less and less responsive in sending signals to the brain for the muscles to initiate movement
- A decrease in the concentrations of some hormones, including growth hormone, testosterone, and insulin-like growth factor
- A decrease in the body's ability to synthesize protein
- Inadequate intake of calories and/or protein to sustain muscle mass [374]

Treatments for Muscle Mass Loss

- **The primary treatment for sarcopenia is exercise.**

Strength training with weights and resistance bands has been shown to be useful for both the prevention and treatment of muscle mass loss. Resistance training has been reported to positively influence the neuromuscular system, hormone concentrations, and protein synthesis rate. Research has shown that a program of progressive resistance training exercises can increase protein synthesis rates in older adults in as little as two weeks.

- **Bio-identical Hormone Replacement Therapy**.

One of the most significant factors to personal injury in those over sixty is weakness due to loss of muscle strength.

The most important and essential treatment for loss of muscle mass is replacing diminishing levels of testosterone.

Men should maintain the same healthy levels of testosterone as they had when they were younger.

Women should have testosterone levels of 80 pg/dL.

When a woman's production of hormones is diminished at menopause, hormone replacement therapy has been shown to increase lean body mass, reduce abdominal fat short-term, and prevent bone loss.

Some may point to theoretical objections to the use of testosterone, saying *we don't need as much testosterone as we had when we were young.* But these objections are without evidence. The evidence points to the many health benefits of maintaining healthy levels of testosterone.

- Other treatments for sarcopenia include testosterone supplementation, growth hormone supplementation, and medication for treatment of metabolic syndrome (insulin-resistance, obesity, hypertension, etc.).

If found useful, all of these would complement the effects of resistance exercise.

Journal thoughts and questions:

_____

_____

_____

_____

_____

_____

_____

_____

_____

_____

_____

_____

_____

_____

_____

_____

_____

_____

_____

_____

CHAPTER 37

Osteoporosis

The Porous Bone Disease

***Women who are postmenopausal are the most prone people to
have osteoporosis.***

Osteoporosis is a disease that weakens bones over time. It causes them to become weak and brittle. Many times, they become so brittle that a fall or even mild stresses like bending over or coughing can cause a bone fracture. If you suffer from osteoporosis, you have an increased chance of breaking a bone. Women who are postmenopausal are the most prone people to have osteoporosis.

One disease common with aging is arthritis. Along with arthritic changes associated with aging is osteoporosis – deterioration of the bones. Most studies show that as muscle mass decreases with loss of testosterone so goes bone loss (osteoporosis). [375] Bone density in the spine is decreased in men with low testosterone. [376] Men with low testosterone are more likely to sustain fractures of the hip than men with normal sex hormones. [377]

All of us have cells that remove old bone and other cells that rebuild new bone. It is through this process that our bones are kept strong.

Postmenopausal osteoporosis occurs when bone-removing cells are more active than the ones that build new bone cells. The result is thinner, weaker bones that can break more easily. This process is accelerated after menopause. Within five to seven years after menopause, women can lose up to twenty percent of their bone mass, which increases the risk for fracture.

Bones are constantly growing, changing, developing, throughout our lives, but they are also dissolving and rebuilding. Osteoclasts are cells in the bone that are constantly searching for old bone cells. When old cells are found, osteoclasts dissolve these. This is called resorption—tearing down old bone.

Calcium, magnesium, vitamin D, strontium and other minerals in these old bone cells that are dissolved are then released back into the circulation. Each year about twenty-five percent of bone is torn down, dismantled and replaced.

Often a fracture may occur without a fall. Just taking a step or twisting and turning when walking can cause a hip bone to fracture. Most osteoporosis-related fractures occur in the hip, spine, and wrist. A fracture due to postmenopausal osteoporosis may never heal, leaving a patient in a wheel chair for the rest of their life.

Hear From Heather

Heather was fifty years old when she had a bone mass densitometry showing that she already had osteoporosis.

My mother was in a wheelchair after a stroke when she was sixty-six years old. She had begun to be humped over before that. When the doctor told me I had osteoporosis the first thought was that I did not want to be like Mother.

The most significant finding at her exam was that Heather weighed ninety-eight pounds. She had the typical *"Nancy Reagan body type,"* which is frequently seen in women who have early osteoporosis. She was somewhat anxious in appearance, but very resistant to take any drugs. The doctor who discovered the osteoporosis had written a prescription for *Fosamax*, but she never filled it.

Heather's sex hormones were extremely low. She had gone through menopause five years earlier, causing a lot of anxiety.

Heather was treated with small doses of pellets of testosterone and estradiol just under the skin. She was given a prescription for a rapid dissolve tablet of progesterone to be placed under the tongue at bedtime.

Heather did very well with her therapy with a return to normal of her sex hormones. Eighteen months from her previous BMD, she returned to the same doctor and had the same exam performed. This time her bone scan showed *"normal bone scan."* Heather was elated. Today, nine years later, she still has maintained healthy bones with no back pain or fractures. Her greatest fear? *"I just didn't want to end up in a wheelchair like my mother."*

"I just didn't want to end up in a wheelchair like my mother."

The Effects of Osteoporosis

Osteoporosis is a very debilitating condition. In the formative years, bones grow rapidly to their maximum density. By age forty, men and women begin losing bone at a rate of .5 percent per year. By age sixty and beyond, both men and women will begin losing bone more rapidly. After menopause the rate of bone loss will increase by ten times. Osteoporosis leads to falls which may cause a hip fracture. The patient may pass the next few months immobile.

Millions of women suffer from symptoms they do not associate with bone loss. Chronic back pain may very well be due to small fractures in the vertebra of the spine. Over years these tiny crush fractures cause the typical hunched back of old age. Especially seen in women is a "dowager's hump." This makes her body form the shape of a question mark – perpetually hunched over.

Osteoporosis occurs after menopause when bones have used up their storehouse of calcium and other minerals. This causes bones to become fragile. Couple this with an elderly person who has weak muscles, poor vision, poor balance, and on drugs that cause drowsiness, this adds up to the painful disaster of a fall causing a fractured hip, spine, wrist, or rib.

The most important hormones that cause bones to grow in women and men are human growth hormones, testosterone, progesterone and DHEA.

Fifty percent of women over fifty years old have the potential of a debilitating fracture. Twenty-five percent of men over fifty are in the same potential danger. By age seventy, one-half of all women will suffer a bone fracture. Twenty-four million Americans have osteoporosis. Twenty-seven million women have osteopenia. The most important hormones that cause bones to grow in women and men are human growth hormones, testosterone, progesterone and DHEA.

Tearing Down / Building Up

At the same time osteoclasts are dissolving old bone cells, osteoblasts are working just as hard to build new bone using calcium phosphate from the old dissolved bone cells to patch up the holes left by the osteoclasts. This process is like a drywall worker patching cracks or holes in a wall. The osteoblasts use the same calcium and other minerals from the circulation to build new bone.

However, as we age, the *tearing down* outpaces the *rebuilding* of the bones, causing more destruction than building. Eventually bones are more fragile and weak. Not only are fractures more likely but healing is very slow and, too frequently, the fracture never heals.

By age thirty-five, most men and women will begin to see a decline in bone mass — the osteoclasts begin outdoing the osteoblasts.

Reversing the Trend: Building New Bone

Bone loss can be stopped with Bio-identical Hormone Replacement Therapy.

Here is a very important point: **Bone loss can be stopped with Bio-identical Hormone Replacement Therapy (BHRT).**

If you have already begun to lose bone mass, this can be reversed with BHRT. When you were in your mid-twenties, you had strong bones because you had high levels of testosterone, progesterone and estradiol. There may be some things that are inevitable as we age: some of our hair turns grey, and some of it falls out. But losing bone mass does not need to be part of aging.

Women will benefit from the supplementation of estradiol as well as testosterone. Estradiol will slow down the rate of bone resorption or destruction. But the process of osteoporosis will continue unless there is stimulation of the osteoblasts with progesterone and testosterone. *To use only estradiol means that one has slowed down the rate of bone loss, but to build new bone requires stimulation of osteoblast — that requires testosterone and progesterone.* [378]

Women who are treated with estradiol 50 mg pellets will have an increase in bone mineral density. However, if a postmenopausal woman is treated with both estradiol 50 mg subcutaneous pellet plus testosterone 50 mg pellet, there will be *even greater increases* in bone density in the hip, lumbar spine and total body. [379]

In a two-year study, thirty-four postmenopausal women were treated with either estradiol implants 50 mg alone or estradiol 50 mg plus testosterone 50 mg, given every three months.

The results? Total body, lumbar vertebrae and hip area increased significantly in both treatment groups. Bone mineral density increased more rapidly in the testosterone treated group. All these women had a significant improvement in sexual parameters; however, the women treated with both estradiol and testosterone reported a greater improvement in sexual activity, satisfaction, pleasure, orgasm and relevancy.

This clearly demonstrates that Bio-identical Testosterone Pellet Hormone Replacement Therapy is extremely helpful for postmenopausal women with diminished estradiol and testosterone. [380]

A 2007 study in Menopause involved women having their bone mineral density checked who were postmenopausal. One group received estradiol plus progesterone. Another group received estradiol plus progesterone plus testosterone. After twelve months, the bone mineral density showed improvement in both groups in spinal bones. But in the hip BMD showed significant increases in women who used testosterone as well as estradiol and progesterone. [381]

The risk of such fractures could be substantially reduced with even low-dose Bio-identical Estradiol Replacement Therapy. The complete absence of estradiol substantially increases the breakdown of bone (resorption) by osteoclasts. [382] Osteoclasts "eat up" or absorb old bone cells. That is a good thing. Osteoblasts stimulate bone cells that build new bone. [383] Osteocytes' purpose is to resorb damaged bone cells imposed by weight bearing. [384]

With the absence of sufficient estradiol osteoblasts, the new bone builders, cannot keep up with the osteoclasts, the cells that absorb old bone. Thereby, osteoporosis develops resulting in a hunched back, Dowager's Hump, and hip fractures seen in the elderly. [385] Thus, low but measurable serum estradiol concentrations may decrease the risk of fracture by decreasing bone resorption or maintaining the viability of osteocytes. A total hysterectomy removes the estradiol, testosterone and progesterone producing ovaries. The risks of a hip fracture have just gone up seven-fold. [386]

This is why women should begin Bio-identical Hormone Replacement Therapy by age thirty-five.

Progesterone is essential for osteoblasts to lay down new bone. Progesterone begins to decline in most women by their mid-thirties. So, the process of osteoporosis begins forty years before she is eventually diagnosed with a hip fracture or osteoporosis. ***This is why women should begin Bio-identical Hormone Replacement Therapy by age thirty-five.***

Estrogen prevents osteoclasts from unrestrained resorption of bone. Progesterone provides for new bone to be deposited by osteoblasts. Without adequate progesterone to counter the accelerated bone resorption secondary to loss of estradiol causes a dramatic loss of our skeletal framework. This is made even worse when there is inadequate nutrition.

Men are more likely to suffer an osteoporotic-related fracture than to have prostate cancer. Men suffer thirty percent of all the hip fractures worldwide. Men over seventy-five years old who experience a hip fracture have a mortality rate of thirty percent as opposed to nine percent for women. [387]

Women who have knee and hip replacement due to osteoarthritis have different patterns of sex hormone concentrations compared with the general population. In a study reported in *Endocrinology Update*, 2,600 middle-aged women with a ten-year follow-up found that higher estradiol concentrations reduced the risk of total knee replacement by about one third. Other studies have demonstrated that women using long-term postmenopausal estrogen therapy had greater knee cartilage volume than non-users. A study in Canada of 10,000 women ages fifty and above demonstrated that sixteen percent of these women had osteoporosis in the spine or hip. [388] Every ten years after menopause the risk of a hip fracture doubles. [389]

There are 300,000 hip fractures in the United States each year. Each year 500,000 Americans are hospitalized with a fracture secondary to osteoporosis. The risk is actually greater for a broken hip than cancer of the cervix, uterus and breast combined. [390]

The cruel fact is that even though there is mortality with cancer of the cervix, uterus and breast, if it is discovered early, these can be cured. ***But often a woman has no clue she has osteoporosis until the fracture occurs.*** At times the fracture occurs when the patient takes a step or turns and she then falls as a result of the broken hip. Too often (one in five) these women will end up in a nursing home for an extended stay, and some will never leave the rest of their life. One in four of these will die within one year as a result of this osteoporotic fracture. [391] Back pain may be the first sign of a fracture of the vertebra of the spine, a dramatic loss of height or development of "dowager's hump."

A study of elderly men provided evidence that an evaluation of serum testosterone was the most accurate indicator of a deficiency of calcium in bones. [392] Men with low estradiol levels are at an increased risk for future hip fracture. Men with both low estradiol and low testosterone levels seem to be at greatest risk for hip fracture. [393]

Bone density improves with *Bio-identical Hormone Replacement Therapy*. One sees increases in spinal bone density that is equivalent to men that are much younger with normal testosterone levels. [394] Most men treated with bio-identical testosterone achieve bone density above the fracture threshold. [395]

Testosterone replacement in men with low testosterone improves support strength and density to bones and the spine. [396]

Using Premarin and Other Synthetic Drugs

Traditional medicine has promoted drugs to prevent osteoclasts from removing old bone cells by the use of *Premarin*. And *Premarin* can provide a small delay of osteoporosis despite the dramatic cardiovascular and cancer-causing side effects. [397]

The problem in using the *Premarin* is that the effectiveness is dose- and duration-dependent. [398] This means that to prevent osteoporosis, the dose must be sufficiently high to prevent osteoclast from running wild tearing down bone and the length of time the patient needs to be on the medication is lifetime. [399] Stopping estrogen means loss of bone begins again and the benefit will disappear to the point that after five years there is no residual protection from fractures. [400]

As the treatment to prevent and restore bone mineral density is a life-long quest beginning at age thirty-five, the options are limited to treatments for a lifetime that do not have such deadly consequences as *Premarin* and *Provera*. No doctor is going to keep a patient on *Premarin* and *Provera* from age thirty-five until they are eighty-five years old to prevent osteoporosis. But bio-identical hormones can be used for far more symptoms than just hot flashes and osteoporosis.

The news story from the *PEPI Study* is that the safer alternative to *Provera* is natural progesterone, but traditional medicine suggests that estrogen, even *Premarin*, protects against osteoporosis ignoring the benefits of natural progesterone. It is difficult to imagine that a physician is going to jump on this and start writing prescriptions for *Premarin* and *Provera* to be taken for the next forty years.

One side effect of progesterone is it can cause drowsiness. This is why it is recommended to be taken at bedtime. Synthetic Provera (MPA) on the other hand can cause breast tenderness, skin irritations, swelling, breakthrough bleeding and depression. Of course, *Provera* is associated with breast cancer, heart attacks, birth defects [401] and heart disease. [402]

The above information discusses the advantages of natural progesterone in the prevention and treatment of osteoporosis. However, the treatment is not just one hormone but includes testosterone, progesterone, estradiol, vitamin C, vitamin D, calcium, strontium, magnesium, DHEA, zinc, copper, vitamin K2, manganese, molybdenum, boron, silicon, a proper diet with leafy green vegetables, and exercise. From this list testosterone, progesterone, estradiol, calcium and strontium are essential for one at risk for osteoporosis.

Two groups of drugs designed to prevent osteoporosis are bisphosphonates and SERMs. The list of biphosphonates includes: *Fosamax, Actonel, Didronel, Boniva,* and *Reclast.* [403] These drugs act by inhibiting osteoclast from resorbing old bone cells. This slows down the rate of loss of bone. These medications do nothing to aid osteoblasts to build new bone. Again, this is an effort by Big Pharma to outdo nature.

We have learned that estradiol delays the overactivity of osteoclasts to break down bone and progesterone and testosterone build new bone by adding osteoblastic function. If nature has kept one healthy from puberty through the formative years with testosterone, progesterone and estradiol, why turn to an artificial drug that tries to mimic estrogen?

Bisphosphonates have significant side effects including delaying of healing of fractures, destruction of the upper digestive system, Jaw Death [404] and a doubling of the chances of developing atrial fibrillation. [405]

So, in summary, you have a choice to use the natural hormones that have protected your bones up until your hormone level dropped. These natural hormones, estradiol, testosterone and progesterone, kept your bone building cells (osteoblasts) healthy and laying down new bone. The medicines pushed by Big Pharma do not do this. They slow down the destruction of bones, osteoporosis, but do nothing to build new bones. It is up to natural bio-identical hormone replacement to build new bone cells and take away old bone cells just as was happening naturally up until you slowed down and then stopped producing your own natural hormones.

Journal thoughts and questions:

_____

_____

_____

_____

_____

_____

_____

_____

_____

_____

_____

_____

_____

_____

_____

_____

_____

_____

_____

_____

CHAPTER 38

Prostate Issues

What Does the Prostate Gland Do?

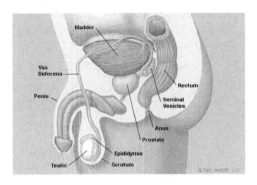

The prostate is a walnut-sized gland located between the bladder and the penis. [406] The prostate is just in front of the rectum. The urethra runs through the center of the prostate, from the bladder to the penis, letting urine flow out of the body.

The gland is not essential for life, but it is necessary for reproduction. The gland secretes a slightly alkaline fluid that supports the sperm. The prostate also prevents the flow of urine during ejaculation.

Testosterone is necessary for the prostate to function properly. Testosterone is produced in the testicles and the adrenal glands.

Problems with the Prostate

Inflammation of the prostate is called *prostatitis*. A bacterial infection may cause acute or chronic prostatitis and is treated with antibiotics.

Older men may suffer from an enlarged prostate.

Older men may suffer from an enlarged prostate. The prostate may enlarge to the point where urination becomes difficult. Symptoms include the need to urinate often (frequency), or taking a while to start the flow of urine (hesitancy). Urgency is the sudden strong sense of needing to urinate. Men may even lose their urine before reaching the bathroom. An enlarged prostate often will cause dribbling at the end of urination causing very prolonged time to finish urinating. Benign prostatic hypertrophy may cause decreased force and volume of ejaculation. The prostate may enlarge to the point the urethra is closed off, making urination difficult and painful and, in extreme cases, completely impossible.

Treatment for BPH may include medication, a minimally invasive surgical procedure or, in extreme cases, surgery that removes the prostate.

Prostate cancer is especially common in older men in developed countries. It is a significant cause of death for elderly men, with some estimates as high as three percent. Because prostate cancer is extremely slow growing in some men, *The American Cancer Society's* position regarding early detection is:

"Research has not yet proven that the potential benefits of testing outweigh the harms of testing and treatment ... that men should not be tested without learning about ... the risks and possible benefits of testing and treatment."

Black men especially, and men of any race who have a father or brother who has acquired prostate cancer before age sixty-five, may need closer surveillance. [407]

This is a very controversial position. The idea is that if a man has tests performed to see if he has prostate cancer, and the results are positive, then he has to make a decision. Does he want treatment or not? Many physicians believe that a man is more likely to die many years later of another cause, not from the prostate cancer.

In other words, he will die *with* prostate cancer, not *from* prostate cancer.

If checks are performed, they can be in the form of a physical rectal exam, measurement of prostate specific antigen level in the blood, or checking for the presence of the protein Engrailed-2 in the urine.

If a man is being treated for prostate cancer, his physician is going to do everything he can to take away testosterone by giving a medication to block testosterone or to remove the testicles. This is very unfortunate, since these men with no health-giving natural testosterone are far more likely to die from not having sufficient testosterone than to die from the prostate cancer.

Many doctors who are very familiar with the use of testosterone will recommend supplemental bio-identical testosterone while going through chemotherapy, radiation therapy or prostatectomy. Men may very well be able to fight and win the disease of prostate cancer if they have the health advantages provided by natural testosterone.

Some physicians still believe that benign prostatic hypertrophy may be made worse with testosterone therapy. Clearly men who have high estrogen levels have greater risk of having an enlarged prostate. Most of these men also have low testosterone. This has been borne out in studies in Japan and in the United States. [408]

The Rectal Exam

On a rectal exam the doctor will be able feel if the prostate is soft (normal) or hard (possibly a sign of an enlarged prostate or prostate cancer).

When a man has a rectal exam, the doctor can touch the back side of the prostate. On a rectal exam the doctor will be able feel if the prostate is soft (normal) or hard (possibly a sign of an enlarged prostate or prostate cancer). The size of the prostate can be estimated with a rectal exam. A normal size prostate is about as large as a walnut, but an enlarged prostate may be the size of a lemon. A more accurate measurement of the size of the prostate is done with an ultrasound probe.

If the patient has prostatitis, an infection of the gland, the rectal exam will cause pain when the physician touches the prostate. The urethra, the tube that carries urine from the bladder, goes through the middle of the prostate. For such a small gland, it surely can cause big problems.

Men over fifty should have a yearly digital rectal and probably a prostate specific antigen test. The PSA test is a blood test. One study found a fifteen-percent-higher-death rate, when compared to men who did not have annual PSA tests performed, possibly due to too many surgeries being done on older men who would not have died from prostate cancer anyway. [409]

Prostate Cancer

Prostate cancer occurrence is increasing in the United States possibly due to men living longer. It is the most common malignancy in American men. One-in-three men will develop prostate cancer, but most will not die of it because it is so slow growing. Less than ten percent of men with prostate cancer will die from it within ten years.

The cause of prostate cancer is not known. For more than sixty years it was thought that testosterone caused it. However, recent research has demonstrated this to be false. If testosterone caused prostate cancer, young men should develop prostate cancer, not old men with very low levels of testosterone.

The risk factors for prostate cancer include:

- Advancing age (the older we are, the greater the chance of developing prostate cancer)
- Smoking
- A genetic tendency (inheritance)
- Hormonal influences (too much estrogen)
- Environmental factors such as toxins, chemicals, and industrial products

There are conflicting recommendations about how to treat prostate cancer—aggressive therapy such as surgery, chemotherapy, and radiation is the best way to go or watch and wait.

I've Heard of BPH – What Is It?

BPH causes symptoms to occur when the gland enlarges to the point that the patient has difficulty urinating.

Benign Prostatic Hypertrophy (BPH) is a condition of the prostate in which the prostate gland has enlarged. The prostate gland normally begins to increase in size at about thirty years of age. By age fifty, about fifty percent of men will have symptoms of BPH, and eighty percent have it by age eighty. BPH causes symptoms to occur when the gland enlarges to the point that the patient has difficulty urinating.

Those symptoms can be:

- Urinary frequency (having to go to the bathroom more often)

- Urgency (the feeling of strong and sudden urge to get to the bathroom quickly)
  - Incontinence (not being able to control the urge)
  - Having to get up at night to urinate
  - Weak flow of urine
  - Difficulty starting the stream (hesitancy)
  - Stopping and starting of the stream during urination (intermittency)
  - Leakage (wetting on oneself)
  - Dribbling at the end of urination
  - Inability to urinate (urinary retention)
  - Incomplete emptying of the bladder
  - Pain with urination or bloody urine—infection [410]

BPH is more likely to develop if the male patient has elevated estrogen levels over a long period of time. Testosterone can convert to estradiol. This happens in all men, as men need some estradiol for good health. The problem occurs if there is an over-production of estradiol. This may occur secondary to testosterone hormone replacement therapy.

This conversion process occurs by an enzyme called aromatase acting on testosterone. If a man's estradiol level is too high, he may need to take an aromatase inhibitor for a few days to block this conversion. This is the reason a patient should have his estradiol level checked regularly.

It is occasionally necessary for a surgeon to remove the prostate to relieve the restriction to urine outflow. A common side effect of that procedure is impotence.

Often the cause of BPH is an infection requiring antibiotics specific for this type of bacteria. Because the prostate has a very tough fibrous covering, antibiotics usually have to be used for a month or longer. With a bacterial infection of the prostate, the patient usually feels tired, nauseated, with fever and chills. If untreated, the patient may develop a chronic bacterial prostatitis that is very difficult to eradicate.

The prostate issues described above are not normal but are common with aging. Nutrients may be beneficial to help maintain prostate health. These nutrients include:

- Saw Palmetto [411]
- Nettle Root
- Pigeon [412]
- Selenium [413]
- Vitamin D [414]
- Beta Sit sterol [415]
- Pumpkin Seed [416]
- Hydrangea [417]
- Lycopene [418]
- Pomegranate [419]
- Zinc [420]
- Copper
- Vitamina E [421]
- Boswell [422]
- Flower Pollen

These ingredients can be found in a product by Medic Select called *"Prostate Revive."* [423]

Gene's Story

Gene was a sixty-eight-year-old healthy-appearing man but complaining of having to go to the bathroom two or three times a night. He said,

I'm having more symptoms of dribbling and taking a long time to urinate. Last week I was at an amateur boxing gym where there was only one bathroom. I had the urge to go out of nowhere. There was a young man moving toward the bathroom door, but I cut him off. I felt bad – but I had to. Then it took me five minutes to go. I was so embarrassed when I walked out and he was still standing there. He didn't say anything. Maybe his dad has the same problem.

I have trouble having good erections. I've tried Viagra but it doesn't work like it did two or three years ago. I've noticed my ejaculation is not as forceful as it was when I was young and it just oozes out. Even after I have an orgasm the semen seems to drip out for the next few minutes onto my shorts.

I feel pretty good and don't have any other health problems except it is harder to keep my weight down now that I'm older.

Gene's testosterone was low. But just as troubling was his high estradiol level. He was slightly anemic, and his hematocrit was low. His prostate was also enlarged.

Gene was treated with ten 200 mg testosterone pellets for a total of 2400 mg. He was given a prescription for *Arimidex* 1 mg to be taken three times a week for one month. He was told to order Prostate *Revive*, one pill to be taken twice a day for ten days, then one each morning. He was given a bottle of *Revive* for erectile dysfunction to be taken one each evening until his next visit. Gene was encouraged to begin an easy exercise program by walking daily. He was told to follow a low glycemic index diet.

When Gene returned in four weeks, he was elated. He now had the energy to walk up to five miles a day.

I could have never done that before the testosterone treatment. I've lost nine pounds since I was here last month. My sex life is great. My wife is twelve years younger than me. We almost never miss a day without having sex. The erections come easier and last longer. The orgasms are stronger like it was when I was thirty. I usually don't have to get up at night to use the bathroom if I'm careful not to drink anything for two or three hours before going to bed. I'm so excited about how I feel I don't ever want it to end. I also started taking saw palmetto twice a day like you suggested.

Gene's testosterone was 1124 ng/dL and his estradiol level was down to 43 pg/ml. His hemoglobin was up to normal at 16.3 g/dL and the same with his hematocrit at 48 %. Gene's wife was with him and confirmed his story. Rae said, *"I'm so glad he came in for treatment. I knew he needed some help. I've been on BHRT for four months now. So he and I are on the same page sexually."*

Journal thoughts and questions:

_____

_____

_____

_____

_____

_____

_____

_____

_____

_____

_____

_____

_____

_____

_____

_____

_____

_____

CHAPTER 39

Restless Leg Syndrome

What Is RLS?

Restless leg syndrome is a neurological disorder characterized by throbbing, pulling, pins and needles, itchy, or creepy crawly feeling or other unpleasant sensations in the legs and an uncontrollable and sometimes overwhelming urge to move them. The sensations are usually worse when sitting still or lying down.

Patients who suffer with restless legs syndrome have uncomfortable sensations in their legs (and sometimes arms or other parts of the body) and an irresistible urge to move their legs to relieve the sensations.

The severity of RLS symptoms ranges from mild to intolerable. Symptoms can come and go and severity can also vary. The symptoms are generally worse in the evening and at night and less severe in the morning. For some people, symptoms may cause severe nightly sleep disruption that can significantly impair a person's quality of life.

Restless legs syndrome may affect up to 10% of the U.S. population.

Restless legs syndrome may affect up to 10 percent of the U.S. population. It affects both sexes, but is more common in women and may begin at any age, even in young children. Most people who are affected severely are hormone-deficient women who are middle-aged or older.

Diagnosing and Treating RLS

RLS is often unrecognized or misdiagnosed. This is especially true if the symptoms are intermittent or mild. A very effective treatment of RLS is replacing lost hormones.

Most doctors are told that the cause of restless leg syndrome is unknown. While it is true that there may be more than one cause of this condition, in the vast majority of cases it attacks women who are menopausal.

About fifty percent of people who have RLS have a family member who suffers from the same malady.

Some other conditions which may contribute to the symptoms of restless leg syndrome include:

- Patients with a chronic conditions such as iron deficiency, Parkinson's disease, kidney failure, diabetes, and peripheral neuropathy. When these conditions are treated, the symptoms of RLS may improve also.
- Some medications seem to exacerbate the symptoms of restless leg syndrome. Medicines such as antinausea drugs, antipsychotic drugs, some

antidepressants, and cold and allergy medications containing sedating antihistamines may worsen symptoms.

- Some women experience an increase in symptoms during pregnancy, especially in the last trimester. Symptoms usually go away within a month after delivery.
- Other factors, including alcohol use and sleep deprivation, may trigger symptoms or make them worse. Improving sleep or eliminating alcohol use in these cases may relieve symptoms.

The only relief is to move the legs, but this relief lasts for only a very short time when there is another need to move. In some there is involuntary leg twitching or jerking while sleeping that occurs every fifteen to forty seconds. This naturally causes difficulty sleeping which causes daytime tiredness, poor concentration and loss of energy. Most patients with RLS have excessive movements of the legs. When they are asleep, they kick in bed. The condition is most likely based on an abnormal central nervous system disturbance in the brain. A secondary cause could be a lack of the normal hormones which previously washed over the brain.

Most patients with RLS say it affects their jobs. They have problems with personal relationships, and daily living is affected because of sleep deprivation.

Most patients say RLS affects their jobs. They have problems with personal relationships, and daily living is affected because of sleep deprivation. They also have trouble concentrating, have faulty memory and have difficulty completing a task. Depression is often seen in patients with RLS.

Long periods of sitting such as on a plane or long car trips, sitting in a movie theater, or having a cast stimulates the symptoms of RLS. Some suggestions to help might include:

- Try wearing compression socks or stockings or wrap your legs in bandages (but not so tight that you cut off circulation). Pressure can help relieve the discomfort of restless legs syndrome.
- Try sleeping with a pillow between your legs. It may prevent nerves in your legs from compressing.
- Try to find a work setting where you can be active. If you work at an office, look into a desk that lets you stand while you type.
- Tell friends, family, and co-workers why you have to move more than others. They'll likely be accommodating and want to help you create a healthy environment.
- Choose an aisle seat at movies and on planes so that you can get up and move.
- Give yourself stretch breaks at work and during long car rides.
- **Sleep better by sticking to a regular sleep schedule.** Fatigue can worsen the symptoms of restless legs syndrome, so doing what it takes to get enough sleep is crucial. Try hitting the sack at the same time every night. Take warm baths or read in bed to make you sleepy. Allow plenty of time for winding down.

RLS cannot be diagnosed by an x-ray, a blood test, a physical exam, an ultrasound, or an MRI. RLS is diagnosed based on clinical history, unless one has an iron deficiency or a vitamin deficiency or low magnesium or folate causing the symptoms.

A physician unfamiliar with *Bio-identical Hormone Replacement Therapy* will usually tell the patient with RLS that all tests are normal. If her hormones had been checked, the diagnosis may have been obvious. However, it is important to perform all studies to make sure there are no other diagnoses that may be causing these symptoms, but usually nothing abnormal is found except of hormone deficiencies. The physical exam should include a detailed exam of the nervous system, but if the patient has restless leg syndrome the neurological exam will be normal.

This strongly suggests that a hormonal issue could be at the heart of the problem.

Twice as many women have restless leg syndrome as men. These women are more likely to be affected in perimenopause or even more so in menopause. This strongly suggests that a hormonal issue could be at the heart of the problem. In spite of this obvious connection, most physicians wrongly tell the patient that the symptoms are due to nervousness, insomnia, stress, arthritis, muscle cramps, or aging. How sad!

Because of this, many women are not treated and suffer in silence. It is so unfortunate to hear a doctor tell the patient that she may have this condition because she may be drinking too much coffee or soft caffeinated drinks, smoking, antidepressants, consuming too much alcohol or taking antihistamines. She may be told that she needs to lose weight; she may be encouraged to **practice relaxation techniques such as yoga or to avoid stress and to do daily stretching or have massage therapy. However, there is no evidence that any of these suggestions relieve the symptoms of RLS.**

There are natural remedies that have proven helpful:

- Valerian Root has been shown to act as a natural relaxant that helps insomnia, relieves muscle pain, reduces nervous twitches, and muscle spasms.
- Chamomile Powder is an herb used to relieve muscle spasms by increasing glycine in the body.
- Potassium is an electrolyte that helps to regulate muscle contraction. It plays a role in nerve and muscle function, muscle contractions and nerve impulses.
- Folate deficiency has been found in RLS, especially in familial inheritance and with pregnancy.
- Magnesium affects muscle contractions throughout the body as a muscle relaxation and reducing muscle tension. Magnesium aids in the transmission of nerve messages to the brain and nervous system.
- It is possible (but rare) that restless leg syndrome may be due to iron deficiency, causing a lack of oxygen to the muscles in the legs.

Medications used for restless leg syndrome may be helpful if you can tolerate the side effects. The list of medications is long because there is no single clear-cut treatment. This leads to doctors trying many different treatments. In other words, if the doctor knows the correct treatment, there would not be such a long list of experimental treatments. This list includes:

- **Dopamine agonists:** These are most often the first medicines used to treat RLS. These drugs, including *Mirapex* (pramipexole), *Neupro* (rotigotine), and *Requip* (ropinirole), act like the neurotransmitter dopamine in the brain. Side effects include daytime sleepiness, nausea, and lightheadedness.
- **Dopaminergic agents:** These drugs, including *Sinemet*—a combination of levodopa and carbidopa—increase the level of dopamine in the brain and may improve leg sensations in RLS. However, they may cause a worsening of symptoms for some people after daily use. Side effects can also include nausea, vomiting, hallucinations, and involuntary movements.
- **Benzodiazepines:** Benzodiazepines, such as *Restoril, Xanax*, and *Klonopin* are sedatives. They do not so much relieve symptoms as help you sleep through the symptoms.
- **Opiates:** These drugs are most often used to treat pain, but they can also relieve RLS symptoms. Because opiates are very addictive, they are usually used only when other drugs don't work. *Vicodin* is one example of this type of drug.
- **Anticonvulsants:** These agents, such as *Neurontin* and *Horizant*, may help relieve the symptoms of RLS as well as any chronic pain or nerve pain.
- **Alpha2 agonists:** These agents stimulate alpha2 receptors in the brain stem. This activates nerve cells that *"turn down"* the part of the nervous system that controls muscle involuntary movements and sensations. The drug *Catapres* is an example.

As I said earlier, probably ten percent of the population suffers from restless leg syndrome. When one reads the above descriptions, it may sound overwhelming and hopeless. No one wants to suffer the drastic side effects of the above medications and most patients stop such treatment within one month. There are no well-done scientific studies that provide evidence that any of the above suggestions are valid.

However, observations from many doctors practicing *Bio-identical Hormone Replacement Therapy* testify that women who suffer from restless leg therapy will receive relief of symptoms in the first 3 to 5 nights after pellet hormone therapy.

Bonnie's Story

Bonnie was generally healthy, though somewhat overweight. She suffered from restless leg syndrome.

I dread going to bed at night because I know it's going to start. It takes me more than an hour to go to sleep. And I wake up all during the night and have to walk around the bedroom. I know it bothers my husband – but I can't help it. I've tried different medicines, but they all make me feel terrible. I can't tolerate the side effects.

Bonnie was a sixty-three-year-old postmenopausal woman who still had her uterus and ovaries. She did not use hormone therapy as she passed through menopause.

I heard about the study that showed hormones cause breast cancer. But a friend at church told me the natural kind don't do that. I have been on Paxil at bedtime to help me sleep but it makes me so tired. My doctor told me that Paxil may help my restless legs, but it doesn't. I have no interest in sex and no matter how much my husband tries, I can't have an orgasm.

Bonnie's blood pressure was very good. The vaginal exam showed a thin lining of the vagina. Her breast exam was normal and her recent Pap smear and mammogram were normal. Bonnie weighed 178 pounds at 5'2" tall. *"I know I should exercise and try to lose weight but I don't have the energy."*

Her blood work showed a significant deficiency in sex hormones. Her estradiol, testosterone and progesterone were almost nonexistent. Her thyroid, lipid panel, and CBC were all normal.

Bonnie was treated with pellet *Bio-identical Hormone Replacement Therapy* to replace lost estradiol and testosterone. She was prescribed oral sublingual rapid dissolve progesterone to be taken at bedtime.

In one month Bonnie was like a different person. When asked how she was feeling, Bonnie raised her hands in celebration saying,

I can sleep all night now. That's the best thing ever.

I can sleep all night now. That's the best thing ever. I stopped having that twitchy legs thing on the third night and haven't had any since.

You know, I can remember my mother having the same thing. When I was still at home, one time I saw mother sitting on the side of the bed rubbing her legs. I asked her what was wrong and she said it was her legs aching and couldn't sleep because they twitched all the time. I asked her if she had mentioned it to her doctor. She said she did and all he did was to give her hydrocodone. After mine went away, I now feel bad for my mother because she suffered for years without the treatment I know would have helped her.

I tell everyone that will listen how much bio-identical hormones have helped me.

Journal thoughts and questions:

_____

_____

_____

_____

_____

_____

_____

_____

_____

_____

_____

_____

_____

_____

_____

_____

_____

_____

CHAPTER 40

Diminished Sex Drive

The Inevitability

There can be no doubt that as sex hormones begin to increase in adolescence, sexual activity begins. This connection continues throughout life. When our hormones are at optimal levels, our sex life usually is optimal (at its best).

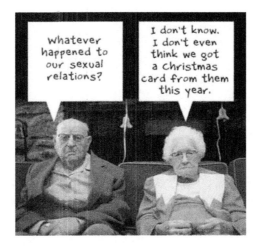

There is also a clear connection between the decline in sex hormones as women enter perimenopause, the stage where she still has her monthly cycle, but with less regularity. This is often accompanied by less sexual drive and less sexual activity.

Then comes menopause. In some cases the sex almost comes to a halt. Instead of three or four times a week, it is three or four times a month ... or even three or four times a year.

Low testosterone in men often causes diminished sex drive and erectile dysfunction. As men experience a dramatic drop in testosterone, there will be fewer sexual thoughts, sexual fantasies and desire. These changes come more gradually and are five to ten years later than as observed in women. This is because testosterone is essential for the brain to respond to sexual stimuli in men and women.

However, men usually have about twenty times more testosterone as women. This is important as the doctor replaces declining testosterone in men as opposed to women — remember the 20:1 ratio. Estradiol is crucial for the health of women for everything from proper brain function, to the skin looking young, to providing for vaginal moisture and less depression. [424]

With testosterone at optimal levels there will be more sexual activity. There will be more orgasms and stronger, longer-lasting orgasms with more pleasure. Men will have sex with a feeling of great satisfaction afterwards.

That's the job of testosterone. It stimulates arousal, sexual desire and motivates us to have sexual fantasies. With testosterone at optimal levels there will be more sexual activity. There will be more orgasms and stronger, longer-lasting orgasms with more pleasure. Men will have sex with a feeling of great satisfaction afterwards. [425]

The Mayo Clinic has done extensive research on the causes of diminished sex drive.[426] They include ...

Physical causes.

A wide range of illnesses, physical changes and medications can cause a low sex drive, including:

- Sexual problems. If you experience pain during sex or an inability to orgasm, it can hamper your desire for sex.
- Medical diseases. Numerous nonsexual diseases can also affect desire for sex, including arthritis, cancer, diabetes, high blood pressure, coronary artery disease and neurological diseases.
- Medications. Many prescription medications — including some antidepressants and antiseizure medications — are notorious libido killers.
- Lifestyle habits. A glass of wine may make you feel amorous, but too much alcohol can spoil your sex drive. The same is true of street drugs. Smoking decreases blood flow, which may dampen arousal.
- Surgery. Any surgery related to your breasts or your genital tract can affect your body image, sexual function and desire for sex.
- Fatigue. Exhaustion from caring for young children or aging parents can contribute to low sex drive. Fatigue from illness or surgery also can play a role in a low sex drive.

Hormone changes

Changes in your hormone levels may alter your desire for sex. This can occur during:

- Menopause. Estrogen levels drop during the transition to menopause. This can cause decreased interest in sex and dryer vaginal tissues, resulting in painful or uncomfortable sex.
- At the same time, women may also experience a decrease in testosterone — a hormone that boosts sex drive in men and women alike, which may lead to decreased libido. Although many women continue to have satisfying sex during menopause and beyond, some women experience a lagging libido during this hormonal change.
- Pregnancy and breast-feeding. Hormone changes during pregnancy, just after having a baby and during breast-feeding can put a damper on sex drive. Of course, hormones aren't the only factor affecting intimacy during these times.

Fatigue, changes in body image, and the pressures of pregnancy or caring for a new baby can all contribute to changes in your sexual desire.

Psychological causes

Your problems don't have to be physical or biological to be real. There are many psychological causes of low sex drive, including:

- Mental health problems, such as anxiety or depression
- Stress, such as financial stress or work stress
- Poor body image
- Low self-esteem
- History of physical or sexual abuse
- Previous negative sexual experiences
- Relationship issues

For many women, emotional closeness is an essential prelude to sexual intimacy. So problems in your relationship can be a major factor in low sex drive. Decreased interest in sex is often a result of ongoing issues, such as:

- Lack of connection with your partner
- Unresolved conflicts or fights
- Poor communication of sexual needs and preferences
- Infidelity or breach of trust

Clair's Story

A young woman of twenty years old will often have a testosterone level of 80 or 90 ng/dL. But a woman who is fifty-five-years-old may have a testosterone of 11 ng/dL or even less. The increase in a woman's sexual response when treated with *Bio-identical Hormone Replacement Therapy* is one of the most dramatic changes seen by physicians practicing BHRT.

Clair was one such patient. She was twenty-two when she married Jim. They enjoyed each other for years until she reached forty-seven.

I'm here today for one thing—I need my sex drive back. My marriage is okay, I think, but my husband is frustrated with me. He has started sleeping in the other bedroom most of the time. He told me that we are more like friends instead of lovers. I tried talking to my doctor about it but she told me that all women go through this and it's just something I would have to live with. She then said most women just use KY Jelly and fake it. A friend of mine at church told me about bio-identical hormones and how it helped her sex life a lot. So I bought a book about it and studied it.

I know that the artificial hormones are dangerous but the book I read says the kind you use are safe and even good for you. I need what my friend has, a good sex life. I don't want to fake it with my husband.

Clair had gained twenty-eight pounds since her marriage twenty-five years earlier. She still had sufficient estradiol but her testosterone and progesterone were very low.

Clair was treated with testosterone according to her symptoms. The goal was to increase her blood level of testosterone up to at least 80 ng.dL and help her with her weight loss. She was also given progesterone 100 mg sublingual tablets to be taken from the first to the 25th of each month.

When Clair returned, her testosterone was up and she said,

My sex life is one-hundred-and-ten percent of what it was twenty-five years ago. I have an orgasm almost every day. I sometimes call my husband at work to see if he can come home at lunch. He likes that. I'm sleeping all night now and feel full of energy the next day. My husband tells everyone how happy he is to have a new wife now.

Testosterone is equally essential for proper functioning of the penis and the brain in men. This is most likely why there has been such a demand for *Viagra, Levitra* and *Cialis*. Nitric oxide is responsible for erections by increasing the blood supply to the penis. Nitric oxide is stimulated by testosterone. [427]

Men who have low testosterone often complain of being tired all the time, not able to concentrate at work and not having the vitality they once had. As testosterone acts on the brain to stimulate sex drive and sexual fantasies. It also increases mental clarity and energy level in men and women.

Journal thoughts and questions:

_____

_____

_____

_____

_____

_____

_____

_____

_____

_____

_____

_____

_____

_____

_____

_____

_____

_____

SECTION THREE

Common Questions

About Bio-Identical

Hormone Replacement Therapy

CHAPTER 41

What Are The Side Effects Of Testosterone Therapy?

Introduction

In this section, I want to answer some of the most-asked questions up front. Most of these chapters will be rather short. A few will be longer, because of the nature of the questions.

This first question deals with the possible side effects of *Bio-identical Testosterone Replacement Therapy*.

The possible side effects:
- In men: acne, testicular atrophy, erythrocytosis, decreased sperm count, hypertension, and increased red blood cell count in men.
- In women the side effects of testosterone can be acne, hypertension (extremely rare), increased red blood cell count (again, extremely rare), deepening of the voice, anxiety, facial hair, and loss of hair on the scalp.

These side effects are generally preventable with proper monitoring of treatment by periodic lab studies, listening to the patient's symptoms and appropriate physical exams.

Acne

Acne is rare in men as a side effect of testosterone therapy. Men are more likely to have an outbreak of acne if they had moderate acne as a youngster. This side effect is usually easily resolved with adjustments in dosing and temporary acne therapy.

Testicular Atrophy

Testicular atrophy usually goes unnoticed by the patient as the degree of atrophy is so minor. The testicles are normally stimulated to produce testosterone by a hormone luteinizing hormone (LH). As a result of aging, there is a decreased production of testosterone. This causes the pituitary gland at the base of the brain to increase its production of LH to *"send a signal"* to the testicles to work harder, to produce more testosterone. This over-stimulation of the testicles may cause the testicles to actually enlarge.

When supplemental testosterone is introduced, the production of LH is reduced as the pituitary gland senses that the body now has enough testosterone. With this reduction in the stimulation of the testicles, they may actually decrease in size compared to the previously enlarged state.

Erythrocytosis

Testosterone stimulates the production of red blood cells (RBCs) primarily from bone marrow. With a decreased production of testosterone secondary to aging it is common for older men to become anemic, registering a low RBC count. This may account for lethargy and tiredness in older men.

Because testosterone replacement causes an increase in red blood cells, normally a good thing in men who have anemia, too much testosterone can cause an over-production of RBCs, or erythrocytosis.

Some use the diagnosis of polycythemia in the same context of an overproduction of RBCs. This side effect can easily be managed by careful monitoring of the patients complete blood count, reducing the dosing of testosterone or, in more extreme cases, may require removal of a unit of blood, a phlebotomy or donating blood at the blood bank.

Lowering of Sperm Count

If one has plans to father a child, this therapy may need to be delayed as it is very common for the sperm count to be considerably diminished.

If testosterone supplementation is used for a relatively short time, the sperm count will return to normal quickly. There are no reliable studies to confirm exactly what constitutes *"short time"* testosterone supplementation, or what time is required for the sperm count to return quickly. A reasonable estimate is to consider not using testosterone supplementation more than five years if fathering a child is considered. After stopping testosterone therapy generally the sperm count will return to adequate levels within six to eighteen months and fertility is reestablished. [428]

Increase in Blood Pressure

Bio-identical Testosterone Replacement Therapy usually causes vasodilatation, thereby reducing blood pressure. However, the initial dose of testosterone has been known in very rare cases to cause a temporary increase in blood pressure. The cause is not known but thought to be possible secondary to temporary fluid retention.

This usually resolves in a few days, especially if a diuretic is given. It is advisable if one has hypertension or borderline hypertension to begin with a reduced dose of testosterone to allow a gradual increase in this hormone.

Breast and Prostate Cancer

Bio-identical Testosterone Replacement Therapy should not be initiated in men who have breast or prostate cancer. However, there is no evidence that testosterone replacement therapy causes prostate cancer or breast cancer. There is much speculation that testosterone may cause a tumor in the prostate to grow more rapidly, but this too has not been proven.

Athletic Performance

Testosterone use to improve athletic performance or to cause an increase in one's height or to correct ambiguous genitalia is dangerous and should not be administered for these reasons.

Male Birth Control

Using testosterone therapy in sufficiently high doses to function as a type of birth control has troublesome and unwanted consequences. [429]

Side Effects for Women

Deepening of the voice in women is rarely seen and usually is not a problem. However, if she notices such changes, the dose of testosterone needs to be reduced or discontinued.

Loss of hair on the scalp may result from too high a dose of testosterone. This hair loss is usually not marked and is noticed only by the patient. The hair loss usually occurs three or four months after her testosterone level was too high. When adjustments are made in the dosing to bring back down her testosterone, the hair will regrow.

Anxiety is extremely rare. Most women experience less anxiety secondary to progesterone and estradiol. However, if the dose of testosterone is too high, she may feel a little jittery until the body is able to adjust itself to the higher range of testosterone in the blood.

Journal thoughts and questions:

_____

_____

_____

_____

_____

_____

_____

_____

_____

_____

_____

_____

_____

_____

_____

_____

_____

_____

CHAPTER 42

What Are The Side Effects Of Estradiol Therapy?

When estradiol is dosed appropriately, there are not evident side effects. Even when estradiol is produced by the ovaries, the effects are natural. Most every woman knows what these are. She may have some swelling of the breast, have a bit more energy and will know her period is not far behind.

However, if there is an excess of estrogen from synthetic estrogen or even estradiol there may be the following side effects:

- Swollen breasts
- Weight gain
- Panic attacks
- Agitation
- Poor sleep
- Spotting
- Tender breasts
- Bleeding
- Bloating
- Headaches
- Low sex drive
- Heavy periods
- Migraine headaches
- Menstrual cramps
- Infertility
- Mood swings
- Ovarian cysts
- Panic attacks
- Depression
- Endometriosis
- Uterine fibroids
- Irregular periods
- Miscarriages
- Fibrocystic breast disease

These side effects are far more often seen with the use of synthetic estrogens. When being treated with bio-identical estradiol, it is important to have regular blood levels of estradiol (E2) and follicular stimulating hormones (FSH) performed.

Estradiol levels of 90 pg/ml to 110 pg/ml and maintaining FSH below 10 mIU/L should relieve menopausal symptoms and provide for protection from health issues such as:

- Osteoporosis
- Dementia
- Coronary artery disease
- Vaginal dryness
- Urinary leakage
- Depression
- Hot flashes
- Night sweats
- Alzheimer's disease
- Fatigue
- Poor sleep
- Loss of sense of well-being
- Mood changes
- Painful intercourse   Loss of bone from the face
- Early degeneration of teeth
- Stroke
- Degeneration of the eyes
- Undue skin wrinkles

Journal thoughts and questions:

_____

_____

_____

_____

_____

_____

_____

_____

_____

_____

_____

_____

_____

_____

_____

_____

_____

_____

CHAPTER 43

What Are The Side Effects Of Progesterone Therapy?

The main side effect of Progesterone is that it can cause drowsiness. This is the reason progesterone is taken at bedtime.

The side effects of progesterone compared to the synthetic *Provera* are minimal. Doctors who use natural progesterone will usually report that they never have seen a side effect. There have been rare reports of mild nausea, mild diarrhea, bloating, stomach cramps, dizziness, acne and breast pain. Increased hair growth has been reported with higher doses.

Most all these side effects are seen just as often as when a patient is given a placebo. So, in truth, drowsiness is about the only side effect one has to be concerned about.

The usual dose of progesterone is 50 mg to 200 mg at bedtime. Adjustments in dosing are made according to the symptoms of the patient and the blood levels. The balance between progesterone and estradiol is extremely important. Without this balance women will experience the side effects of excess estrogen. Again, it is important to understand that bio-identical progesterone has no side effects in the vast majority of women except for some sleepiness.

If you read a comment from the FDA or Wyeth (the manufacture of *Provera*) that there is no difference in the side effects or safety of *Provera* and natural progesterone, they are wrong. Why? Neither the FDA or Wyeth can give even one scientific study to support their claim. They just say it. If Wyeth says it – so *"it must be true."*

Wrong!! As we discussed earlier, the PEPI study sponsored by the *National Institute of Health* compared synthetic *Provera* to natural progesterone. Bio-identical progesterone virtually never caused any adverse side effects.

Some supporters of Big Pharma have said that without any clinical studies, natural progesterone might not protect the endometrial lining of the uterus in women using *Premarin* as much as *Provera* does. This is absurd! There are at least a dozen well-done studies confirming that natural progesterone protects the uterine lining as well as *Provera* without the dangerous side effects of *Provera* such as blood clots, heart attacks, strokes, breast cancer and dementia.

The only side effect those who want to boost sales of the patented drug *Provera* can come up with is it may cause a calming of stress.

Journal thoughts and questions:

_____

_____

_____

_____

_____

_____

_____

_____

_____

_____

_____

_____

_____

_____

_____

_____

_____

_____

CHAPTER 44

I Want My Skin To Look As Young As Possible.
Will Bhrt Help Me Avoid Skin Wrinkles?

It is no secret that women want to look young as long as possible. But menopause changes all that. [430]

Skin cells are prolific with receptor sites for estradiol. This means the skin is very sensitive to changes in estrogen levels.

What will aging do to our skin?

- Aging causes loss of elastin, hyaluronic acid and collagen.
- Elastin is a protein in connective tissue that is elastic and allows many tissues in the body to resume their shape after stretching or contracting. Elastin helps skin to return to its original position.
- Collagen is the main structural protein of the various connective tissues including the skin, bone, tendons and cartilage.
- Because of this protein, these structures have increased strength. Therefore, they can withstand great pressure without breaking. [431]
- Menopause results in a decrease in estradiol in the skin.
- This causes the skin to become thinner and dryer with less elasticity. The skin bruises more easily and heals slower.
- Loss of natural estradiol results in the sagging of the skin with deep wrinkles.

Women will begin to lose collagen by age forty, even before menopause. It is well known that old skin cells slough off and new skin cells form, keeping our skin looking fresh and young. With the loss of estrogen, the old cells do not turn over as quickly. The skin sometimes takes on a "leathery" appearance.[432]

In 1999, a German physician performed an interesting experiment. The doctor and his staff made a guess of what they thought the age of one hundred new women patients were as they entered the clinic. This estimation of the women's ages was done before their actual ages was known.

As a new patient, each woman had blood drawn checking their estradiol levels along with noting their actual age, ranging from thirty-five to fifty-five years old. After collecting this data, the actual ages were compared to the estimated ages with the estradiol levels noted for each.

It is no surprise that the women who looked younger had higher levels of estradiol. Some women had a discrepancy between the actual age and the estimated age of eight years. [433]

However, with bio-identical estradiol replacement, collagen acts as a filler to the skin and adds water to the skin by increasing hyaluronic acid. This occurs because the protein in cells that is prolific with estrogen receptors attract and attach estrogen to skin cells. Estrogen increases the elastin in skin cells causing an increase in blood supply with resulting increase in skin thickness and water and a decrease in the depth of wrinkles. [434]

Bio-identical estradiol cream used on the face of postmenopausal women who had the typical signs of aging showed remarkable improvement in almost one hundred percent of these women. There were objective measurements to confirm the results.

- The positive changes were:
- Fewer wrinkles
- Firmness of the skin with an increase in elasticity
- More hydration
- More moisture
- An increase in blood supply

The depth of the wrinkles improved to as much as complete disappearance. Also the size of the pores of the skin improved. [435]

Bio-identical hormone replacement with estradiol can double the thickness of the skin to a menopausal woman. Omega-3-fish oil can hydrate the skin as well. [436]

Journal thoughts and questions:

_____

_____

_____

_____

_____

_____

_____

_____

_____

_____

_____

_____

_____

_____

_____

_____

_____

_____

CHAPTER 45

How Do Hormones Protect Against Breast Cancer?

Breast cancer is one of the biggest fears among women today. It is generally known that women who give birth to multiple children have a lower risk for breast cancer.Progesterone escalates to one hundred times more during pregnancy than is seen in a non-pregnant female. In societies where women commonly bear six or more children, studies show they are far less likely to experience breast cancer.

Menopause produces a state of very low serum levels of progesterone. Normal progesterone in a young female is usually 15 to 25 ng/ml. That same woman in menopause may have only ten percent of what she did when she was young and healthy. And some have even less than that.

There are doctors who believe that progesterone supplementation is meant for just one thing, to protect the inside lining of the uterus from cancer. For those physicians, progesterone is administered only if she is using estrogen supplementation and has a uterus. If she has no uterus she has no need of progesterone, they propose. This is ridiculous when one reviews the benefits of natural progesterone.

Most physicians who are knowledgeable in the discipline of *Bio-identical Hormone Replacement Therapy* will recommend that women in perimenopause, menopause and who are postmenopausal need to be supplemented with natural progesterone daily or at least twenty-one days a month. Before menopause, progesterone rises and falls monthly. During the first ten days or so of a menstrual cycle progesterone is low. Nearing ovulation at mid-cycle progesterone begins to rise. The purpose of progesterone in this part of the cycle is to prepare the uterus for implantation of a fertilized egg. If there is no fertilized egg to implant into the wall of the uterus progesterone drops and a menstrual flow follows. If there is a fertilized egg implanted in the uterus, progesterone continues to increase greatly to provide for a healthy environment to nourish the implanted embryo.

Progesterone has many advantages beyond preparing the uterus for implantation of a fertilized egg and protecting the uterus from endometrial cancer. Progesterone functions as an antidepressant. It is noteworthy that so many women, as they enter the perimenopausal and menopausal years will be placed on an antidepressant. The reason for their depression most likely is loss of the natural progesterone they once had. Progesterone is an antioxidant, protects the nervous system, protects the cardiovascular system and increases sex drive.

Whether one takes progesterone daily or less frequently is the decision of the doctor and the patient, but to deny this great hormone to a woman suffering in the menopausal years is unfortunate. Women who deliver a child before age twenty-four have a decreased risk of developing breast cancer in their lifetime. And the more pregnancies you have, the more protection from breast cancer you will have because of the progesterone that is produced. [437]

Journal thoughts and questions:

CHAPTER 46

How Does Bhrt Help With Inflammation In My Body?

Aging brings with it a host of changes to our bodies. One of those that is most prevalent is a chronic low-grade inflammation in the body.

Inflammation is the body's response to injury or infection. It can be classified as either acute or chronic. Acute inflammation is the initial inflammatory response that occurs almost immediately after minor injuries like burns and cuts as well as major trauma such as myocardial infarction. Chronic inflammation as seen in aging is a continuous process of tissue breakdown and attempted repair. Protein is released from the site of inflammation. These proteins can be detected in the blood and are therefore referred to as inflammatory markers. Perhaps the most commonly used marker of inflammation is C-reactive protein (CRP). Chronic inflammatory diseases can be monitored with serial CRP measurements.

Measuring C-reactive protein is a strong measure of frailty, disability, and cardiovascular disease. [438]

Inflammation is an important factor that causes loss of muscle mass. [439] Low-grade inflammatory seen in aging is caused by hormonal changes. [440] Testosterone treatment aids in the prevention of the release of inflammatory cytokines such as tumor necrosis factor-α, interleukin-6, and interleukin-1β. [441]

Beyond this action, testosterone treatment causes the release of interleukin-10 which is an anti-inflammatory cytokine to fight inflammation. [442] However, in older women, testosterone and estradiol levels that are unduly elevated are associated with insulin resistance and diabetes, conditions characterized by low-grade inflammation. This is the reason careful monitoring of blood levels of these hormones is important. [443]

The loss of natural sex hormones allows the development of chronic inflammation throughout the body. This inflammation resulting from debilitating hormonal changes affects various chronic conditions, such as atherosclerosis, cardiovascular diseases, metabolic syndrome, and type 2 diabetes.

Normal aging is associated with loss of muscle mass. The reason is loss of life-giving hormones: testosterone, progesterone and estradiol. At least seven proteins which are growth factors are involved in our immune response, as well as proteins involved in the production of collagen are all reduced in older men. When men are treated with testosterone lean muscle mass is increased, and there is an increase in the appetite as the hormone leptin is suppressed. This means men will have more muscle mass and less fat.

Estrogen treatment increases the energy produced from these cellular power plants while at the same time acting as antioxidants. When these tiny mitochondrial power plants are not working right this causes age-related disorders. This leads to loss of energy. Almost all cells in the body have mitochondria which produce the body's essential energy. How estrogen works to prevent age-related cardiovascular diseases, including stroke, may result from how hormones affect mitochondrial function. This process of estrogen promoting mitochondrial efficiency may also be a contributing factor to the longer lifespan of women. [444]

Endothelial cells make up the inside lining of arteries in the entire circulatory system, from the heart to the smallest capillaries. A key component to vascular disease is when there is dysfunction of the endothelial lining causing cardiovascular disease and aging. Hormonal therapy, exercise and a diet low in calories such as fruits and vegetables protect against cardiovascular disease. Endothelial cells function as fluid filtration, such as in the glomeruli of the kidney, blood vessel tone, hemostasis, neutrophil recruitment, and hormone trafficking. Endothelial dysfunction is a major contributor to atherosclerotic disease which is a direct consequence of estrogen deficiency. Estrogen supplementation may help prevent endothelial dysfunction which causes high blood pressure and coronary artery disease. [445]

Symptoms of hormone deficiency leading to endothelial dysfunction associated with aging include:

- Poor growth
- Loss of muscle coordination
- Muscle weakness
- Visual problems
- Hearing problems
- Learning disabilities
- Heart disease
- Liver disease
- Kidney disease
- Gastrointestinal disorders
- Respiratory disorders
- Neurological problems
- Autonomic dysfunction
- Dementia

Scientific Research

In November 2007, a large prospective study by Dr. Khaw demonstrated that high endogenous levels of testosterone are seen in men who live longer. They are less likely to die at an earlier age from any disease. This was especially true when looking at cardiovascular disease. [446]

A study by Dr. Shores and colleagues followed 858 men for eight years and described their risk of death. **Men with low testosterone had an eighty-eight percent increased risk of dying than men with higher testosterone.** [447]

In a study reported in *Heart* in 2010, a high percentage of the men who have low testosterone have cardiovascular disease. This gives evidence that there is a positive relationship between low testosterone and cardiovascular disease. The death rate of those who have low testosterone was approximately forty-seven percent higher than men with normal testosterone. [448]

Low testosterone levels in men are associated with several cardiovascular risk factors including a lipid profile that deposits fat and cholesterol to the walls of arteries (hardening of the arteries), insulin resistance (may lead to type 2 diabetes), obesity and a condition promoting blood clots. [449] Studies in male animals have shown that castration or induced hypogonadism increases atherosclerosis. Testosterone replacement nullifies this. [450]

Testosterone therapy has beneficial effects for men with cardiovascular disease. Testosterone is a potent coronary vasodilator—opens up blood vessels acting as a calcium channel blocker as seen in certain medications (*Norvasc, Procardia, Calan, Cardizem*), and by this action helps prevent angina (chest pain on exertion), especially in men with low testosterone. [451] Testosterone therapy reduces cholesterol, excess body fat, waist circumference and blood products that promote atherosclerosis, diabetes and the metabolic syndrome all contributing to coronary artery disease. [452] In men with heart failure, testosterone therapy increases one's ability to be functional (move about) and decrease insulin resistance—makes cells more sensitive to insulin. [453]

It is extremely rare to find a man over sixty years old to have a testosterone level to be at the lower level of normal for a young man. It is even rarer for such a man to be at the upper level of normal. Thirty per cent of men over the age of 60 years suffer from this debilitating condition. [454]

The undesirable effects of testosterone deficiency include osteoporosis, loss of muscle mass, weight gain in the form of fat, decreased energy, loss of functional ability and decreased sexual function. Up until recently, these have been considered the natural part of aging. But more studies are evolving demonstrating that low testosterone causes men to be more likely to die at an earlier age than men with higher levels of testosterone. [455]

The *EPIC-Norfolk* study is one of the most well-known trials describing the effects of testosterone on mortality. [456] *EPIC-Norfolk* excluded men with cardiovascular disease and cancer to assure accuracy of the study.

The results confirmed that for every degree of reduction in testosterone, there was a corresponding increase in death rate in men. The increase in mortality was found in men with cardiovascular disease but also for any other cause of death. This is an especially important study since this group represents patients who are more likely to have testosterone deficiency. Men with symptoms of diabetes mellitus, chronic heart failure or cardiovascular disease may be helped by testosterone replacement therapy. [457]

Conclusions

Based on a multitude of studies, there can now be no doubt that ***testosterone deficiency is associated with premature death in men with cardiovascular disease.***

Even with so much evidence to the contrary, some doctors doubt the benefits of testosterone replacement therapy. Until this therapy is adapted by physicians caring for men with coronary artery disease, many will continue to die from the effects of low testosterone.

There has been a huge increase in testosterone therapy in the last twenty years – despite the voices of the naysayers. [458] Most of the resistance to the use of testosterone supplementation is fear of side effects from excess testosterone seen in the abuse of this hormone. However, there is a plethora of scientific trials demonstrating that with correct monitoring of blood levels, testosterone replacement therapy is safe. [459]

If one accepts the well-done studies confirming that testosterone deficiency is part of the underlying cause of atherosclerotic disease in men, then the serum testosterone should be seen as something that can be modified to the advantage of these men. ***Bio-identical Testosterone Replacement Therapy is inexpensive with very few easily managed side effects with careful monitoring.*** [460]

Journal thoughts and questions:

CHAPTER 47

How Do I Deal With Incontinence, Urinary Tract Infections, And Vaginal Dryness?

Bio-identical Hormone Replacement Therapy is not only beneficial in alleviating such disease processes as heart disease, osteoporosis, and memory loss – but also urinary incontinence and urinary tract infections.

BHRT keeps the vagina moist. Vaginal dryness not only is very uncomfortable and causes painful intercourse, but it also causes a ripe environment for infections. *Premarin* in studies actually increased the risk of urinary incontinence. [461]

In another study menopausal women using both *Premarin* and *Provera*, women had a sixty-four percent chance of having urinary incontinence compared to forty-nine percent in women using placebo. [462] Urinary incontinence (leakage) bothers about forty to fifty percent of menopausal women. [463]

It is also interesting to note that women who are without hormones are far more likely to have depression and these same women are more likely to have urinary incontinence. [464]

Leakage is most often to occur when a woman is laughing, sneezing, coughing, or exercising. This happens because there is stress applied to the bladder. Often there is a strong urge to use the bathroom quickly, even though the bladder is not full. What is important to know is that low estradiol can be responsible for weak muscles in postmenopausal women and replacing estradiol can provide great relief.

With hormonal balance using bio-identical estradiol, progesterone and testosterone, the vagina maintains a balanced pH helping to resist infections and keeping the pelvic muscles strong helping a woman from having embarrassing leakage from the bladder. This occurs secondary to increased blood flow to surrounding tissues including those that control the bladder and the urethra (the passage from the bladder to the outside). [465] *Premarin* increases the risk of UTI. [466]

Bea, a fifty-two-year-old school teacher, complained of having at least five urinary tract infections a year.

I've had bladder infection after bladder infection starting when I went through menopause. Before then I never had this trouble. I have to go to the bathroom every few minutes. When this happens it hurts to urinate. It is a major problem when I have to leave my classroom in the middle of a lesson. My doctor gives me Bactrim and Pyridium for a few days and it goes away. But two weeks later I have a yeast infection that causes a lot of itching and burning and a white discharge. I take a pill, just one, I can't remember the name, and it goes away. But a month later, I end up with a bacterial vaginal infection that hurts in a different way than the yeast infection. I'm just going around in circles. I don't know why this is happening to me.

When Bea had normal hormone levels everything *"down there"* was working fine. Bea began having menopausal symptoms when she was forty-four years old. She was offered *Premarin* for her hot flashes which meant she also had to take *Provera* to protect the uterus from the side effects of *Premarin*. Bea remembered,

After eighteen months she told me I could not take the hormones any longer. She said a report showed that the two hormones I was on caused breast cancer and blood clots. When I stopped Premarin I began to have hot flashes every hour. It was so embarrassing. After that is when the infections began.

Bea's complaints were of being tired, poor sleep, depression, low sex drive, painful intercourse and weight gain.

When my doctor stopped my hormones she gave me *Lexapro*. She said it was for symptoms of menopause. All it did was make me numb all over, killed my desire for sex and made me gain thirty-five pounds. When I hit 185 pounds, I knew I had to do something different. I stopped the *Lexapro*, but haven't been able to drop any weight.

She wanted me to try a different antidepressant but I knew better than to do that because on the internet the side effects were the same as with the one I was on.

The exam was as is often seen in menopausal women. Bea was 5'4" and had maintained 125 to 135 pounds since she was married at twenty-seven years old. She was frustrated over her fifty-pound weight gain.

Her blood pressure was good, as well as her blood work except for her hormones. Her testosterone, progesterone, estradiol were all low. And her FSH was 76 mIU/L (normal 1 to 4 mIU/L). Her recent mammogram and Pap smear were normal. The pap showed atrophic cells indicating hormone deficiency.

Bea was very pleased to know her hormone levels.

I asked my doctor to check my hormones. She said it was just something I would have to go through. Most all women have this. I told her I had read one of Suzanne Somers' books. I asked her what she thought of bio-identical hormones. She said those kinds of hormones have the same risks as Premarin and Provera. She told me there were no studies that showed they were any different than what she had given me. I knew that was not true, but I didn't argue. I looked up some of the references from Suzanne Somers' book and found lots of studies showing that bio-identical hormones are safer. Then I read a couple more books all saying the same thing.

Needless to say, because Bea was a teacher, she did her homework.

She was confident the problem was her hormones.

Bea was treated with bio-identical hormones according to her symptoms, her weight, and her lab work. She spoke to a dietitian about portion control and a low glycemic diet. She joined a gym with a personal trainer and works with him at least 3 times a week. For her poor sleep, she was given melatonin 15 mg at bedtime even though low progesterone was probably the reason for poor sleep. Melatonin is a good natural antioxidant and is very inexpensive.

One month later Bea said,

I have so much more energy. I haven't had a bladder infection or vaginal infection since the hormones. I have absolutely no hot flashes, none! What a relief. I actually look forward to having sex with my husband. There is no pain. He has noticed how much vaginal moisture I have and it makes it easier for him too. I go to the gym five times a week. My trainer has increased my workout. It makes me sore but I've lost 9 and ½ pounds in one month. I never want to do without my hormones. My husband has an appointment with you next week.

Bea has been on bio-identical hormones for the last five years. She now weighs 138 pounds at fifty-seven years old. She and her husband say,

We are more in love today than we were twenty-five years ago. We are always together and like it that way. We have told everyone about how we feel. We want to spread the word that you don't have to suffer from growing older.

Sometimes women will say, *"I am so dry down there it feels like it's going to crack open."* This seems to happen quickly after a total hysterectomy. Most will notice changes in their personality, and skin and vagina within one month after losing their ovaries.

Joyce was a worried forty-nine-year-old executive secretary who just had a total hysterectomy nine months earlier. Her complaint was vaginal pain and terrible hot flashes. Her husband of twenty-two years was so frustrated with his wife. Her husband did not come home until late at night saying he had to work late, which was unusual.

I love my husband very much and I believe he loves me. But when we have sex it hurts so much," raising her hands up in the air in an expression of I CAN'T DO IT, *"it hurts so bad I can't stand it even with Vaseline. One of my friends told me she thought my husband might be seeing someone. I don't want to lose my husband. He's a good man."*

Estrogen deficiency was the cause of her pain. Her doctor was afraid to give her estrogen so she was given *Paxil* 10 mg, an SSRI. If having vaginal pain was not enough, she now had no desire for sex and was completely unable to have an orgasm.

Her lab values confirmed that her sex hormones were extremely low. She was treated with bio-identical pellets of low dose testosterone and estradiol. She was given bio-identical progesterone sublingual rapid dissolve at bedtime. She was encouraged to gradually reduce her SSRI.

When Joyce returned in 4 weeks for her follow-up visit she had a glow about her that expressed such relief.

This is so difficult to imagine. I have no pain with intercourse now. None! I've not had a hot flash in 3 weeks. I have as much vaginal moisture as I did when I was 18. And my sex drive is like a teenager. My husband is home every evening now. Doctor, you saved my marriage.

At this point, both Joyce and I needed a tissue to dry the tears.

What Joyce and Bea learned was how effective hormone treatment could be when it came to issues such as Incontinence, Urinary tract infections, and vaginal dryness.

Journal thoughts and questions:

_____

_____

_____

_____

_____

_____

_____

_____

_____

_____

_____

_____

_____

_____

_____

_____

_____

_____

_____

CHAPTER 48

How Does Testosterone Supplementation Help Weight Loss?

While testosterone supplementation does not ensure weight loss, it does give you more energy. Usually the increase in energy both in the brain and the muscles promotes a desire and ability to exercise.

Testosterone increases a natural hormone in the brain, norepinephrine, which acts as an antidepressant. Testosterone certainly increases muscle mass instead of fat storage. Testosterone gives more youthful shape to the body. And it is the most important independent hormonal determinant of HDL-C levels. [467]

Patients who have at least a fifty percent narrowing of an artery of at least one vessel had low testosterone and also high blood pressure, elevated causes of blood clots, high triglycerides, a decreased ability of the heart to pump, and low HDL-C (good cholesterol). [468]

It is probably better to ask your doctor what your testosterone level is than what your cholesterol is. Your testosterone is a better predictor of longevity than cholesterol.

Other studies report the same conclusions that testosterone deficiency contributes to the metabolic syndrome and mortality.

Low testosterone precedes the development of central obesity, the metabolic syndrome, and diabetes over the following ten to fifteen years in non-obese men without these conditions at baseline. In this study, lower total testosterone levels were associated with central obesity and established cardiovascular disease risk factors including insulin and insulin resistance, glycemia, lipid profile, and blood pressure.

This same study notes that older men with low levels of circulating total testosterone had a forty percent increased risk of death over the following twenty years, compared with men with normal testosterone. [469]

Men are more than twice as likely to die of coronary artery disease as women. Men with low testosterone are almost twice as likely to die of this disease as men with normal testosterone. [470]

It is commonly accepted that excess use of any anabolic steroid use – such as testosterone seen with those who self-inject in high doses – is dangerous. [471] However, high testosterone levels from an outside source are not harmful if the levels are within the normal range are within the normal range for young men.

Journal thoughts and questions:

_____

_____

_____

_____

_____

_____

_____

_____

_____

_____

_____

_____

_____

_____

_____

_____

_____

CHAPTER 49

Why Do Doctors Continue To Prescribe Dangerous Synthetic Hormones?

You've read a lot of information so far. You've seen the dangers of synthetic drugs. You've seen the studies that have been done on these drugs, including the *Women's Health Initiative Trial.*

You've also read about the safety and "naturalness" of *Bio-identical Hormone Replacement Therapy.* No one has ever gotten cancer from BHRT. No one has ever suffered the severe side effects from it like they do from *Premarin* and *Provera.*

Unfortunately, there are still doctors prescribing these dangerous synthetic hormones to unsuspecting women without being told of the risks ... risks that include increased risk of breast cancer, cardiovascular disease, stroke, dementia, and blood clots. We've known conclusively about these risks since 2002.

So the logical question is ... **why do doctors continue to prescribe dangerous synthetic hormones** to these women?

Some contend that the risks of bio-identical hormones are the same as the risks from traditional hormones. The argument is that *"estrogen is estrogen is estrogen."*

That argument may be answered by comparing two chemicals, H2O2 and H2O. One is hydrogen peroxide (H2O2) and the other water (H2O). There is just one molecule difference between the two of them. These two chemicals are so similar that the effects should be similar. Wrong! When you are thirsty, would you rather be offered a glass of hydrogen peroxide to drink or a glass of water?

The reason so many women are living without hormones is the errant interpretation of the *Women's Health Initiative Study* by doctors that all hormones are the same. The reasoning goes like this: *"If traditional hormones like Premarin and Provera cause breast cancer, heart attacks, strokes, and blood clots, surely bio-identical hormones do the same."*

That is simply WRONG!!!

Controlled studies and most observational studies published over the last five years suggest that the addition of synthetic progestins like Provera to estrogen in hormone replacement therapy increases the breast cancer risk compared to estrogen alone. By contrast, a recent study suggests that the addition of bio-identical progesterone in cyclic regimens does not affect breast cancer risk.

However, in contrast to natural bio-identical progesterone, **Provera has some non-progesterone-like effects, which can increase the side effects of estrogen.** These side effects include stimulating the breast tissue. *Provera* has negative effects on the liver causing decreased insulin sensitivity, increased levels and activity of insulin-like growth factor-I, and decreased levels of SHBG, which is the opposite effect induced by oral estrogen. [472]

Randomized controlled studies demonstrate that when a synthetic progestin like *Provera* is added to estrogen, this combination increases the breast cancer risk much more than estrogen alone. [473]

However, a very authoritative study known as E3N-EPIC proved that **when bio-identical progesterone is used instead of synthetic Provera in hormone replacement therapy, breast cancer is not increased.** [474]

In addition, a Danish study found an increase in ovarian cancer in women who used synthetic hormone replacement. [475]

Who is to blame? I can think of four potential sources:

- **First, Big Pharma is to blame.** In chapter eleven, we saw their agenda and evidence of their cover-ups and manipulation.
- **Second, physicians are to blame.** They have, for the most part, remained uneducated about BHRT. They have also allowed themselves to be duped by Big Pharma. Instead of putting patient interests in first place, they have allowed their own interests to reign supreme. And millions have suffered as a result.
- **Third, the public is to blame.** Instead of investigating everything thoroughly, they have remained uninformed, although there has been growing literature about BHRT out there.
- **Fourth and finally, we – the physicians who use and promote BHRT – are to blame.** Our voice has not been heard. We have not been loud enough. That is one reason I've written this book. I've tried to be as clear and forthright as I can be. May our silence never again be the cause for lack of information.

The medical community must wake up. We must hear the truth about BHRT – so our patients don't suffer anymore.

Journal thoughts and questions:

CHAPTER 50

How Are Men And Women Different
When It Comes To Bhrt?

The Perfect Husband?

Several men are in the locker room of a golf club. A cell phone on a bench rings and a man engages the hands-free speaker function and begins to talk. Everyone else in the room stops to listen.

MAN: *"Hello"*
WOMAN: *"Hi Honey, it's me. Are you at the club?"*
MAN: *"Yes."*
WOMAN: *"I'm at the shops now and found this beautiful leather coat. It's only $2,000; is it OK if I buy it?"*
MAN: *"Sure, go ahead if you like it that much."*
WOMAN: *"I also stopped by the Lexus dealership and saw the new models. I saw one I really liked.*
MAN: *"How much?"*
WOMAN: *"$90,000."*
MAN: *"OK, but for that price I want it with all the options."*
WOMAN: *"Great! Oh, and one more thing... I was just talking to Janie and found out that the house I wanted last year is back on the market. They're asking only $980,000 for it."*
MAN: *"Well, then go ahead and make an offer of $900,000. They'll probably take it. If not, we can go the extra eighty-thousand if it's what you really want."*
WOMAN: *"OK. I'll see you later! I love you so much!"*
MAN: *"Bye! I love you, too."*

The man hangs up. The other men in the locker room are staring at him in astonishment, mouths wide open.

He turns and asks, *"Anyone know whose phone this is?"*

We laugh ... and we should. Because we all know men and women are different.

In this chapter, I would like to focus on how men and women are different from the perspective of a hormone doctor.

This is going to be a fairly long chapter – but one that I think you will really appreciate because of its important implications.

How Are Women Unique?

The term "postmenopause" is somewhat a misnomer. This word suggests that a woman has gone through menopause and now things are going to be okay. As one gynecologist commented to her patient who was complaining of severe symptoms of hormone loss after a hysterectomy, *"Don't worry. You'll get over this in six months."* You don't *"get over"* the loss of vital-to-a-healthy-life hormones.

The term perimenopause refers to the period when women begin to lose the sex hormones, testosterone, progesterone and estradiol—all produced by the ovaries. Menopause is the period when women stop having a period—almost complete loss of all the sex hormones, especially estradiol and progesterone. Postmenopause is the period of time after menopause. Again, this suggests that you have gone through the hard part, like going through drug withdrawal or getting off alcohol. Now you are okay because you are not using these drugs any more.

When one is off drugs such as cocaine, heroin, and alcohol, the patient is better off. But when a woman goes through menopause and passes into postmenopause, she is far from being better off. It is beyond argument that women's health begins to decline quickly during this transition.

Postmenopausal women have an increase in cardiovascular disease—heart attacks, strokes, poor circulation, blood clots, high blood pressure, lipid abnormalities (elevated cholesterol and triglycerides). These cardiovascular attacks on the heart cause marked changes to the heart muscle.

The injuries to the heart are due to acute myocardial infarction, volume overload (excess fluid), chronic hypertension (high blood pressure), congenital heart disease, and valvular heart disease. These damages to the heart cause scar tissue (cardiac remodeling) which causes changes in size, shape, structure and function of the heart. This leads to a decline in the performance of the heart, and eventually results in congestive heart failure and death. [476]

Replacing these lost hormones has been shown to have cardio-protective effects.

Bio-identical estradiol therapy can prevent some of these changes. [477] Certainly 17β-estradiol is protective from damages brought on during menopause but the addition of natural progesterone limits even more changes to the heart that occur as a woman ages.

In women, 17β-estradiol protects the heart from damages. This is known because:

- Women in the reproductive age group are protected against cardiovascular disease and hardening of the arteries compared to men.[478]
- When women go through menopause, there is ovarian dysfunction—the ovaries stop producing the hormones that keep a woman healthy through the child-bearing years.
- There is a decrease in circulating estradiol and as a result there is an increased incidence of cardiovascular disease. [479]
- Replacing lost estradiol with bio-identical estradiol markedly reduces the risk of cardiovascular disease in postmenopausal women. [480]

- Because coronary artery disease is the most frequent cause of death among women, [481] the importance of understanding the influence estradiol has on the walls of blood vessels cannot be overstated.

The role estradiol plays in the cardiovascular system is as follows:

- Hormone receptors for 17β-estradiol are on the walls of the blood vessels and the smooth muscle cells in the vascular walls. [482]
- 17β-estradiol has direct effects on vascular cells. [483]
- 17β-estradiol improves the function of the arteries (contracting and dilating) and prevents damage to the arteries. [484]
- 17β-estradiol prevents overgrowth of smooth muscle cells into the intima, the inside lining of blood vessels causing narrowing of arteries and depositing plaque such as collagen. [485]

Estradiol exerts its protective effect on the cardiovascular system (the heart and blood vessels) by preventing scar tissue formation in the heart muscle, by preventing occlusion of the coronary arteries (blood vessels around the heart), and by prevention of collagen buildup in the form of plaque inside the arteries. [486] It is well known that there is increased atherosclerosis in the arteries in the absence of estradiol and estradiol inhibits these damages. [487]

In menopause there is ovarian insufficiency/dysfunction and a decrease in estrogen levels. [488]

Progesterone enhances the protective effects of 17β-estradiol. [489] In contrast to natural progesterone, synthetic progestins such as *Provera*, which is used by many doctors, reduce the various cardioprotective effects of 17β-estradiol. [490] *Provera* has also been shown to stop the beneficial effects of 17β-estradiol. [491]

The possibility of excess mortality secondary to not using hormone therapy was examined in 2013 in the *American Journal of Public Health*. In the 1990s, estrogen therapy was the standard treatment for 600,000 women in the United States who had a hysterectomy. At that time doctors were told that *Prempro* was effective for treatment of menopausal symptoms and appeared to be bone protective and cardio protective. More than 90% of women who had a hysterectomy in their fifties used estrogen therapy. Most of these women used this drug for four to five years, but many used *Prempro* for twenty or thirty years. [492]

While it is true that oral *Premarin* is not safe because any kind of estrogen taken by mouth increases the risk for blood clots, not taking any kind of estrogen causes an increase in mortality. If lack of hormones causes early death and oral estrogen causes an increased risk of strokes and heart attacks, what can you do?

Answer: Why not use a non-synthetic natural bio-identical hormone that is not taken by mouth ... such as Bio-identical 17 beta estradiol? [493]

Despite the benefits of estrogen-only therapy, only one in three women who have had a hysterectomy are using estrogen. [494] Because of the avoidance of any kind of hormone therapy, many women will die prematurely.

How many women who have had a hysterectomy are dying because they are afraid to use any kind of hormone?

It is so unfortunate that so many women and their physicians are not aware of the lifesaving benefits of bio-identical hormones. There does not have to be a choice between not taking any hormones and taking dangerous hormones. [495]

There is even evidence that sex hormones (testosterone, progesterone and estradiol) act on damaged nerves to help repair especially peripheral nerves. Sex hormones are probably protective from nerve damage (peripheral neuropathy) and may be beneficial in the aging process to prevent many degenerative diseases. [496]

Without hormones we cannot function well. But the key is which hormone replacement to use. Remember, the *Women's Health Initiative* used *Prempro*. It turned out to be a bad drug. But just because *Prempro* was bad, this indictment cannot be applied to bio-identical hormones no matter had hard Big Pharma tries to say, "*If ours is bad, theirs must be as bad.*" Not true.

Women are different from men. They are far more complicated and clearly respond differently to sex hormones. Do not believe that you don't need the complete complement of testosterone, progesterone and estradiol. ***Healthy women need all three!***

The Delivery System Makes the Difference

We talked briefly about the various delivery systems for hormones back in chapter 25. I would like to highlight some of the applications for women here.

Bio-identical hormones are vastly different and superior to the artificial synthetic hormones advertised by Big Pharma. However, the method of the delivery of bio-identical hormones is the key to achieving maximal benefit.

Bio-identical hormones may be found in various formulations: oral (by mouth) tablets, topical on the skin creams, topical patches, injections, vaginal creams, nasal sprays, buccal (placed on the gums) patches and pellets inserted under the skin. Each has its advantages and disadvantages.

Tablets—Estradiol

Any hormone tablet taken by mouth, including a bio-identical hormone, enters into a hostile environment. The stomach is very acidic. Acid in the stomach breaks down the tablet preparing it for digestion. Natural hormones produced in the body as well as bio-identical hormones are composed of a chain of molecules arranged in a specific order. If even one link in the chain is altered, it is no longer a functional hormone.

These changes from the original contribute to the vast number of side effects from such hormonal therapy. The long chain of molecules connected in a certain order is what makes hormones different from other chemicals. Such a hormone carries instructions from many different endocrine glands and cells all over the body. There are about fifty different hormones, all of which vary in structure, action and response controlling a variety of biological processes – including muscle growth, heart rate, menstrual cycles and hunger. If the hormone is changed in such a drastic manner, it cannot function correctly.

Creams—estrogen, progesterone and testosterone

Bio-identical creams are much safer with fewer side effects than oral tablets. At issue is the fact that you have to determine what the dose will be for that particular day.

This can be problematic in that the cream must be applied daily or twice a day to an area of the skin that is relatively thin. This may mean one has to carry the cream to work and apply it to a sensitive area at work. Usually creams are only effective for eight to ten hours. Often you begin noticing the loss of benefits of the hormone cream after ten hours. The symptoms return—hot flashes, night sweats, vaginal dryness, anxiety, and depression. Finally, a fairly large amount of cream is necessary to prevent menopausal symptoms.

Another negative effect of creams is the resistance to creams that are applied to the skin. Frequently the patient will notice the cream that gave marginal benefit when first started now doesn't help at all. This requires discontinuing the treatment for a month or so, or changing to a different treatment plan.

The Transdermal Patch—Alora, Climara, Estraderm, Estradiol Patch, Menostar, Minivelle, Vivelle, Vivelle-DotVivella-DOT

This medication is a female hormone estradiol. It is used by women to help reduce symptoms of menopause such as hot flashes, vaginal dryness and night sweats caused by the ovaries not producing enough estradiol. This type of hormonal treatment is intended for systemic (total body effects) use and not for a local problem such as only vaginal dryness.

The patch is usually replaced twice a week.

Side effects include:

- Skin redness/irritation at the application site
- Nausea/vomiting
- Bloating
- Breast tenderness
- Increased or new vaginal irritation/itching/odor/discharge
- Weight changes
- Mental/mood changes (such as depression, memory loss)
- Breast lumps
- Unusual vaginal bleeding (such as spotting, breakthrough, severe stomach pain, bleeding, prolonged/recurrent bleeding)
- Headache

The most common complaint with the use of the skin patches is the patch falling off in the shower. The second is the lack of relief of symptoms especially if they are severe, such as hot flashes and vaginal dryness.

Injections—testosterone

Hormonal liquids that are made for injections are not bio-identical. They may produce similar responses in the body, but they have an entirely different chemical makeup. The limitation of an injectable is the need for an injection every week to ten days. The usual response is a quick positive effect for three to four days by the male patient feeling more energy and sexual function. But within seven days a man will have a drop off of energy and feel the need for another injection.

What about the Men?

Low Testosterone in men will display itself with these symptoms:

- Low sex drive (libido)
- Erectile dysfunction
- Fatigue and poor energy level
- Difficulty concentrating
- Depression
- Irritability
- Low sense of well-being

More than 90% of men who are low in testosterone will experience benefits for the above symptoms if their testosterone level is brought to the level of a young man.

Many "failures" to testosterone therapy are a result of the patient not reaching blood levels of that of a much younger man. Reaching these levels may require large and more frequent injections than can be easily tolerated.

Concerns about Testosterone Replacement Therapy

Testosterone replacement seems to be generally safe. Some lists of side effects of testosterone therapy may include an enlarged prostate. You may read that

The prostate grows naturally under the stimulation of testosterone. For many men, their prostates grow larger as they age, squeezing the tube (urethra) carrying urine. The result is difficulty urinating. This condition, benign prostatic hypertrophy, can be made worse by testosterone therapy.

The truth is that an elevated estradiol in men is the reason for enlargement of the prostate in most men, not elevated testosterone. It is very difficult to find any well-done study that confirms that testosterone causes the prostate to enlarge.

Another misconception is that testosterone therapy may cause prostate cancer.

This is an "old wives tale" and not confirmed by the latest studies. Some experts suggest that low testosterone may actually contribute to the development of prostate cancer.

In his book, *Testosterone Syndrome,* Eugene Shippen, MD, states, there *is "no connection between testosterone levels and PSA levels. And, since PSA is the most reliable lab marker for prostate cancer risk, the absence of any relationship to testosterone is reassuring."* [497]

Finally, a Japanese study demonstrated that men with the least prostate enlargement had higher testosterone levels. And men with an enlarged prostate had higher levels of estrogen. [498]

Journal thoughts and questions:

_____

_____

_____

_____

_____

_____

_____

_____

_____

_____

_____

_____

_____

_____

_____

_____

_____

_____

_____

CHAPTER 51

What Are The Misconceptions Associated With Bhrt?

This chapter specifically addresses misinformation about *Bio-identical Hormone Replacement Therapy*. I will discuss thirteen specific charges made against BHRT ... and give some honest and forthright responses.

First, some background.

Sex hormones are very powerful substances that are made inside the body. Without these hormones, symptoms develop indicating that something is not right within our body. When a car will not start or the motor is missing it is usual to take it to a mechanic to correct the problem. The chances are the problem will not correct itself. The same is true with our body. A symptom is the body saying, *"Something is wrong."* The symptoms of hormone deficiency should not be ignored.

It is very true that when one is young, the body produces hormones naturally. An example is hormones produced by the ovaries primarily estradiol, progesterone and testosterone.

The ovaries contain follicles or sacs with an egg in each one. When a young girl reaches her first menstrual period, she may have as many as 500,000 follicles each with an egg inside. When she gets her first period, she may have had only 400 to 480 to actually mature and be expelled from the ovary. Each month one follicle (containing an egg) will mature – the first month from the right ovary and the next one from the left ovary.

During the early stage of a menstrual cycle, day one through five, her hormones are inactive allowing for menstruation. Two hormones produced by the pituitary, LH and FSH, stimulate the ovaries to secrete their own hormones, estradiol and progesterone.

By days five to seven of the cycle, a follicle will respond to the stimulation from the pituitary hormone FSH causing the follicle to mature. By day fourteen, the other pituitary hormone, LH, stimulates the ovary to release the egg from the follicle into the fallopian tube (ovulation). As the follicle is maturing, it produces a large amount of estradiol which causes the inside lining of the uterus to thicken, preparing for the egg that is coming down the fallopian tube to be implanted into the wall of the uterus if it is fertilized.

As the follicle ruptures releasing the egg, the empty sac remaining is called the corpus luteum. The corpus luteum immediately begins producing large amounts of progesterone and estradiol which cause the endometrial lining of the uterus to thicken even more preparing for implantation of a fertilized egg.

A fertilized egg passes through the fallopian tube and eventually imbeds itself into the uterus. A fertilized egg causes the release of human chorionic gonadotropin (HCG) which can be detected by a pregnancy test within seven days of pregnancy. HCG helps keep the corpus luteum viable which continues the production of estradiol and progesterone.

If the egg is not fertilized, the empty follicle sac in the ovary ceases the production of hormones which results in the shedding of the inside lining of the uterus called menstruation.

It is important to understand the above process that occurs monthly for forty years in order to comprehend what happens in perimenopause and menopause.

The balance between just the right amount of LH and FSH that stimulates the production of the follicle which produces just the right amount of estradiol and progesterone provides for good health. Without this balance between LH, FSH, progesterone and estradiol, the wheels begin coming off. Women recognize this by experiencing hot flashes, night sweats, vaginal dryness, depression, weight gain, fatigue, mental lapses, etc.

In women FSH stimulates the follicle to produce estradiol. If there are no more follicles to reach maturity there is no more production of estradiol. If there is no production of estradiol in the ovary the pituitary gland continues sending out more and more FSH in the serum trying to persuade the ovaries to produce more estradiol. If the patient's FSH begins to rise as measured by blood tests this is an indication that she is entering into menopause. Normal FSH in a woman twenty years old is around 1 to 4 mIU/mL, but it will rise to 10 mIU/ml and continue over the next few months to rise to 60 or 80 or even above 100 mIU/mL.

This is the reason checking the serum for these hormones is essential. These hormones cannot be accurately checked by hair analysis or sputum analysis.

So what happens to the 495,600 follicles that are not used? Little by little the follicles in the ovaries become resistant to the stimulatory effects of FSH. The follicles never mature and will atrophy by the time of perimenopause. Because a follicle fails to develop, there is less production of estradiol. As estradiol declines FSH increases. This increase in FSH found in the serum is the body's effort to stimulate the follicles in the ovaries to produce more estradiol and progesterone as it did before.

As the old adage says, *"It's like beating a dead horse."* At this point the ovaries are not going to respond to the stimulus of FSH.

As the ovaries stop producing estradiol, the body increases its production of a different type of estrogen, estrone. Estrone has been shown to increase the risk of breast cancer. This type of estrogen is not produced in the ovaries but in fat cells and the adrenal glands. The ovaries continue producing testosterone, but in small amounts.

Testosterone production in the ovaries begins to decline in the late twenties or thirties. This decline is not sudden, as is the case with estradiol and progesterone. The decline in testosterone may contribute to a gradual increase in weight and a decrease in energy and sex drive in women.

Even though estradiol production in the ovaries may continue until women reach their mid-forties or early fifties, the production of progesterone begins to decline in the mid-thirties. A thirty-five-year-old woman may have only twenty-five percent of the progesterone she had when she was twenty.

From her first period until the mid-thirties, there is a balance between estrogen and progesterone production. However, as progesterone declines and estrogen production remains relatively normal, there becomes an imbalance of hormones called estrogen dominance or perhaps more accurately called progesterone deficiency.

This causes a host of symptoms during this period: [499]

- Excess vaginal bleeding
- Premenstrual syndrome (PMS)
- Water retention
- Depression
- Anxiety
- Osteoporosis
- Forgetfulness
- Stroke
- Fibrocystic breast disease
- Breast tenderness
- Migraine headaches
- Uterine fibroids
- Infertility
- Decreased libido
- Increased chance of breast cancer [500]

The above symptoms can be easily remedied by the addition of natural progesterone for two or three weeks of the menstrual cycle.

Thirteen Misconceptions about BHRT

1. Some argue that menopausal symptoms can be cured with nutritional balance.

While good nutrition is certainly beneficial to overall health, eating a better diet is not going to cause the ovaries to produce more estradiol or progesterone.

As discussed above, the follicles in the ovaries produce estradiol secondary to the stimulation by FSH. As the follicle ruptures, at which time it is now known as the corpus luteum, progesterone is produced.

There is not any credible scientific evidence that eating a good diet will cause the ovaries or any other part of the body to continue producing estradiol and progesterone.

2. It has been said that hormone therapy can cause cancer.

This statement begs for clarification. There is an abundance of evidence that synthetic hormones like *Premarin* can cause heart attacks, strokes, blood clots and heart attacks. When synthetic progesterone look-alike *Provera* is added to *Premarin*, as in *Prempro*, there is a marked increase in cancer especially of the breast.

Since there is very little production of estradiol after menopause, estrone becomes the predominant estrogen which stimulates the type of breast cells that are more likely to become cancerous. No one can predict that a woman will not develop breast cancer.

However, we know that women in their younger years have very little chance of breast cancer even though they have an abundance of estradiol. But we also know that when natural hormones decline in the late forties and fifties, there is an increased risk of breast cancer.

The key is to supplement with natural bio-identical estradiol and the correct balance of natural progesterone.

3.   Some point out that bio-identical hormones are delivered in ways that are totally unnatural.

While a majority of hormones (both synthetic and bio-identical) are far from natural, the next question would be, *"How can bio-identical hormones be delivered in the closest way possible to nature?"*

It has been pointed out that our bodies produce hormones as they are needed using a complex feedback system that involves the pituitary gland and the hypothalamus. How true this is. The body is magnificent. But when the body stops producing these wonderful hormones, science has produced the next best solution, bio-identical hormones.

The advantages and disadvantages of each different delivery system have been presented elsewhere—oral, injections, buccal, creams, skin patches, vaginal creams, and pellets. None is perfect. You have to choose which is best for yourself.

But to do nothing because it is not exactly like it was when the ovaries were working is like denying a cardiac pacemaker when the heart is beating too slowly, or to refuse an artificial limb after an amputation, or to not take insulin injections for diabetes because it is not made by the patient himself.

4.   It has been pointed out that hormone replacement seriously upsets the delicate hormone feedback systems in the body and may do more harm than good.

My question is, *"Is not this delicate hormone feedback system seriously upset when the ovaries stop producing estradiol or progesterone that has been part of her body for forty years or the testicles stop producing testosterone?"*

An obvious example of a seriously upset biofeedback system would be the elevation of FSH from 4 to 100 mIU/mL with the decline of estradiol. When bio-identical estradiol is administered FSH will decline to normal levels.

Even though the body may not produce its own hormones as it did when you were younger, this does not mean that the body has lost its ability to monitor itself and adjust the many body systems when bio-identical hormones are administered.

5.   It has been written that hormone therapy rarely addresses the root cause of illness. It treats mainly symptoms.

It has been suggested that hormone imbalances include nutrient deficiencies, toxic metal excesses, toxic chemicals and the effects of radiation, emotional imbalances and stress from other causes.

Some say that the only time hormone replacement addresses a root cause is when the gland that produces the hormone has been surgically removed or is damaged so that it cannot function.

So is it appropriate to replace lost hormones if the gland that produced these hormones has been removed, but not if the gland simply stops producing estradiol and progesterone because of menopause? I say yes.

Whatever the reason the patient has lost the normal amount of hormones he/she had at the prime of life, these hormones have to be replaced.

6.   Some believe bio-identical hormone therapy does not address the root causes of menopause.

These critics believe that women who are having menopausal symptoms have nutrient deficiencies, toxic metal excesses, toxic chemicals and the effects of radiation, emotional imbalances and stress from other causes.

One hundred percent of women will go through menopause at about the same general time period. It seems strange that these women have been able to avoid all these nutrient deficiencies and toxic chemicals until they turn forty-five, and then suddenly all these environmental hazards occur to one hundred percent of these women. Coincidence? I don't think so. Bio-identical hormone replacement therapy addresses the root cause of loss of hormones by replacing lost hormones.

7.   Some contend that when men or women go through andropause or menopause, the body handles this change of life very well.

In other words, they argue that menopause should not be a disease that requires treatment. It has been suggested that hot flashes, vaginal dryness or other symptoms are caused by the adrenal glands and perhaps thyroid.

But, when a woman is having hot flashes, vaginal dryness, night sweats, low libido, depression, poor sleep, etc., wouldn't it be natural for a doctor to first think that she may have a deficiency of the sex hormones that have been part of her life for four decades?

8.   An argument may be made that hormone replacement therapy often masks underlying problems such as heavy metal toxicity, nutrient deficiencies or chemical toxicity.

There is a saying in medicine, *"When you hear hoof beats, think first of horses, not elephants."* In other words, when she is at the age of menopause, her serum estradiol, testosterone and progesterone levels are low and she has the typical symptoms of menopause, think menopause first.

It may be appropriate to test for heavy metal toxicity, nutrient deficiencies or chemical toxicity, but treating menopausal symptoms has nothing to do with masking underlying problems.

9.   You may have read that even bio-identical hormones are toxic.

If you accept the definition that toxicity is the degree to which a substance can damage an organism, certainly most anything taken in excess can be toxic – including bio-identical hormones. That is precisely why blood work along with a careful history of the patient and monitoring symptoms is crucial to proper care of the patient being treated with bio-identical hormones.

10. An ambiguous statement may be made that one cannot provide the correct dosage of replacement hormones.

It is impossible to duplicate the hormones that anyone had when they were twenty with natural hormone replacement therapy of any kind.

To understand the ignorance of this statement, one has to know that the body changes many hormones back and forth from DHEA to progesterone to testosterone to estradiol and back again to a previous hormone as the feedback mechanisms see fit.

In other words, just because the ovaries have stopped producing estradiol and progesterone and have gradually reduced the production of testosterone does not mean the feedback loops that control the delicate balance of hormones in the body have stopped functioning.

If one hormone is administered, the body has the ability to convert that hormone into another as the body demands. If the correct dose of replacement hormones upsets the body severely, how much more would the body be upset from a complete absence of these life-giving natural hormones?

11. It has been estimated that a hormone's metabolic effect is what is most important, not its serum, urine or saliva level. A hair mineral analysis may give more information about the circulating hormone.

By this argument a patient should request a hair mineral analysis for a hormone's metabolic effect rather than checking the actual circulating hormone in the serum.

Now does that make sense to you?

A hair has been dead for weeks. But a doctor is going to use the analysis of minerals instead of the actual hormone that is circulating throughout the body at that moment? Some people will believe anything!

12. Hormone replacement therapy may be costly.

Some point out that the costs include the hormones and repeated testing and that you may need to use hormone replacement therapy for years. An individual may become dependent on the tests and doctors. That can get *expensive!*

Some suggest that it is less expensive to turn to nutritional balancing instead.

It is difficult to imagine how nutritional balancing is going to replace testosterone, estradiol and progesterone, all extremely powerful hormones essential for good health.

The question really is, *"How important is our health?"* With all the positive benefits laid out in this book, isn't it worth it? Ask any of my patients. They will tell you the honest truth about what matters most.

13. If the hormones are not produced naturally in the body, then any replacement therapy should be suspect.

To deny a hormone-deficient patient *Bio-identical Hormone Replacement Therapy* because hormones are supposed to be produced within the body may be the height of incompetence. If one argues that blood pressure is supposed to be controlled within the body, does that mean treating hypertension should be banned.

A patient should be able to produce antibodies to fight off pneumonia. Therefore administering an antibiotic is inappropriate. The list goes on and on.

But even the concept that hormones are supposed to be produced within the body is bogus because as time goes on the one constant is that hormones decline as we age. The same denial of the true is found when one says the only natural approach to hormone correction is to rebuild the organ or gland that produces the hormone.

The obvious question is, *"How would you propose to rebuild the ovaries or testicles in a patient in which these organs stop functioning or are functioning at only ten percent of what they were forty years before?"*

Journal thoughts and questions:

_____

_____

_____

_____

_____

_____

_____

_____

_____

_____

_____

_____

_____

_____

_____

_____

_____

_____

CHAPTER 52

A Final Appeal

This has been a long journey. Thank you, my friend, for taking the journey with me. **I've shared with you my passion** for how *Bio-identical Hormone Replacement Therapy* can make a difference in your life. The lifesaving truth about BHRT is that they can indeed make you feel younger, stronger and sexier.

I've laid out the truthful facts:

- Synthetic hormones pose a grave danger to our health.
- Big Pharma has an agenda that puts profits first and disregards patients' health.
- I've shown the research that BHRT is safe, beneficial and appropriate.
- I've told you many stories of patients whose lives have been changed because of BHRT. Their health has improved, and perhaps most importantly, their outlook and emotional health have benefitted as well.

It's at this point that **I must issue a challenge to you:**

What are you going to do with what you have heard and read?

- Will you put this book on your bookshelf and say, *"That was informative?"* but do nothing else? If so, you are cheating your health – and missing out on a wonderful opportunity.
- Do you still have questions? Will you investigate further? Good for you!
- That's one reason I've included all the endnotes in this book. Do your own research – if that's what is needed. Talk with others who have had BHRT. Talk with BHRT practitioners.
- Are you ready to take that step and receive BHRT if tests show that's what you need? Call a BHRT physician today.

If you are looking for a physician who specializes in natural *Bio-identical Hormone Replacement Therapy,* a good first place is to find a doctor who is a member of the world's largest association of such physicians, *the American Association of Anti-Aging Medicine* (A4M).

This organization was established in 1992 and now has over 26,000 members including physicians, health practitioners, scientists, governmental officials, and members of the general public, representing over 110 nations.

A4M is a global medical education provider. Through the *Anti-Aging Academy,* Anti-Aging breakthroughs are provided, practical knowledge is shared, treatment modalities and skills for the practicing are taught to physician and health practitioners through live conferences and online programming.

Simply go to their web site (www.a4m.com) and click on Directory and type in your zip code or your country, state and city to find someone who understands what this book teaches.

Don't wait. Don't let another week ... or another month ... or, God forbid, another year go by without taking action.

Would you make a phone call if you were bleeding profusely? Would you rush to the emergency room if you were having a heart attack? Would you call your doctor if your blood pressure skyrocketed?

If you suspect that BHRT is right for you, make that phone call. Do it today. Don't wait.

You'll never regret that decision.

Journal thoughts and questions:

_____

_____

_____

_____

_____

_____

_____

_____

_____

_____

_____

_____

_____

_____

_____

_____

_____

_____

ENDNOTES

Chapter One

[1] Lab values showed loss of hormones with a low total testosterone of 9.1 ng/dL (normal 60 to 90 ng/dL), estradiol of 12.6 pg/ml (normal 100 pg/ml or higher), very high follicular stimulating hormone 63 mIU/mL (normal 1 to 4 mIU/mL) and progesterone was .8 ng/ml (normal 15 to 25 mg/ml).

[2] Resnick SM, Espeland MA, Jaramillo SA, et al. Postmenopausal hormone therapy and regional brain volumes: the WHIMS-MRI Study. Neurology. 2009; 72:135-142.

[3] Estrogen protects neuronal cells from amyloid beta-induced apoptosis via regulation of mitochondrial proteins and function. Jon Nilsen, Shuhu Chen, Ronald W Irwin, Sean Iwamoto and Roberta D Brinton Department of Pharmacology and Pharmaceutical Sciences, School of Pharmacy, University of Southern California, Los Angeles, California, 2006.

[4] Rocca WA, Bower JH, Maraganore DM, et al. Increased risk of cognitive impairment or dementia in women who underwent oophorectomy before menopause. Neurology: 2007; 69:1074-1083.

[5] Rocca WA, Bower JH, Maraganore DM, et al. Increased risk of Parkinsonism in women who underwent oophorectomy before menopause. Neurology 2007.

[6] Rocca WA, Grissardt BR, de Andrade M, Malkasian GD, Melton LJ, 3rd. Survival patterns after oophorectomy in premenopausal women: a population-based cohort study. Lancet Oncol. 2006; 7:821-828.

[7] Hogervorst E, Williams J, Budge M, Riedel W, Jolles J. The nature of the effect of female gonadal hormone replacement therapy on cognitive function in postmenopausal women: a meta-analysis. Neuroscience. 2000; 101:485-512.

[8] Gleason CE, Schmitz TW, Hess T, et al. Hormone effects of fMRI and cognitive measures of encoding: importance of hormone preparation. Neurology. 2006; 67:2039-2041.

[9] Rasgon NL, Magnusson C, Johansson AL, Pedersen NL, Elman S, Gatz M. Endogenous and exogenous hormone exposure and risk of cognitive impairment in Swedish twins: a preliminary study. Psychoneuroendocrinology: 2005; 30:558-567.

[10] Schumaker M, Guennoun R, Ghoumari A, et al. Novel perspectives for progesterone in HRT, with special reference to the nervous system. Endocr Rev. 2007; 28:387-439.

[11] Stay Young & Sexy with Bio-identical Hormone Replacement: The Science Explained by Dr. Jonathan V. Wright, Lane Lenard, PhD, SmartPublications, copyright 2010. Page 83.

Chapter Two

[12] As estradiol drops, the follicle stimulating hormone (FSH) increases. This hormone is secreted from the pituitary gland to stimulate the ovaries to produce more estradiol. The normal FSH of a young female may be 1 to 4 mIU/mL, but with the loss of ovarian production of estradiol, the FSH will increase to 60 to 80 and sometimes over 100 mIU/mL – demonstrating that the pituitary is trying to stimulate the ovaries to produce more estradiol. When estradiol is administered to such a

menopausal patient her FSH will gradually decline to 10 mIU/mL or lower as her estradiol increases to 80 pg/ml or even 100 pg/ml.

[13] Testosterone Syndrome: The Critical Factor for Energy, Health, and Sexuality—Reversing the Male Menopause Eugene Shippen, MD and William Fryer Publisher M. Evans copyright 2007.

[14] Ibid.

Chapter Three

[15] Gobinet J, Poujol N, Sultan C. Molecular action of androgens. Mol Cell Endocrinol. 2002; 198(1–2):15–24.

[16] The Role of Androgens and Estrogens on Healthy Aging and Longevity J Gerontol A Biol Sci Med Sci. Nov 2012; 67(11): 1140–1152. Published online Mar 26, 2012. Astrid M. Horstman, E. Lichar Dillon, Randall J. Urban, and Melinda Sheffield-Moore.

[17] The Hormone Solution, Stay Younger Longer with Natural Hormone and Nutrition Therapies Thierry Hertoghe, MD Copyright 2002 Three Rivers Press page 17.

[18] Ageless The Naked Truth about Bio-identical Hormones, Three Rivers Press, copyright 2006.

[19] Anxiety, Hypnotic Medications May Triple Mortality Risk, Deborah Brauser, British Medical Journal BMJ Published on line March 19, 2014.

Chapter Four

[20] Heiss G, Wallace R, Anderson GL, et al. Health risks and benefits 3 years after stopping randomized treatment with estrogen and progestin. JAMA. 2004; 291:1701-1712.

[21] Stay Young & Sexy with Bio-identical Hormone Replacement: The Science Explained by Dr. Jonathan V. Wright, Lane Lenard, PhD, SmartPublications, copyright 2010.

[22] Berger L. Hormone Therapy: The Dust I Still Settling. The New York Times. June 6, 2004.

[23] Radvin PM, Cronin KA, Howlander N, et al. The decrease in breast-cancer Incidence in 203 in the United States. New England Journal of Medicine 2007; 356:1670-1674.

[24] Glass AG, Lacey JV, Carreon JD, Hoover RN. Breast cancer incidence, 1980-2006: Combined role of menopausal hormone therapy, screening mammography, and estrogen receptor status. Journal of Cancer Inst. 2007; 99:1152-1161.

[25] Anderson GL, Limacher M, Assaf AR, et al. Effects of conjugated equine estrogen in postmenopausal women with hysterectomy: the Women's Health Initiative randomized controlled trial. JAMA. 2003; 289:2663-2672.

[26] Premarin (conjugated estrogen tablets). Wyeth Pharmaceuticals, Inc. 2004; Philadelphia, PA 19101: Full Prescribing Information.

[27] Crandall C, Low-dose estrogen therapy for menopausal women: a review of efficacy and safety. Journal of Women's Health (Larchmt). 2003; 12:723-747.

[28] Head KA, Estriol: safety and efficacy. Alternative Medical Review: 1998; 3:101-113.

Chapter Five

[29] Mäkinen J., Jarvisalo M., Pollanen P., Perheentupa A., Irjala K., Koskenvuo M., Mäkinen J., Huhtaniemi I., Raitakari O.. Increased carotid atherosclerosis in andropausal middle-aged men. J Am Coll Cardiol. 2005;45: 1603–1608.

[30] Traish AM, Guay AT, Feeley R., Saad F.. The dark side of testosterone deficiency: I. Metabolic syndrome and erectile dysfunction. J Androl. 2009a;30(1): 10–22.

[31] What You Must Know About Women's Hormones" Pamela Wartian Smith, MD., MPH Square One Publishers copyright 2010 page 6.

Chapter Six

[32] "Menopause and Postmenopause" Doctors Lauren Nathan and Howard Judd, chapter 59.

[33] The Hormone Solution, Stay Younger Longer with Natural Hormone and Nutrition Therapies Thierry Hertoghe, MD Copyright 2002 Three Rivers Press page 22.

[34] The Hormone Solution, Stay Younger Longer with Natural Hormone and Nutrition Therapies Thierry Hertoghe, MD Copyright 2002 Three Rivers Press.

[35] Stay Young and Sexy with Bio-identical Hormone Replacement page 110 Jonathon Wright, MD and Simon, JA Testosterone therapy in women: its role in the management of hypoactive sexual desire disorder. International Journal of Impotence Research 2007; 19; 458-463. Page 17.

Chapter Eight

[36] For more information, see http://www.pcab.org/consumers

Chapter Nine

[37] Mudali S, Dobs AS. Effects of testosterone on body composition of the aging male. Mech Ageing Dev. 2004; 125(4):297–304.)

[38] Ferrando AA, Sheffield-Moore M, Paddon-Jones D, Wolfe RR, Urban RJ. Differential anabolic effects of testosterone and amino acid feeding in older men. J Clin Endocrinol Metab. 2003; 88(1):358–362.

Page ST, Amory JK, Bowman FD, et al. Exogenous testosterone (T) alone or with finasteride increases physical performance, grip strength, and lean body mass in older men with low serum T. J Clin Endocrinol Metab. 2005; 90(3):1502–1510.

Harman SM, Blackman MR. The effects of growth hormone and sex steroid on lean body mass, fat mass, muscle strength, cardiovascular endurance and adverse events in healthy elderly women and men. Horm Res. 2003; 60 (suppl 1):121–124.

Wittert GA, Chapman IM, Haren MT, Mackintosh S, Coates P, Morley JE. Oral testosterone supplementation increases muscle and decreases fat mass in healthy elderly males with low-normal gonadal status. J Gerontol A Biol Sci Med Sci. 2003; 58(7):618–625.

Ferrando AA, Sheffield-Moore M, Yeckel CW, et al. Testosterone administration to older men improves muscle function: molecular and physiological mechanisms. Am J Physiol Endocrinol Metab. 2002; 282(3):E601–E607.

Urban RJ, Bodenburg YH, Gilkison C, et al. Testosterone administration to elderly men increases skeletal muscle strength and protein synthesis. Am J Physiol. 1995; 269(5 Pt 1):E820–E826.

Bhasin S, Storer TW, Berman N, et al. Testosterone replacement increases fat-free mass and muscle size in hypogonadal men. J Clin Endocrinol Metab. 1997; 82(2):407–413.

Kenny AM, Prestwood KM, Gruman CA, Marcello KM, Raisz LG. Effects of transdermal testosterone on bone and muscle in older men with low bioavailable testosterone levels. J Gerontol Med Sci. 2001; 56(5):M266–M272.

Bhasin S, Storer TW, Berman N, et al. The effects of supraphysiologic doses of testosterone on muscle size and strength in normal men. N Engl J Med. 1996; 335(1):1–7.

Dillon EL, Durham WJ, Urban RJ, Sheffield-Moore M. Hormone treatment and muscle anabolism during aging: androgens. Clin Nutr. 2010; 29(6):697–700.

Urban RJ. Effects of testosterone and growth hormone on muscle function. J Lab Clin Med. 1999; 134(1):7–10.

[39] Worboys S, Kotsopoulos D, Teede H, McGrath B, Davis SR. Evidence that parenteral testosterone therapy may improve endothelium-dependent and -independent vasodilation in postmenopausal women already receiving estrogen. J Clin Endocrinol Metab. 2001; 86(1):158–161.

[40] Burckart K, Beca S, Urban RJ, Sheffield-Moore M. Pathogenesis of muscle wasting in cancer cachexia: targeted anabolic and anticatabolic therapies. Curr Opin Clin Nutr Metab Care. 2010; 13(4):410–416.

[41] Canguven O, Albayrak S. Do low testosterone levels contribute to the pathogenesis of asthma? Med Hypotheses. 2011; 76(4):585–588.

Mason A, Wong SC, McGrogan P, Ahmed SF. Effect of testosterone therapy for delayed growth and puberty in boys with inflammatory bowel disease. Horm Res Paediatr. 2011; 75(1):8–13.

Cutolo M. Androgens in rheumatoid arthritis: when are they effective? Arthritis Res Ther. 2009; 11(5):126.

[42] Maggio M, Lauretani F, Ceda GP, et al. Relationship between low levels of anabolic hormones and 6-year mortality in older men: the aging in the Chianti Area (InCHIANTI) study. Arch Intern Med. 2007; 167(20):2249–2254.

[43] Laughlin GA, Barrett-Connor E, Bergstrom J. Low serum testosterone and mortality in older men. J Clin Endocrinol Metab. 2008; 93(1):68–75.

Khaw KT, Dowsett M, Folkerd E, et al. Endogenous testosterone and mortality due to all causes, cardiovascular disease, and cancer in men: European prospective investigation into cancer in Norfolk (EPIC-Norfolk) Prospective Population Study. Circulation. 2007; 116(23):2694–2701.

Shores MM, Matsumoto AM, Sloan KL, Kivlahan DR. Low serum testosterone and mortality in male veterans. Arch Intern Med. 2006; 166(15):1660–1665.

Jones TH, Saad F. The effects of testosterone on risk factors for, and the mediators of, the atherosclerotic process. Atherosclerosis. 2009; 207(2):318–327.

[44] Bonora E, Kiechl S, Willeit J, et al. Insulin resistance as estimated by homeostasis model assessment predicts incident symptomatic cardiovascular disease in Caucasian subjects from the general population: the Bruneck study. Diabetes Care. 2007; 30(2):318–324.

de Simone G, Devereux RB, Chinali M, et al. Prognostic impact of metabolic syndrome by different definitions in a population with high prevalence of obesity and diabetes: the Strong Heart Study. Diabetes Care. 2007; 30(7):1851–1856.

Saely CH, Aczel S, Marte T, Langer P, Hoefle G, Drexel H. The metabolic syndrome, insulin resistance, and cardiovascular risk in diabetic and nondiabetic patients. J Clin Endocrinol Metab. 2005; 90(10):5698–5703.

Traish AM, Saad F, Feeley RJ, Guay A. The dark side of testosterone deficiency: III. Cardiovascular disease. J Androl. 2009; 30(5):477–494.

[45] Stay Young and Sexy with Bio-identical Hormone Replacement page 110 Jonathon Wright, MD and Simon, JA Testosterone therapy in women: its role in the management of hypoactive sexual desire disorder. International Journal of Impotence Research 2007; 19; 458-463. Page 36.

[46] Stay Young and Sexy with Bio-identical Hormone Replacement page 110 Jonathon Wright, MD and Simon, JA Testosterone therapy in women: its role in the management of hypoactive sexual desire disorder. International Journal of Impotence Research 2007; 19; 458-463. Page 38.

[47] Katzenellenbogen BS, Montano MM, Le Goff P, et al. Antiestrogens: mechanisms and actions in target cells. J Steroid Biochem Mol Biol. 1995; 53(1–6):387–393.

[48] Kendall B, Eston R. Exercise-induced muscle damage and the potential protective role of estrogen. Sports Med. 2002; 32(2):103–123.

Tiidus PM. Can estrogens diminish exercise induced muscle damage? Can J Appl Physiol. 1995; 20(1):26–38.

Tiidus PM. Oestrogen and sex influence on muscle damage and inflammation: evidence from animal models. Curr Opin Clin Nutr Metab Care. 2001; 4(6):509–513.

Vina J, Sastre J, Pallardo FV, Gambini J, Borras C. Role of mitochondrial oxidative stress to explain the different longevity between genders: protective effect of estrogens. Free Radic Res. 2006; 40(12):1359–1365.

[49] MacNeil LG, Baker SK, Stevic I, Tarnopolsky MA. 17beta-estradiol attenuates exercise-induced neutrophil infiltration in men. Am J Physiol Regul Integr Comp Physiol.

[50] Calmels P, Vico L, Alexandre C, Minaire P. Cross-sectional study of muscle strength and bone mineral density in a population of 106 women between the ages of 44 and 87 years: relationship with age and menopause. Eur J Appl Physiol Occup Physiol. 1995; 70(2):180–186.

[51] Carville SF, Rutherford OM, Newham DJ. Power output, isometric strength and steadiness in the leg muscles of pre- and postmenopausal women; the effects of hormone replacement therapy. Eur J Appl Physiol. 2006; 96(3):292–298.

Cooper R, Mishra G, Clennell S, Guralnik J, Kuh D. Menopausal status and physical performance in midlife: findings from a British birth cohort study. Menopause. 2008; 15(6):1079–1085.

Greeves JP, Cable NT, Reilly T, Kingsland C. Changes in muscle strength in women following the menopause: a longitudinal assessment of the efficacy of hormone replacement therapy. Clin Sci (Lond) 1999; 97(1):79–84.

Kurina LM, Gulati M, Everson-Rose SA, et al. The effect of menopause on grip and pinch strength: results from the Chicago, Illinois, site of the Study of Women's Health Across the Nation. Am J Epidemiol. 2004; 160(5):484–491.

Samson MM, Meeuwsen IB, Crowe A, Dessens JA, Duursma SA, Verhaar HJ. Relationships between physical performance measures, age, height and body weight in healthy adults. Age Ageing. 2000; 29(3):235–242.

Skelton DA, Phillips SK, Bruce SA, Naylor CH, Woledge RC. Hormone replacement therapy increases isometric muscle strength of adductor pollicis in post-menopausal women. Clin Sci (Lond) 1999; 96(4):357–364.

52 Phillips SK, Rook KM, Siddle NC, Bruce SA, Woledge RC. Muscle weakness in women occurs at an earlier age than in men, but strength is preserved by hormone replacement therapy. Clin Sci (Lond) 1993; 84(1):95–98.

53 Sipila S. Body composition and muscle performance during menopause and hormone replacement therapy. J Endocrinol Invest. 2003; 26(9):893–901.

54 Sipila S. Body composition and muscle performance during menopause and hormone replacement therapy. J Endocrinol Invest. 2003; 26(9):893–901.

55 Grumbach MM, Auchus RJ. Estrogen: consequences and implications of human mutations in synthesis and action. J Clin Endocrinol Metab. 1999; 84(12):4677–4694.

Jankowska EA, Rozentryt P, Ponikowska B, et al. Circulating estradiol and mortality in men with systolic chronic heart failure. JAMA. 2009; 301(18):1892–1901.

56 Jankowska EA, Rozentryt P, Ponikowska B, et al. Circulating estradiol and mortality in men with systolic chronic heart failure. JAMA. 2009; 301(18):1892–1901.

Arnlov J, Pencina MJ, Amin S, et al. Endogenous sex hormones and cardiovascular disease incidence in men. Ann Intern Med. 2006; 145(3):176–184.

Abbott RD, Launer LJ, Rodriguez BL, et al. Serum estradiol and risk of stroke in elderly men. Neurology. 2007; 68(8):563–568.

Pinkerton JV, Stovall DW. Reproductive aging, menopause, and health outcomes. Ann N Y Acad Sci. 2010; 1204:169–178.

57 Birkhauser MH. Quality of life and sexuality issues in aging women. Climacteric. 2009; 12(suppl 1):52–57.

58 What You Must Know About Women's Hormones" Pamela Wartian Smith, MD., MPH Square One Publishers copyright 2010 page 5.

Chapter Eleven

59 Bio-identical Hormone Therapy Mayo Clinic Procedure July 2011.

60 The Hormone Solution, Stay Younger Longer with Natural Hormone and Nutrition Therapies Thierry Hertoghe, MD Copyright 2002 Three Rivers Press.

Chapter Twelve

61 Heiss G, Wallace R, Anderson GL, et al. Health risks and benefits 3 years after stopping randomized treatment with estrogen and progestin. JAMA 2008; 299:1036-1045.

62 What You Must Know About Women's Hormones" Pamela Wartian Smith, MD., MPH Square One Publishers copyright 2010.

63 Chlebowski RT, Hendrix SL, Langer RD, Stefanick ML, Gass M, Lane D, Rodabough RJ, Gilligan MA, Cyr MG, Thomson CA, Khandekar J, Petrovitch H,

McTiernan A. Influence of estrogen plus progestin on breast cancer and mammography in healthy postmenopausal women: the Women's Health Initiative Randomized Trial. JAMA. 2003; 289(24):3243–3253.

[64] Ross RK, Paganini-Hill A, Wan PC, Pike MC. Effect of hormone replacement therapy on breast cancer risk: estrogen versus estrogen plus progestin. J Natl Cancer Inst. 2000; 92(4):328–332.

Chen CL, Weiss NS, Newcomb P, Barlow W, White E. Hormone replacement therapy in relation to breast cancer. JAMA. 2002; 287(6):734–741.

Schairer C, Lubin J, Troisi R, Sturgeon S, Brinton L, Hoover R. Menopausal estrogen and estrogen-progestin replacement therapy and breast cancer risk. JAMA. 2000; 283(4):485–491.

Magnusson C, Baron JA, Correia N, Bergstrom R, Adami HO, Persson I. Breast-cancer risk following long-term oestrogen- and oestrogen-progestin-replacement therapy. Int J Cancer. 1999; 81(3):339–344.

Stahlberg C, Pedersen AT, Lynge E, Andersen ZJ, Keiding N, Hundrup YA, Obel EB, Ottesen B. Increased risk of breast cancer following different regimens of hormone replacement therapy frequently used in Europe. Int J Cancer. 2004; 109(5):721–727.

Kerlikowske K, Miglioretti DL, Ballard-Barbash R, Weaver DL, Buist DS, Barlow WE, Cutter G, Geller BM, Yankaskas B, Taplin SH, Carney PA. Prognostic characteristics of breast cancer among postmenopausal hormone users in a screened population. J Clin Oncol. 2003; 21(23):4314–4321.

Willett WC, Colditz G, Stampfer M. Postmenopausal estrogensopposed, unopposed, or none of the above. JAMA. 2000; 283(4):534–535.

Bakken K, Alsaker E, Eggen AE, Lund E. Hormone replacement therapy and incidence of hormone-dependent cancers in the Norwegian women and cancer study. Int J Cancer. 2004; 112(1):130–134.

[65] Foidart JM, Colin C, Denoo X, Desreux J, Beliard A, Fournier S, de Lignieres B. Estradiol and progesterone regulate the proliferation of human breast epithelial cells. Fertil Steril. 1998; 69(5):963–969.

[66] Grattarola R. The premenstrual endometrial pattern of women with breast cancer. A study of progestational activity. Cancer. 1964; 17(5):1119–1122.

[67] Bentel JM, Birrell SN, Pickering MA, Holds DJ, Horsfall DJ, Tilley WD. Androgen receptor agonist activity of the synthetic progestin, medroxyprogesterone acetate, in human breast cancer cells. Mol Cell Endocrinol. 1999; 154(1–2):11–20.

Kaaks R. Nutrition, hormones, and breast cancer: is insulin the missing link? Cancer Causes Contr. 1996; 7(6):605–625.

Progestins and progesterone in hormone replacement therapy and the risk of breast cancer Carlo Campagnoli, Françoise Clavel-Chapelon, Rudolf Kaaks, Clementina Peris, and Franco Berrino, J Steroid Biochem Mol Biol. Author manuscript; available in PMC 2007 September 25. Published in final edited form as: J Steroid Biochem Mol Biol. 2005 July; 96(2): 95–108.

[68] Campagnoli C, Biglia N, Peris C, Sismondi P. Potential impact on breast cancer risk of circulating insulin-like growth factor I modifications induced by oral HRT in menopause. Gynecol Endocrinol. 1995; 9(1):67–74.

[69] Fournier A, Berrino F, Riboli E, Avenel V, Clavel-Chapelon F. Breast cancer risk in relation to different types of hormone replacement therapy in the E3N-EPIC cohort. Int J Cancer. 2005; 114:448–454.

[70] Progestins and progesterone in hormone replacement therapy and the risk of breast cancer Carlo Campagnoli, Françoise Clavel-Chapelon, Rudolf Kaaks, Clementina Peris, and Franco Berrino, J Steroid Biochem Mol Biol. Author manuscript; available in PMC 2007 September 25. Published in final edited form as: J Steroid Biochem Mol Biol. 2005 July; 96(2): 95–108.

[71] What You Must Know About Women's Hormones. Pamela Warten Smith, MD, MPH Square One Publishers copyright 2010.

Chapter Thirteen

[72] She had a low total testosterone of 8.2 ng/dL (normal 60 to 80 ng/dL), estradiol of 11.4 pg/ml (normal 100 pg/ml or higher), follicular stimulating hormone 49 mIU/mL (normal 1 to 4 mIU/mL) and progesterone was .6 ng/ml (normal 15 to 25 mg/ml).

[73] MPA Medroxy-Progesterone Acetate Contributes to Much Poor Advice for Women by Cynthia L. Bethea Copyright © 2011 by The Endocrine Society.

Chapter Fourteen

[74] Gobinet J, Poujol N, Sultan C. Molecular action of androgens. Mol Cell Endocrinol. 2002; 198(1–2):15–24.

[75] The Role of Androgens and Estrogens on Healthy Aging and Longevity J Gerontol A Biol Sci Med Sci. Nov 2012; 67(11): 1140–1152. Published online Mar 26, 2012. Astrid M. Horstman, E. Lichar Dillon, Randall J. Urban, and Melinda Sheffield-Moore.

[76] www.healthline.com/health/low-testosterone/effects-on-body

[77] This is not a prescription drug. These natural supplements come from Harmony Spring out of Tampa, Florida. Check them out at www.harmonyspring.com. Their phone number is 888-515-1885.

Chapter Sixteen

[78] DeKosky ST, Kaufer DI, Hamilton RL, Wolk DA, Lopez OL. The dementias. In: Bradley WG, Daroff RB, Fenichel GM, Jankovic J, eds. Bradley: Neurology in Clinical Practice. 5th ed. Philadelphia, Pa: Butterworth-Heinemann Elsevier; 2008: chap 70.

Knopman DS. Alzheimer's disease and other dementias. In: Goldman L, Schafer AI, eds. Cecil Medicine. 24th ed. Philadelphia, Pa: Saunders Elsevier; 2011: chap 409.

Mayeux R. Early Alzheimer's disease. N Engl J Med. 2010 Jun 10; 362(4):2194-2201.) (Peterson RC. Clinical practice. Mild cognitive impairment. N Engl J Med 2011 Jun 9; 364(23):2227-2234.

Querfurth HW, LaFerla FM. Alzheimer's disease. N Engl J Med. 2010 Jan 28; 362(4):329-44.

[79] DeKosky ST, Kaufer DI, Hamilton RL, Wolk DA, Lopez OL. The dementias. In: Bradley WG, Daroff RB, Fenichel GM, Jankovic J, eds. Bradley: Neurology in Clinical Practice. 5th ed. Philadelphia, Pa: Butterworth-Heinemann Elsevier; 2008: chap 70.

Knopman DS. Alzheimer's disease and other dementias. In: Goldman L, Schafer AI, eds. Cecil Medicine. 24th ed. Philadelphia, Pa: Saunders Elsevier; 2011: chap 409.

Mayeux R. Early Alzheimer's disease. N Engl J Med. 2010 Jun 10; 362(4):2194-2201. (145)Peterson RC. Clinical practice. Mild cognitive impairment. N Engl J Med 2011 Jun 9; 364(23):2227-2234.

Querfurth HW, LaFerla FM. Alzheimer's disease. N Engl J Med. 2010 Jan 28; 362(4):329-44.

[80] Impact of Progestins on Estrogen-Induced Neuroprotection: Synergy by Progesterone and 19-Norprogesterone and Antagonism by Medroxyprogesterone Acetate JON NILSEN AND ROBERTA DIAZ BRINTON Department of Molecular Pharmacology and Toxicology and the Program in Neuroscience, University of Southern California, Pharmaceutical Sciences Center, Los Angeles, California 90033.

[81] Brinton RD 1999 A Women's Health Issue: Alzheimer's disease and strategies for maintaining cognitive health. Int J Fertil Womens Med 44:174–185.

Henderson VW 1997 Estrogen, cognition, and a woman's risk of Alzheimer's disease. Am J Med 103:11S – 18S.

[82] Halliwell, Barry (2007). "Oxidative stress and cancer: have we moved forward?." Biochem. J. 401 (1): 1–11.)

Valko, M., Leibfritz, D., Moncol, J., Cronin, MTD., Mazur, M., Telser, J. (August 2007). "Free radicals and antioxidants in normal physiological functions and human disease". International Journal of Biochemistry & Cell Biology 39 (1): 44–84.)

Singh, N., Dhalla, A.K., Seneviratne, C., Singal, P.K. (June 1995). "Oxidative stress and heart failure". Molecular and Cellular Biochemistry 147 (1): 77–81.

Ramond A, Godin-Ribuot D, Ribuot C, Totoson P, Koritchneva I, Cachot S, Levy P, Joyeux-Faure M. (December 2011). "Oxidative stress mediates cardiac infarction aggravation induced by intermittent hypoxia." Fundam Clin Pharmacol.

Dean OM, van den Buuse M, Berk M, Copolov DL, Mavros C, Bush AI. (July 2011). "N-acetyl cysteine restores brain glutathione loss in combined 2-cyclohexene-1-one and D-amphetamine-treated rats: relevance to schizophrenia and bipolar disorder". Neurosci Lett. 499 (3): 149–53.

de Diego-Otero Y, Romero-Zerbo Y, el Bekay R, Decara J, Sanchez L, Rodriguez-de Fonseca F, del Arco-Herrera I. (March 2009). "Alpha-tocopherol protects against oxidative stress in the fragile X knockout mouse: an experimental therapeutic approach for the Fmr1 deficiency." Neuropsychopharmacology 34 (4): 1011–26.

Amer, J., Ghoti, H., Rachmilewitz, E., Koren, A., Levin, C. and Fibach, E. (January 2006). "Red blood cells, platelets and polymorphonuclear neutrophils of patients with sickle cell disease exhibit oxidative stress that can be ameliorated by antioxidants". British Journal of Haematology 132 (1): 108–113.

Aly, D. G.; Shahin, R. S. (2010). "Oxidative stress in lichen planus". Acta dermatovenerologica Alpina, Panonica, et Adriatica 19 (1): 3–11.

Arican, O.; Kurutas, EB. (Mar 2008). "Oxidative stress in the blood of patients with active localized vitiligo." Acta Dermatovenerol Alp Panonica Adriat 17 (1): 12–6.

James, SJ.; Cutler, P.; Melnyk, S.; Jernigan, S.; Janak, L.; Gaylor, DW.; Neubrander, JA. (Dec 2004). "Metabolic biomarkers of increased oxidative stress and impaired methylation capacity in children with autism." Am J Clin Nutr 80 (6): 1611–7.

Gwen Kennedy, Vance A. Spence, Margaret McLaren, Alexander Hill, Christine Underwood & Jill J. F. Belch (September 2005). "Oxidative stress levels are raised in chronic fatigue syndrome and are associated with clinical symptoms". Free radical biology & medicine 39 (5): 584–9.

Behl C, Holsboer F 1999 The female sex hormone oestrogen as a neuroprotectant. Trends Pharmacol Sci 20:441–444.

Brinton RD, Chen S, Montoya M, Hsieh D, Minaya, J 2000 The estrogen replacement therapy of the Women's Health Initiative promotes the cellular mechanisms of memory and neuronal survival in neurons vulnerable to Alzheimer's disease. Maturitas 34 (Suppl 2):S35–S52.

[83] Estrogen replacement therapy is associated with improvement of cognitive deficits and reduced incidence of Alzheimer's disease. Published by The Endocrine Society in 2002.

[84] Impact of progestins on estrogen-induced neuroprotection: Synergy by progesterone and 19-norprogesterone and antagonism by medroxyprogesterone acetate The Endocrine Society 2002 Archive January 2002 Nilsen and Brinton.

[85] Kirkland JL, Murthy L, Stancel GM 1992 Progesterone inhibits the estrogen-induced expression of c-fos messenger ribonucleic acid in the uterus. Endocrinology 130:3223–3230.

Kraus WL, Katzenellenbogen BS 1993 Regulation of progesterone receptor gene expression and growth in the rat uterus: modulation of estrogen action by progesterone and sex steroid hormone antagonist. Endocrinology 132:2371–2379.

[86] Gambrell Jr RD 1986 Prevention of endometrial cancer with progestogens. Maturitas 8:159 5. Hirvonen E 1996 Progestins. Maturitas 23(Suppl):S13–S18.

[87] Gambrell Jr RD 1989 Use of progestogens in postmenopausal women. Int J Fertil 34:315 –321.

[88] Schairer C, Lubin J, Troisi R, Sturgeon S, Brinton L, Hoover R 2000 Menopausal estrogen and estrogen-progestin replacement therapy and breast cancer risk. J Am Med Assoc 283:485–491.

[89] Henderson VW, Paganini-Hill A, Emanuel CK, Dunn ME, Buckwalter JG 1994 Estrogen replacement therapy in older women: comparisons between Nilsen and Brinton •Progestins Impact Neuroprotection Endocrinology, January 2002, 143(1):205–212.

Brenner DE, Kukull WA, Stergachis A, van Belle G, Bowen JD, McCormickWC, Teri L, Larson EB 1994 Postmenopausal estrogen replacement therapy and the risk of Alzheimer's disease: a population-based case-control study. Am J Epidemiol 140:262–267.

Paganini-Hill A1996 Oestrogen replacement therapy and Alzheimer's dis-ease. Br J Obstet Gynecol 103:80–86.

Tang M-X, Jacobs D, Stern Y, Marder K, Schofield P, Gurland B 1996 Effect of oestrogen during menopause on risk and age at onset of Alzheimer's disease. Lancet 348:429–432.

[90] Hormonal treatment, mild cognitive impairment and Alzheimer's disease Joanne Ryan, Jaqueline Scali, Isabelle Carriere, Karen Ritchie, and Marie-Laure Ancelin Int Psychogeriatr. 2008 February; 20(1): 47–56.

[91] Testosterone improves spatial memory in men with Alzheimer disease and mild cognitive impairment. Neurology. 2005 Jun 28; 64(12):2063-8. Cherrier MM, Matsumoto AM, Amory JK, Asthana S, Bremner W, Peskind ER, Raskind MA, Craft S.

[92] Lu P, Masterman D. Effects of testosterone on cognition, and mood in male patients with mild Alzheimer disease and healthy elderly men. Archives of Neurology 2006; 63: 177–85.

Chapter Seventeen

[93] Ferrucci L, Maggio M, Bandinelli S, et al. Low testosterone predicts anemia in older adults. Arch Intern Med 2006; 166:1380–8.

Hormones in Wellness and Disease Prevention: Common Practices, Current State of the Evidence, and Questions for the Future Erika T. Schwartz, MD, Kent Holtorf, MD 10 West 74 Street, Suite 1A, New York, NY 10023, USA 23456 Hawthorne Boulevard, Suite 160, Torrance, CA 90505, USA Corresponding author. E-mail address: erika@drerika.com (E. Schwartz). Prim Care Clin Office Pract 35 (2008) 669–705 primarycare.theclinics.com 2008 Elsevier Inc.

Chapter Eighteen

[94] The Role of Androgens and Estrogens on Healthy Aging and Longevity J Gerontol A Biol Sci Med Sci. Nov 2012; 67(11): 1140–1152. Astrid M. Horstman E. Lichar Dillon, Randall J. Urban, and Melinda Sheffield-Moore.

[95] Birkhauser MH. Quality of life and sexuality issues in aging women. Climacteric. 2009; 12(suppl 1):52–57.

The Role of Androgens and Estrogens on Healthy Aging and Longevity J Gerontol A Biol Sci Med Sci. Nov 2012; 67(11): 1140–1152. Published online Mar 26, 2012. Astrid M. Horstman, E. Lichar Dillon, Randall J. Urban, and Melinda Sheffield-Moore.

[96] The Role of Androgens and Estrogens on Healthy Aging and Longevity J Gerontol A Biol Sci Med Sci. Nov 2012; 67(11): 1140–1152. Published online Mar 26, 2012. Astrid M. Horstman, E. Lichar Dillon, Randall J. Urban, and Melinda Sheffield-Moore.

[97] Goodman-Gruen D, Barrett-Connor E. Sex differences in the association of endogenous sex hormone levels and glucose tolerance status in older men and women. Diabetes Care. 2000; 23(7):912–918.

Daniel SAJ, Armstrong ST. Androgens in the ovarian micro environment. Semin Reprod Endocrinol. 1986; 4:89–100.

[98] van Geel TA, Geusens PP, Winkens B, Sels JP, Dinant GJ. Measures of bioavailable serum testosterone and estradiol and their relationships with muscle mass, muscle strength and bone mineral density in postmenopausal women: a cross-sectional study. Eur J Endocrinol. 2009; 160(4):681–687.

Cappola AR, Xue QL, Fried LP. Multiple hormonal deficiencies in anabolic hormones are found in frail older women: the Women's Health and Aging studies. J Gerontol A Biol Sci Med Sci. 2009; 64(2):243–248.

Bachmann G, Bancroft J, Braunstein G, et al. Female androgen insufficiency: the Princeton consensus statement on definition, classification, and assessment. Fertil Steril. 2002; 77(4):660–665.

van der Made F, Bloemers J, Yassem WE, et al. The influence of testosterone combined with a PDE5-inhibitor on cognitive, affective, and physiological sexual functioning in women suffering from sexual dysfunction. J Sex Med. 2009; 6(3):777–790.

Davis SR, McCloud P, Strauss BJ, Burger H. Testosterone enhances estradiol's effects on postmenopausal bone density and sexuality. Maturitas. 2008; 61(1–2):17–26.

[99] Zumoff B, Strain GW, Miller LK, Rosner W. Twenty-four-hour mean plasma testosterone concentration declines with age in normal premenopausal women. J Clin Endocrinol Metab. 1995; 80(4):1429–1430.

[100] Longcope C. Androgen metabolism and the menopause. Semin Reprod Endocrinol. 1998; 16(2):111–115.

[101] Chakravarti S, Collins WP, Forecast JD, Newton JR, Oram DH, Studd JW. Hormonal profiles after the menopause. Br Med J. 1976; 2(6039):784–787.

The Role of Androgens and Estrogens on Healthy Aging and Longevity J Gerontol A Biol Sci Med Sci. Nov 2012; 67(11): 1140–1152. Published online Mar 26, 2012. Astrid M. Horstman, E. Lichar Dillon, Randall J. Urban, and Melinda Sheffield-Moore.

[102] Feldman HA, Longcope C, Derby CA, et al. Age trends in the level of serum testosterone and other hormones in middle-aged men: longitudinal results from the Massachusetts male aging study. J Clin Endocrinol Metab. 2002; 87(2):589–598.

[103] Harman SM, Metter EJ, Tobin JD, Pearson J, Blackman MR. Longitudinal effects of aging on serum total and free testosterone levels in healthy men. Baltimore Longitudinal Study of Aging. J Clin Endocrinol Metab. 2001; 86(2):724–731.

[104] Orwoll ES, Oviatt SK, McClung MR, Deftos LJ, Sexton G. 1990 The rate of bone mineral loss in normal men and the effects of calcium and cholecalciferol supplementation. Ann Intern Med. 112:29–34.

Marcus R. 1991 Skeletal aging. Understanding the functional and structural basis of osteoporosis. Trends Endocrinol Metab. 2:53–58.

[105] Forbes GB, Reina JC. 1970 Adult lean body mass declines with age: some longitudinal observations. Metabolism. 19:653–663.

Gallagher D, Visser M, De Meersman RE, et al. 1997 Appendicular skeletal muscle mass: effects of age, gender, and ethnicity. J Appl Physiol. 83:229–239.

[106] Kallman DA, Plato C, Tobin J. 1990 The role of muscle loss in age-related decline in grip strength: A cross-sectional and longitudinal analysis. J Gerontol. 45:M82–M88.

Bruce SA, Newton D, Woledge RC. 1989 Effects of age on voluntary force and cross-sectional area of human adductor policis muscle. Q J Exp Physiol. 74:359–362.

[107] Fleg JL, Lakatta EG. 1990 Role of muscle loss in the age-associated reduction in VO2max in older men. J Appl Physiol. 68:329–333.

[108] Horber FF, Gruber B, Thomi F, Jensen EX, Jaeger P. 1997 Effect of sex and age on bone mass, body composition and fuel metabolism in humans [see Comments]. Nutrition. 13:524–534.

Siervogel RM, Wisemandle W, Maynard LM, et al. 1998 Serial changes in body composition throughout adulthood and their relationships to changes in lipid and lipoprotein levels. The Fels Longitudinal Study. Arterioscler Thromb Vasc Biol. 18:1759–1764.)

Kreisberg RA, Kasim S. 1987 Cholesterol metabolism and aging. Am J Med. 82:54–60.

Couillard C, Lemieux S, Moorjani S, et al. 1996 Associations between 12 year changes in body fatness and lipoprotein- lipid levels in men and women of the Quebec Family Study. Int J Obes Relat Metab Disord. 20:1081–1088.

[109] Mauras N, Hayes V, Welch S, et al. 1998 Testosterone deficiency in young men: marked alterations in whole body protein kinetics, strength, and adiposity. J Clin Endocrinol Metab. 83:1886–1892.

Katznelson L, Rosenthal DI, Rosol MS, et al. 1998 Using quantitative CT to assess adipose distribution in adult men with acquired hypogonadism. AJR Am J Roentgenol. 170:423–427.

[110] Kannus P, Parkkari J, Sievanen H, et al. 1996 Epidemiology of hip fractures. Bone. [1 Suppl] 18:57S–63S.

[111] Deslypere JP, Vermeulen A. 1984 Leydig cell function in normal men: effect of age, life-style, residence, diet, and activity. J Clin Endocrinol Metab. 59:955–962.

Harman SM, Metter EJ, Tobin JD, Pearson J, Blackman MR. Longitudinal effects of aging on serum total and free testosterone levels in healthy men. Baltimore Longitudinal Study of Aging. J Clin Endocrinol Metab. 2001; 86(2):724–731.

[112] Mauras N, Hayes V, Welch S, et al. Testosterone deficiency in young men: marked alterations in whole body protein kinetics, strength, and adiposity. J Clin Endocrinol Metab. 1998; 83(6):1886–1892.

[113] Brodsky IG, Balagopal P, Nair KS. Effects of testosterone replacement on muscle mass and muscle protein synthesis in hypogonadal men—a clinical research center study. J Clin Endocrinol Metab. 1996; 81(10):3469–3475.

[114] Sheffield-Moore M, Dillon EL, Casperson SL, et al. A randomized pilot study of monthly cycled testosterone replacement or continuous testosterone replacement versus placebo in older men. J Clin Endocrinol Metab. 2011; 96(11):E1831–E1837.

Ferrando AA, Sheffield-Moore M, Yeckel CW, et al. Testosterone administration to older men improves muscle function: molecular and physiological mechanisms. Am J Physiol Endocrinol Metab. 2002; 282(3):E601–E607.

Urban RJ, Bodenburg YH, Gilkison C, et al. Testosterone administration to elderly men increases skeletal muscle strength and protein synthesis. Am J Physiol. 1995; 269(5 Pt 1):E820–E826.

[115] Tenover JS. Effects of testosterone supplementation in the aging male. J Clin Endocrinol Metab. 1992; 75(4):1092–1098.

[116] Roy TA, Blackman MR, Harman SM, Tobin JD, Schrager M, Metter EJ. Interrelationships of serum testosterone and free testosterone index with FFM and strength in aging men. Am J Physiol Endocrinol Metab. 2002; 283(2):E284–E294.

Perry HM, 3rd, Miller DK, Patrick P, Morley JE. Testosterone and leptin in older African-American men: relationship to age, strength, function, and season. Metabolism. 2000; 49(8):1085–1091.

Baumgartner RN, Waters DL, Gallagher D, Morley JE, Garry PJ. Predictors of skeletal muscle mass in elderly men and women. Mech Ageing Dev. 1999; 107(2):123–136.

Iannuzzi-Sucich M, Prestwood KM, Kenny AM. Prevalence of sarcopenia and predictors of skeletal muscle mass in healthy, older men and women. J Gerontol Med Sci. 2002; 57(12):M772–M777.

[117] Onder G, Penninx BW, Lapuerta P, et al. Change in physical performance over time in older women: the Women's Health and Aging Study. J Gerontol Med Sci. 2002; 57(5):M289–M293.

Leveille SG, Penninx BW, Melzer D, Izmirlian G, Guralnik JM. Sex differences in the prevalence of mobility disability in old age: the dynamics of incidence, recovery, and mortality. J Gerontol B Psychol Sci Soc Sci. 2000; 55(1):S41–S50.)

Laughlin GA, Barrett-Connor E, Bergstrom J. Low serum testosterone and mortality in older men. J Clin Endocrinol Metab. 2008; 93(1):68–75.

Ding EL, Song Y, Malik VS, Liu S. Sex differences of endogenous sex hormones and risk of type 2 diabetes: a systematic review and meta-analysis. JAMA. 2006; 295(11):1288–1299.

Zarrouf FA, Artz S, Griffith J, Sirbu C, Kommor M. Testosterone and depression: systematic review and meta-analysis. J Psychiatr Pract. 2009; 15(4):289–305.

Dhindsa S, Prabhakar S, Sethi M, Bandyopadhyay A, Chaudhuri A, Dandona P. Frequent occurrence of hypogonadotropic hypogonadism in type 2 diabetes. J Clin Endocrinol Metab. 2004; 89(11):5462–5468.

Bhasin S, Cunningham GR, Hayes FJ, et al. Testosterone therapy in adult men with androgen deficiency syndromes: an endocrine society clinical practice guideline. J Clin Endocrinol Metab. 2006; 91(6):1995–2010.

[118] Khaw KT, Dowsett M, Folkerd E, et al. Endogenous testosterone and mortality due to all causes, cardiovascular disease, and cancer in men: European prospective investigation into cancer in Norfolk (EPIC-Norfolk) Prospective Population Study. Circulation. 2007; 116(23):2694–2701.

Shores MM, Matsumoto AM, Sloan KL, Kivlahan DR. Low serum testosterone and mortality in male veterans. Arch Intern Med. 2006; 166(15):1660–1665.

[119] Sheffield-Moore M, Paddon-Jones D, Casperson SL, et al. Androgen therapy induces muscle protein anabolism in older women. J Clin Endocrinol Metab. 2006; 91(10):3844–3849.

Saad F. The role of testosterone in type 2 diabetes and metabolic syndrome in men. Arq Bras Endocrinol Metabol. 2009; 53(8):901–907.

[120] Saad F. The role of testosterone in type 2 diabetes and metabolic syndrome in men. Arq Bras Endocrinol Metabol. 2009; 53(8):901–907.

Saad F, Gooren LJ. The role of testosterone in the etiology and treatment of obesity, the metabolic syndrome, and diabetes mellitus type 2. J Obes. 2011; 2011 pii:471584.

[121] Fink HA, Ewing SK, Ensrud KE, et al. Association of testosterone and estradiol deficiency with osteoporosis and rapid bone loss in older men. J Clin Endocrinol Metab. 2006; 91(10):3908–3915.

[122] Meier C, Nguyen TV, Handelsman DJ, et al. Endogenous sex hormones and incident fracture risk in older men: the Dubbo Osteoporosis Epidemiology Study. Arch Intern Med. 2008; 168(1):47–54.

[123] Tuck SP, Francis RM. Testosterone, bone and osteoporosis. Front Horm Res. 2009; 37:123–132.

Chapter Nineteen

[124] Helmick, CG; Felson, DT; Lawrence, RC; Gabriel, S; Hirsch, R; Kwoh, CK; Liang, MH; Kremers, HM; Mayes, MD; Merkel, PA; Pillemer, SR; Reveille, JD; Stone, JH; National Arthritis Data, Workgroup (January 2008). "Estimates of the prevalence of arthritis and other rheumatic conditions in the United States. Part I". *Arthritis and rheumatism* 58 (1): 15–25.

[125] "Handout on Health: Rheumatoid Arthritis". National Institute of Arthritis and Musculoskeletal and Skin Diseases. April 2009. Retrieved 2013-03-26.

[126] Turesson C, O'Fallon WM, Crowson CS, Gabriel SE, Matteson EL (2003). "Extra-articular disease manifestations in rheumatoid arthritis: incidence trends and risk factors over 46 years". *Ann. Rheum. Dis.* 62 (8): 722–7.

[127] *Davidson's principles and practice of medicine.* (21st ed.). Edinburgh: Churchill Livingstone/Elsevier. 2010.

[128] Majithia V, Geraci SA (2007). "Rheumatoid arthritis: diagnosis and management". *Am. J. Med.* 120 (11): 936–9.

[129] Wolfe F; Mitchell DM; Sibley JT; Fries, James F.; Bloch, Daniel A.; Williams, Catherine A.; Spitz, Patricia W.; Haga, May et al. (April 1994). "The mortality of rheumatoid arthritis". *Arthritis Rheum.* 37 (4): 481–94.

Aviña-Zubieta JA; Choi HK; Sadatsafavi M; Etminan, Mahyar; Esdaile, John M.; Lacaille, Diane (2008). "Risk of cardiovascular mortality in patients with rheumatoid arthritis: a meta-analysis of observational studies". *Arthritis Rheum.* 59 (12): 1690–1697.

[130] de Groot K (August 2007). "[Renal manifestations in rheumatic diseases]". *Internist (Berl)* 48 (8): 779–85.

[131] Sugiyama D, Nishimura K, Tamaki K, Tsuji G, Nakazawa T, Morinobu A, Kumagai S (2010). "Impact of smoking as a risk factor for developing rheumatoid arthritis: a meta-analysis of observational studies". *Ann Rheum Dis.* 69 (1): 70–81.

[132] Wen, H; Baker, JF (March 2011). "Vitamin D, immunoregulation, and rheumatoid arthritis". *Journal of clinical rheumatology: practical reports on rheumatic & musculoskeletal diseases* 17 (2): 102–7.

[133] Hooyman JR, Melton LJ, 3rd, Nelson AM, O'Fallon WM, Riggs BL. Fractures after rheumatoid arthritis. A population-based study. Arthritis Rheum. 1984 Dec; 27(12):1353–1361.

Spector TD, Hall GM, McCloskey EV, Kanis JA. Risk of vertebral fracture in women with rheumatoid arthritis. BMJ. 1993 Feb 27; 306(6877):558–558.

Sambrook PN, Reeve J. Bone disease in rheumatoid arthritis. Clin Sci (Lond) 1988 Mar; 74(3):225–230.

Lindsay R, Hart DM, Forrest C, Baird C. Prevention of spinal osteoporosis in oophorectomised women. Lancet. 1980 Nov 29; 2 (8205):1151–1154.

Weiss NS, Ure CL, Ballard JH, Williams AR, Daling JR. Decreased risk of fractures of the hip and lower forearm with postmenopausal use of estrogen. N Engl J Med. 1980 Nov 20; 303(21):1195–1198.

Hazes JM, Dijkmans BA, Vandenbroucke JP, de Vries RR, Cats A. Pregnancy and the risk of developing rheumatoid arthritis. Arthritis Rheum. 1990 Dec; 33(12):1770–1775.

Vandenbroucke JP, Valkenburg HA, Boersma JW, Cats A, Festen JJ, Huber-Bruning O, Rasker JJ. Oral contraceptives and rheumatoid arthritis: further evidence for a preventive effect. Lancet. 1982 Oct 16; 2(8303):839–842.

Hernandez-Avila M, Liang MH, Willett WC, Stampfer MJ, Colditz GA, Rosner B, Chang RW, Hennekens CH, Speizer FE. Exogenous sex hormones and the risk of rheumatoid arthritis. Arthritis Rheum. 1990 Jul; 33(7):947–953.

Bijlsma JW, Huber-Bruning O, Thijssen JH. Effect of oestrogen treatment on clinical and laboratory manifestations of rheumatoid arthritis. Ann Rheum Dis. 1987 Oct; 46(10):777–779.

Hunt SM, McKenna SP, McEwen J, Williams J, Papp E. The Nottingham Health Profile: subjective health status and medical consultations. Soc Sci Med A. 1981 May; 15(3 Pt 1):221–229.

Stevenson JC, Cust MP, Gangar KF, Hillard TC, Lees B, Whitehead MI. Effects of transdermal versus oral hormone replacement therapy on bone density in spine and proximal femur in postmenopausal women. Lancet. 1990 Aug 4; 336(8710):265–269.

Sambrook P, Birmingham J, Champion D, Kelly P, Kempler S, Freund J, Eisman J. Postmenopausal bone loss in rheumatoid arthritis: effect of estrogens and androgens. J Rheumatol. 1992 Mar; 19(3):357–361.

van den Brink HR, Lems WF, van Everdingen AA, Bijlsma JW. Adjuvant oestrogen treatment increases bone mineral density in postmenopausal women with rheumatoid arthritis. Ann Rheum Dis. 1993 Apr; 52(4):302–305.

Selby PL, Peacock M. Dose dependent response of symptoms, pituitary, and bone to transdermal oestrogen in postmenopausal women. Br Med J (Clin Res Ed) 1986 Nov 22; 293(6558):1337–1339.

Effects of hormone replacement therapy in rheumatoid arthritis a double blind placebo-controlled study. Ann Rheum Dis. 1994 January; 53(1): 54–57. A G MacDonald, E A Murphy, H A Capell, U Z Bankowska, and S H Ralston.

[134] Androgen replacement therapy in male patients with rheumatoid arthritis. Arthritis Rheum. 1991 Jan; 34(1):1-5. Cutolo M, Balleari E, Giusti M, Intra E, Accardo S.

The Effects of Gonadotropin Treatment on the Immunological Features of Male Patients with Idiopathic Hypogonadotropic Hypogonadism Volume 85 Issue 1 | January 1, 2000. Zeki Yesilova, Metin Ozata, Ismail H. Kocar, Mustafa Turan, Aysel Pekel, Ali Sengul and I. Caglayan Ozdemír.

[135] Ahmed SA, Penhale WJ, Talal N. 1985 Sex hormones, immune responses and autoimmune diseases. *Am J Pathol.* 121:531–551.

Beeson PB. 1994 Age and sex associations of 40 autoimmune diseases. *Am J Med.* 96:457–62.

French MAH, Hughes P. 1983 Systemic lupus erythematosus and Klinefelter's syndrome. *Ann Rheum Dis.* 42:471–473.

[136] Lahita RG, Bradlow HL, Fishman J, Kunkel HG. 1982 Abnormal estrogen and androgen metabolism in the human with systemic lupus erythematosus. *Am J Kidney Dis.* 2:206–211.

[137] Olsen NJ, Kovacks WJ. 1995 Case report, testosterone treatment of SLE in a patient with Klinefelter's syndrome. *Am J Med Sci.* 310:158–160.

Lahita RG, Bradlow HL, Fishman J, Kunkel HG. 1982 Abnormal estrogen and androgen metabolism in the human with systemic lupus erythematosus. *Am J Kidney Dis.* 2:206–211.

Ariga H, Edwards J, Sullivan DA. 1989 Androgen control of autoimmune expression in lacrimal glands of MRL/Mp-lpr/LPR mice. *Clin Immunol Immunopathol.* 53:499–508.

[138] Cutolo M, Balleari E, Giusti M, Intra E, Accardo S 1991 Androgen replacement therapy in male patients with rheumatoid arthritis. Arthritis Rheum 34:1–5.

Bizzarro A, Valentini G, Di Martino G, DaPonte A, De Bellis A, Iacono G 1987 Influence of testosterone therapy on clinical and immunological features of autoimmune diseases associated with Klinefelter's syndrome. J Clin Endocrinol Metab 64:32–36.

Olsen NJ, Kovacs WJ 1995 Case report: testosterone treatment of systemic lupus erythematosus in a patient with Klinefelter's syndrome. Am J Med Sci 310:158–160.

[139] The Journal of Clinical Endocrinology & MetabolismThe Endocrine Society |2004 Archive |July 2004 |Malkin et al. 89 (7): 3313 Endocrine Care The Effect of Testosterone Replacement on Endogenous Inflammatory Cytokines and Lipid Profiles in Hypogonadal Men Chris J. Malkin, Peter J. Pugh, Richard D. Jones, Dheeraj Kapoor, Kevin S. Channer and T. Hugh Jones.

[140] Androgen supplementation in eugonadal men with osteoporosis-effects of 6 months of treatment on bone mineral density and cardiovascular risk factors. Bone. 1996 Feb; 18(2):171-7. Anderson FH, Francis RM, Faulkner K.

[141] Comparison of the effects of oral and transdermal oestradiol administration on oestrogen metabolism, protein synthesis, gonadotrophin release, bone turnover and climacteric symptoms in postmenopausal women. Clin Endocrinol (Oxf). 1989 Mar; 30(3):241-9. Selby P, McGarrigle HH, Peacock M.

[142] Could transdermal estradiol + progesterone be a safer postmenopausal HRT? A review. L'hermite M, Simoncini T, Fuller S, Genazzani AR. Maturitas. 2008 Jul-Aug; 60(3-4):185-201.

[143] Effects of estrogen and progesterone on tibia histomorphometry in growing rats. Schmidt IU, Wakley GK, Turner RT. Calcif Tissue Int. 2000 Jul; 67(1):47-52.

[144] Progesterone as a bone-trophic hormone. Prior JC. Endocr Rev. 1990 May; 11(2):386-98.

[145] Taken from the National Institute of Health.

[146] *THE MIRACLE OF BIO-IDENTICAL HORMONES, How I lost my: fatigue, hot flashes, ADHD, ADD, Fibromyalgia, PMS, osteoporosis, weight, sexual dysfunction, anger, migraines.....* Michael E. Platt, M.D. Clancy Lane Publishing, California, Copyright @ 2007 Michael E. Platt, M.D.

Chapter Twenty-One

[147] Zhou J, Ng S, Adesanya-Famuiya O, Anderson K and Bondy CA (2000) Testosterone inhibits estrogen-induced mammary epithelial proliferation and suppresses estrogen receptor expression. FASEB J 14, 1725–1730.

Dimitrakakis C, Zhou J and Bondy CA (2002) Androgens and mammary growth and neoplasia. Fertil Steril 77, S26–S33.

Somboonporn W and Davis SR (2004a) Testosterone effects on the breast: implications for testosterone therapy for women. Endocrine Rev 25, 374–388.

[148] Androgen insufficiency in women diagnostic and therapeutic implications Oxford Journals Medicine Human Reproduction Update Volume 10, Issue 5 Pp. 421-432.

[149] Bergkvist L, Adami H, Persson I, et al. The risk of breast cancer after estrogen and estrogen-progestin replacement. NEJM 1989; 321(5):293–7.

Glass A, Hoover R. Rising incidence of breast cancer: relationship to stage and receptor status. Natl Can Inst 1990; 82:693–6. Testosterone prevents the over-growth of breast cancer cells when the patient has her own natural estrogen or is treated with bio-identical estradiol.

Ando S, De Amicis F. Breast cancer from estrogen to androgen receptor. V Mol Molecular and Cellular Endocrinology 2002; 193:121–8.

[150] Fournier A, Berrino F, Clavel-Chapelon F. Unequal risks for breast cancer associated with different hormone replacement therapies: results from the E3N cohort study. Breast Cancer Res Treat 2008; 107(1):103–11.

[151] De Lignie`res B, de Vathaire F, Fournier S, et al. Combined hormone replacement therapy and risk of breast cancer in a French cohort study of 3175 women. Climacteric 2002; 5:332–40.

[152] Stahlberg C, Pedersen A, Lynge E, et al. Increased risk of breast cancer following different regimens of hormone replacement therapy frequently used in Europe. Int J Cancer 2004; 109:721–7.

[153] Nelson HD. Commonly used types of postmenopausal estrogen for treatment of hot flashes. JAMA 2004; 291(13):1610–20.

[154] Hormones in Wellness and Disease Prevention: Common Practices, Current State of the Evidence, and Questions for the Future Erika T. Schwartz, MD , Kent Holtorf, MD 10 West 74 Street, Suite 1A, New York, NY 10023, USA b 23456 Hawthorne Boulevard, Suite 160, Torrance, CA 90505, USA Corresponding author. E-mail address: erika@drerika.com (E. Schwartz). Prim Care Clin Office Pract 35 (2008) 669–705 primarycare.theclinics.com 0095-4543/08/$ – see front matter 2008 Elsevier Inc.

[155] Stanczyk FZ. All progestins are not created equal. Steroids 2003; 68:879–90.

Fournier A, Berrino F, Clavel-Chapelon F. Unequal risks for breast cancer associated with different hormone replacement therapies: results from the E3N cohort study. Breast Cancer Res Treat 2008; 107(1):103–11.

De Lignie`res B, de Vathaire F, Fournier S, et al. Combined hormone replacement therapy and risk of breast cancer in a French cohort study of 3175 women. Climacteric 2002; 5:332–40. And many other studies demonstrated that the use of either Premarin or bio-identical estradiol plus Provera caused a significant increased risk of breast cancer.

Maxson W, Hargrove J. Bioavailability of oral micronized progesterone. Fertil Steril 1985; 44(5):622–6.

Santen RJ. Risk of breast cancer with progestins: critical assessment of current data. Steroids 2003; 68:953–64.

Schairer C, Lubin J, Troisi R, et al. Menopausal estrogen and estrogen-progestin replacement therapy and breast cancer risk. JAMA 2000; 283:485–91.

Campagnali C, Abba C, Ambroggio S, et al. Breast cancer and hormone replacement therapy: putting the risk into perspective. Gynecol Endocrinol 2001; 15:53–60.

Lyytinen H, Pukkala E, Ylikorkala O. Breast cancer risk in postmenopausal women using estrogen-only therapy. Obstet Gynecol 2006; 108(6):1354–60.

Li C, Malone K, Porter P, et al. Relationship between long durations and different regimens of hormone therapy and risk of breast cancer. JAMA 2003; 289(24):3254–63.

[156] Hormones in Wellness and Disease Prevention: Common Practices, Current State of the Evidence, and Questions for the Future Erika T. Schwartz, MD , Kent Holtorf, MD 10 West 74 Street, Suite 1A, New York, NY 10023, USA b 23456 Hawthorne Boulevard, Suite 160, Torrance, CA 90505, USA Corresponding author. E-mail address: erika@drerika.com (E. Schwartz). Prim Care Clin Office Pract 35 (2008) 669–705 primarycare.theclinics.com 2008 Elsevier Inc.) (Schindler A. European Progestin Club. Differential effects of progestins. Maturitas 2003; 46:S3–5.

[157] Stanczyk FZ. All progestins are not created equal. Steroids 2003; 68:879–90.

Stahlberg C, Pedersen A, Lynge E, et al. Increased risk of breast cancer following different regimens of hormone replacement therapy frequently used in Europe. Int J Cancer 2004; 109:721–7.

Schindler A. European Progestin Club. Differential effects of progestins. Maturitas 2003; 46:S3–5.

Fournier A, Berrino F, Clavel-Chapelon F. Unequal risks for breast cancer associated with different hormone replacement therapies: results from the E3N cohort study. Breast Cancer Res Treat 2008; 107(1):103–11.

De Lignie`res B, de Vathaire F, Fournier S, et al. Combined hormone replacement therapy and risk of breast cancer in a French cohort study of 3175 women. Climacteric 2002; 5:332–40.

Santen RJ. Risk of breast cancer with progestins: critical assessment of current data. Steroids 2003; 68:953–64.

Schairer C, Lubin J, Troisi R, et al. Menopausal estrogen and estrogen-progestin replacement therapy and breast cancer risk. JAMA 2000; 283:485–91.

[158] Schindler A. European Progestin Club. Differential effects of progestins. Maturitas 2003; 46:S3–5.

Grady D, Vittinghoff E, Lin F, et al. Effect of ultra-low-dose transdermal estradiol on breast density in postmenopausal women. Menopause J North Am Men Soc 2007; 14(3):1–6.

Simon JA, Bouchard C, Waldbaum A, et al. Low dose of transdermal estradiol (E2) gel for treatment of symptomatic postmenopausal women. Obstet Gynecol 2007; 109(2):1–10.

Montplaisir J, Lorrain J, Denesle R, et al. Sleep in menopause: differential effects of two forms of hormone replacement therapy. Menopause 2001; 8(1):10–6.

Gambacciani M, Ciaponi M, Cappagli B, et al. Effects of low-dose, continuous combined hormone replacement therapy on sleep in symptomatic postmenopausal women. Maturitas 2005; 50:91–7.

Zegura B, Guzic-Salobir B, Sebestjen M, et al. The effect of various menopausal hormone therapies on markers of inflammation, coagulation, fibrinolysis, lipids, and lipoproteins in healthy postmenopausal women. Menopause 2006; 13(4):643–50.

[159] Hormones in Wellness and Disease Prevention: Common Practices, Current State of the Evidence, and Questions for the Future Erika T. Schwartz, MD, Kent Holtorf, MD 10 West 74 Street, Suite 1A, New York, NY 10023, USA 23456 Hawthorne Boulevard, Suite 160, Torrance, CA 90505, USA Corresponding author. E-mail address: erika@drerika.com (E. Schwartz). Prim Care Clin Office Pract 35 (2008) 669–705 primarycare.theclinics.com 2008 Elsevier Inc.

[160] Gammon M, Thompson W. Polycystic ovaries and the risk of breast cancer. Am J Epidemiol 1991; 134:818–24.

[161] The Hormone of Desire, Susan Rako, MD, 1999.

[162] Foidart J, Colin C, Denoo X, et al. Estradiol and progesterone regulate the proliferation of human breast epithelial cells. Fertil Steril 1998; 69(5):963–9.

[163] Place V, Powers M, Schenkel L, et al. A double-blind comparative study of estraderm and premarin in the amelioration of postmenopausal symptoms. Am J Obstet Gynecol 1985; 152(8):1092–9.

[164] Hormones in Wellness and Disease Prevention: Common Practices, Current State of the Evidence, and Questions for the Future Erika T. Schwartz, MD, Kent

Holtorf, MD 10 West 74 Street, Suite 1A, New York, NY 10023, USA 23456 Hawthorne Boulevard, Suite 160, Torrance, CA 90505, USA Corresponding author. E-mail address: erika@drerika.com (E. Schwartz). Prim Care Clin Office Pract 35 (2008) 669–705 primarycare.theclinics.com 2008 Elsevier Inc.

[165] Foidart J, Colin C, Denoo X, et al. Estradiol and progesterone regulate the proliferation of human breast epithelial cells. Fertil Steril 1998; 69(5):963–9.

[166] Stanczyk FZ. All progestins are not created equal. Steroids 2003; 68:879–90.

Fournier A, Berrino F, Clavel-Chapelon F. Unequal risks for breast cancer associated with different hormone replacement therapies: results from the E3N cohort study. Breast Cancer Res Treat 2008; 107(1):103–11.

De Lignie`res B, de Vathaire F, Fournier S, et al. Combined hormone replacement therapy and risk of breast cancer in a French cohort study of 3175 women. Climacteric 2002; 5:332–40.

[167] Maxson W, Hargrove J. Bioavailability of oral micronized progesterone. Fertil Steril 1985; 44(5):622–6.

Santen RJ. Risk of breast cancer with progestins: critical assessment of current data. Steroids 2003; 68:953–64.

Schairer C, Lubin J, Troisi R, et al. Menopausal estrogen and estrogen-progestin replacement therapy and breast cancer risk. JAMA 2000; 283:485–91.

Campagnali C, Abba C, Ambroggio S, et al. Breast cancer and hormone replacement therapy: putting the risk into perspective. Gynecol Endocrinol 2001; 15:53–60.

Lyytinen H, Pukkala E, Ylikorkala O. Breast cancer risk in postmenopausal women using estrogen-only therapy. Obstet Gynecol 2006; 108(6):1354–60.

Li C, Malone K, Porter P, et al. Relationship between long durations and different regimens of hormone therapy and risk of breast cancer. JAMA 2003; 289(24): 3254–63.

[168] Schindler A. European Progestin Club. Differential effects of progestins. Maturitas 2003; 46:S3–5.

[169] Grady D, Vittinghoff E, Lin F, et al. Effect of ultra-low-dose transdermal estradiol on breast density in postmenopausal women. Menopause J North Am Men Soc 2007; 14(3):1–6.

Simon JA, Bouchard C, Waldbaum A, et al. Low dose of transdermal estradiol (E2) gel for treatment of symptomatic postmenopausal women. Obstet Gynecol 2007; 109(2):1–10., in improving sleep patterns

Montplaisir J, Lorrain J, Denesle R, et al. Sleep in menopause: differential effects of two forms of hormone replacement therapy. Menopause 2001; 8(1):10–6.

Gambacciani M, Ciaponi M, Cappagli B, et al. Effects of low-dose, continuous combined hormone replacement therapy on sleep in symptomatic postmenopausal women. Maturitas 2005; 50:91–7., and lipid profiles

Zegura B, Guzic-Salobir B, Sebestjen M, et al. The effect of various menopausal hormone therapies on markers of inflammation, coagulation, fibrinolysis, lipids, and lipoproteins in healthy postmenopausal women. Menopause 2006; 13(4):643–50.

[170] Hormones in Wellness and Disease Prevention: Common Practices, Current State of the Evidence, and Questions for the Future Erika T. Schwartz, MD, Kent Holtorf, MD 10 West 74 Street, Suite 1A, New York, NY 10023, USA 23456 Hawthorne

Boulevard, Suite 160, Torrance, CA 90505, USA Corresponding author. E-mail address: erika@drerika.com (E. Schwartz). Prim Care Clin Office Pract 35 (2008) 669–705 primarycare.theclinics.com 2008 Elsevier Inc.

[171] Could transdermal estradiol + progesterone be a safer postmenopausal HRT? A review. L'hermite M, Simoncini T, Fuller S, Genazzani AR. Maturitas. 2008 Jul-Aug; 60(3-4):185-201.

[172] Russo J, Gusterson BA, Rogers AE, Russo IH, Welling SR, Van Zwieten MJ. Comparative study of human and rat mammary tumorigenesis. Lab Invest. 1990; 62:244–278.

Srivastava P, Russo J, Russo IH. Inhibition of rat mammary tumorigenesis by human chorionic gonadotropin is associated with increased expression of inhibin. Mol Carcinogen. 1999; 26:1–10.

Ginger MR, Gonzalez-Rimbau MF, Gay JP, Rosen JM. Persistent changes in gene expression induced by estrogen and progesterone in the rat mammary gland. Mol Endocrinol. 2001; 15:1993–2009.

[173] Ginger MR, Rosen JM. Pregnancy-induced changes in cell-fate in the mammary gland. Breast Cancer Res. 2003; 5:192–197.

[174] Progesterone receptor activation. An alternative to SERMs in breast cancer. Eur J Cancer. 2000 Sep; 36 Suppl 4:S90-1. Desreux J, Kebers F, Noël A, Francart D, Van Cauwenberge H, Heinen V, Thomas JL, Bernard AM, Paris J, Delansorne R, Foidart JM.

[175] Estradiol progesterone interaction in normal and pathologic breast cells. Ann N Y Acad Sci. 1986; 464:152-67. Mauvais-Jarvis P, Kuttenn F, Gompel A.

[176] Progesterone inhibits growth and induces apoptosis in breast cancer cells: inverse effects on Bcl-2 and p53. Ann Clin Lab Sci. 1998 Nov-Dec; 28(6):360-9.Formby B, Wiley TS.

[177] Influences of percutaneous administration of estradiol and progesterone on human breast epithelial cell cycle in vivo. Fertil Steril. 1995 Apr; 63(4):785-91. Chang KJ, Lee TT, Linares-Cruz G, Fournier S, de Ligniéres B.

Chapter Twenty-Two

[178] With normal being 1.0

[179] Atsma F, Bartelink ML, Grobbee DE, van der Schouw YT. Postmenopausal status and early menopause as independent risk factors for cardiovascular disease: a meta-analysis. Menopause. 2006; 13:265–279.

[180] Lokkegaard E, Jovanovic Z, Heitmann BL, et al. The association between early menopause and risk of ischaemic heart disease: influence of hormone therapy. Maturitas. 2006; 53:226–233.

[181] J Clin Endocrinol Metab 86, 158–161.

[182] Estrogen and Progesterone Inhibit Vascular Smooth Muscle Proliferation The Endocrine Society Received September 26, 1996. Anjali K. Morey, Ali Pedram, Mahnaz Razandi, Bruce A. Prins, Ren-Ming Hu, Elzbieta Biesiada and Ellis R. Levin Intracellular Signal Systems Division of Endocrinology, Long Beach Veteran Affairs Medical Center, Long Beach, California 90822; and Departments of Medicine (A.P., M.R., R.-M.H., E.B., E.R.L.) and Pharmacology (A.K.M., B.A.P., E.R.L.), University of California, Irvine, Irvine, California 92717.

[183] Castelli W 1984 Epidemiology of coronary heart disease: The Framingham Study. Am J Med 76:4–12.

[184] Stampfer MJ, Willett WC, Colditz GA, Rosner B, Speizer FE, Hennekens CH 1991 Postmenopausal estrogen therapy and cardiovascular disease: ten year follow-up from the Nurses' Health Study. N Engl J Med 325:756–762.

Stampfer MJ, Colditz GA 1991 Estrogen replacement and coronary heart disease: a quantitative assessment of the epidemiologic evidence. Prev Med 20:47–63.

Henriksson P, Angelin B, Berglund L 1992 Hormonal regulation of serum Lp(a) levels. J Clin Invest 89:1166–1171.

[185] Effectiveness of Compounded Bio-identical Hormone Replacement Therapy An Observational Cohort Study Andres D Ruiz, Kelly R Daniels, Jamie C Barner, John J Carson, and Christopher R Frei BMC Womens Health. 2011; 11: 27. Published online 2011 June 8. BMC Womens Health v.11; 2011.

[186] Kalin MF, Zumoff B. Sex hormones and coronary disease: a review of the clinical studies. Steroids. 1990; 55: 330 –352. Heart, and Stroke Facts. Dallas: American Heart Association, 1992.

[187] Age at menopause as a risk factor for cardiovascular mortality. Lancet. 1996 Mar 16; 347(9003):714-8. van der Schouw YT, van der Graaf Y, Steyerberg EW, Eijkemans JC, Banga JD.

[188] Rosano GMC, Sarrel PM, Poole-Wilson PA, Collins P 1993 Beneficial effect of oestrogen on exercise-induced myocardial ischaemia in women with coronary artery disease. Lancet 342:133–136.

[189] Hormones in Wellness and Disease Prevention: Common Practices, Current State of the Evidence, and Questions for the Future Erika T. Schwartz, MD, Kent Holtorf, MD 10 West 74 Street, Suite 1A, New York, NY 10023, USA 23456 Hawthorne Boulevard, Suite 160, Torrance, CA 90505, USA Corresponding author. E-mail address: erika@drerika.com (E. Schwartz). Prim Care Clin Office Pract 35 (2008) 669–705 primarycare.theclinics.com 2008 Elsevier Inc.

[190] Kontoleon PE, Anastasiou-Nana MI, Papapetrou PD, et al. Hormonal profile in patients with congestive heart failure Int J Cardiol 20A3;87:179-183.

Anker SD, Chua TP, Ponikowski P, et al. Hormonal changes and catabolic/anabolic imbalance in chronic heart failure and their importance for cardiac cachexia Circulation 1997;96:526-534.

Moriyama Y, Yasue H, Yoshimura M, et al. The plasma levels of dehydroepiandrosterone sulfate are decreased in patients with chronic heart failure in proportion to the severity J Clin EndocrinolMetab 2000;85: 1834-1M0.

[191] Pugh PJ, Jones RD, West JN, Jones TH, Channer KS. Testosterone treatment for men with chronic heart failure Heart 2004; 90:446-447.

[192] Malkin CJ, Pugh PJ, West JN, Van Beek EJR, Jones TH, Channer KS. Testosterone therapy in men with moderate severity heart failure: a double-blind randomized placebo controlled trial Eur Heart J 2A06; 27:57-64.

Malkin CJ, Jones TH, Channer KS. The effect of testosterone on insulin sensitivity in men with heart failure Eur J Heart Fail 2007; 9:44.

[193] Swan JW, Anker SD, Walton C, et al. Insulin resistance in chronic heart failure: relation to severity and etiology of heart failure J Am Coll Cardiol 1997; 30:527-532.

Ingelsson E, Sundstr0m J, Arnlov J,Zethelius B, Lind L. Insulin resistance and risk of congestive heart failure JAMA A05;294:334-34L.

[194] Testosterone Therapy in Women with Chronic Heart Failure: A Pilot Double-blind, Randomized, Placebo-controlled Study Ferdinando Iellamo, MD, Maurizio

Volterrani, MD, Giuseppe Caminiti, MD, Roger Karam, MD, Rosalba Massaro, MD, Massimo Fini, MD, Peter Collins, MD, PhD, Giuseppe M.C. Rosano, MD J Am Coll Cardiol. 2010; 56(16):1310-1316. Journal of the American College of Cardiology.

[195] Maggio M., Lauretani F., Ceda GP, Bandinelli S., Ling SM, Metter EJ, Artoni A., Carassale L., Cazzato A., Ceresini G., Guralnik JM, Basaria S., Valenti G., Ferrucci L. Relationship between low levels of anabolic hormones and 6-year mortality in older men: the aging in the Chianti Area (InCHIANTI) study. Arch Intern Med. 2007; 167: 2249–2254.

[196] Shores MM, Matsumoto AM, Sloan KL, Kivlahan DR. Low serum testosterone and mortality in male veterans. Arch Int Med. 2006; 166: 1660–1665.

[197] Laughlin GA, Barrett-Connor E., Bergstrom J. Low serum testosterone and mortality in older men. J Clin Endocrinol Metab. 2008; 93: 68–75.

[198] Jones RD, Nettleship JE, Kapoor D, et al. Testosterone and atherosclerosis in aging men: purported association and clinical implications. Am J Cardiovasc Drugs 2005; 5:141–54.

Kapoor D, Aldred H, Clark S, et al. Clinical and biochemical assessment of hypogonadism in men with type 2 diabetes: correlations with bioavailable testosterone and visceral adiposity. Diabetes Care 2007; 30:911–17.

[199] Acute Anti-Ischemic Effect of Testosterone in Men With Coronary Artery Disease Clinical Investigation and Reports Accepted December 29, 1998. Giuseppe M. C. Rosano, MD, PhD; Filippo Leonardo, MD; Paolo Pagnotta, MD; Francesco Pelliccia, MD; Gaia Panina, MD; Elena Cerquetani, MD; Paola Lilla della Monica, MD; Bruno Bonfigli, MD; Massimo Volpe, MD; Sergio L. Chierchia, MD From the Department of Cardiology, Istituto H. San Raffaele, Roma and Milano, Italy.

[200] Testosterone replacement in hypogonadal men with angina improves ischaemic threshold and quality of life Heart 2004;90:871-876 doi:10.1136/hrt.2003.021121 Cardiovascular medicine C J Malkin, P J Pugh, P D Morris, K E Kerry, R D Jones, T H Jones,K S Channer.

[201] Hormones in Wellness and Disease Prevention: Common Practices, Current State of the Evidence, and Questions for the Future Erika T. Schwartz, MD, Kent Holtorf, MD 10 West 74 Street, Suite 1A, New York, NY 10023, USA 23456 Hawthorne Boulevard, Suite 160, Torrance, CA 90505, USA Corresponding author. E-mail address: erika@drerika.com (E. Schwartz). Prim Care Clin Office Pract 35 (2008) 669–705 primarycare.theclinics.com 2008 Elsevier Inc.

[202] Kapoor D, Goodwin E, Channer KS, et al. Testosterone replacement therapy improves insulin resistance, glycaemic control, visceral adiposity and hypercholesterolaemia in hypogonadal men with type 2 diabetes. Eur J Endocrinol 2006; 154:899–906.

Saad F, Gooren L, Haider A, et al. Effects of testosterone gel followed by parenteral testosterone undecanoate on sexual dysfunction and on features of the metabolic syndrome. Andrologia 2008; 40:44–8.

Allan CA, Strauss BJG, Burger HG, et al. Testosterone therapy prevents gain in visceral adipose tissue and loss of skeletal muscle in nonobese aging men. J Clin Endocrinol Metab 2008; 93:139–46.

[203] Hormones in Wellness and Disease Prevention: Common Practices, Current State of the Evidence, and Questions for the Future Erika T. Schwartz, MD, Kent Holtorf, MD 10 West 74 Street, Suite 1A, New York, NY 10023, USA 23456 Hawthorne

Boulevard, Suite 160, Torrance, CA 90505, USA Corresponding author. E-mail address: erika@drerika.com (E. Schwartz). Prim Care Clin Office Pract 35 (2008) 669–705 primarycare.theclinics.com 2008 Elsevier Inc.

Chapter Twenty-Three

[204] Cholesterol is a precursor for the production of steroid hormones, bile acids, and vitamin D. Hanukoglu I (Dec 1992). "Steroidogenic enzymes: structure, function, and role in regulation of steroid hormone biosynthesis." J Steroid Biochem Mol Biol 43 (8): 779–804.

[205] Weingärtner O, Pinsdorf T, Rogacev KS, Blömer L, Grenner Y, Gräber S, Ulrich C, Girndt M, Böhm M, Fliser D, Laufs U, Lütjohann D, Heine GH (2010). "The relationships of markers of cholesterol homeostasis with carotid intima-media thickness". In Federici, Massimo. PLoS ONE 5 (10): e13467.

[206] Tymoczko, John L.; Stryer Berg Tymoczko; Stryer, Lubert; Berg, Jeremy Mark (2002). Biochemistry. San Francisco: W.H. Freeman. pp. 726–727.

[207] Lewis GF, Rader DJ (June 2005). "New insights into the regulation of HDL metabolism and reverse cholesterol transport". Circ. Res. 96 (12): 1221–32.

[208] Gordon DJ, Probstfield JL, Garrison RJ, Neaton JD, Castelli WP, Knoke JD, Jacobs DR, Bangdiwala S, Tyroler HA (January 1989. "High-density lipoprotein cholesterol and cardiovascular disease. Four prospective American studies". Circulation 79 (1): 8–15.

[209] Brunzell JD, Davidson M, Furberg CD, Goldberg RB, Howard BV, Stein JH, Witztum JL (April 2008). "Lipoprotein management in patients with cardiometabolic risk: consensus statement from the American Diabetes Association and the American College of Cardiology Foundation". Diabetes Care 31 (4): 811–22.

[210] Aging, hormones, body composition, metabolic effects. World J Urol. 2002 May; 20(1):23-7. Vermeulen A.

[211] Beneficial effect of hormone replacement therapy on weight loss in obese menopausal women. Maturitas. 1999 Aug 16; 32(3):147-53. Chmouliovsky L, Habicht F, James RW, Lehmann T, Campana A, Golay A.

[212] Cardiovascular pharmacology of estradiol metabolites Raghvendra K. Dubey, Stevan P. Tofovic and Edwin K. Jackson Received October 29, 2003. Accepted December 1, 2003. The American Society for Pharmacology and Experimental Therapeutics.

[213] Conjugated equine estrogens alone, but not in combination with medroxyprogesterone acetate, inhibit aortic connective tissue remodeling after plasma lipid lowering in female monkeys. Arterioscler Thromb Vasc Biol. 1998 Jul; 18(7):1164-71. Register TC, Adams MR, Golden DL, Clarkson TB.

[214] Effect of hormone replacement therapy on age-related increase in carotid artery intima-media thickness in postmenopausal women. Atherosclerosis. 2000 Nov; 153(1):81-8. Tremollieres FA, Cigagna F, Alquier C, Cauneille C, Pouilles J, Ribot C.

[215] Effect of hormone replacement therapy on cardiovascular events in recently postmenopausal women: randomised trial BMJ 2012; (Published 9 October 2012) Cite this as: BMJ 2012;345:e6409 Louise Lind Schierbeck, registrar, Lars Rejnmark, associate professor, consultant, Charlotte Landbo Tofteng, staff specialist, Lis Stilgren, consultant, Pia Eiken, consultant, senior endocrinologist, Leif Mosekilde, professor,

senior consultant, Lars Køber, professor, consultant, Jens-Erik Beck Jensen, associate professor, consultant.

216 Simoncini T, Mannella P, Fornari L, Caruso A, Varone G, Genazzani AR. In vitro effects of progesterone and progestins on vascular cells. Steroids2003; 68(10-13):831-6.

217 Effects of estrogen or estrogen/progestin regimens on heart disease risk factors in postmenopausal women. The Postmenopausal Estrogen/Progestin Interventions (PEPI) Trial. The Writing Group for the PEPI Trial. JAMA1995; 273:199-208.)

Hodis HN, Mack WJ, Lobo RA, Shoupe D, Sevanian A, Mahrer PR, et al. Estrogen in the prevention of atherosclerosis. A randomized, double-blind, placebo-controlled trial. Ann Intern Med2001; 135:939-53.)

Hulley S, Grady D, Bush T, Furberg C, Herrington D, Riggs B, et al. Randomized trial of estrogen plus progestin for secondary prevention of coronary heart disease in postmenopausal women. Heart and Estrogen/progestin Replacement Study (HERS) Research Group. JAMA1998; 280:605-13.

218 Effect of hormone replacement therapy on cardiovascular events in recently postmenopausal women: randomised trial BMJ 2012; (Published 9 October 2012) Cite this as: BMJ 2012;345:e6409 Louise Lind Schierbeck, registrar1, Lars Rejnmark, associate professor, consultant2, Charlotte Landbo Tofteng, staff specialist, Lis Stilgren, consultant, Pia Eiken, consultant, senior endocrinologist, Leif Mosekilde, professor, senior consultant, Lars Køber, professor, consultant, Jens-Erik Beck Jensen, associate professor, consultant.

219 Effects of oestradiol administration via different routes on the lipid profile in women with bilateral oophorectomy. Maturitas. 1994 Mar; 18(3):239-44. Palacios S, Menendez C, Jurado AR, Vargas JC.

220 Castelli W 1984 Epidemiology of coronary heart disease: The Framingham Study. Am J Med 76:4–12.

221 Colditz GA, Willett WC, Stampfer MJ, Rosner B, Speizer FE, Hennekens CH 1987 Menopause and the risk of coronary heart disease in women. N Engl J Med 316:1105–1110.

Stampfer MJ, Willett WC, Colditz GA, Rosner B, Speizer FE, Hennekens CH 1985 A prospective study of postmenopausal estrogen therapy and coronary heart disease. N Engl J Med 313:1044–1049.

Stampfer MJ, Willett WC, Colditz GA, Rosner B, Speizer FE, Hennekens CH 1991 Postmenopausal estrogen therapy and cardiovascular disease: ten year follow-up from the Nurses' Health Study. N Engl J Med 325:756–762.

Stampfer MJ, Colditz GA 1991 Estrogen replacement and coronary heart disease: a quantitative assessment of the epidemiologic evidence. Prev Med 20:47–63.

222 Effects of testosterone supplementation in the aging male. J Clin Endocrinol Metab. 1992 Oct; 75(4):1092-8. Tenover JS.

Low serum testosterone and increased mortality in men with coronary heart disease Volume 96, Issue 22 Heart 2010;96:1821-1825 doi:10.1136/hrt.2010.195412 Coronary artery disease Chris J Malkin, Peter J Pugh, Paul D Morris, Sonia Asif, T Hugh Jones, Kevin S Channer, Department of Cardiology, Royal Hallamshire Hospital, Sheffield, UK.

223 Jones RD, Nettleship JE, Kapoor D, et al. Testosterone and atherosclerosis in aging men: purported association and clinical implications. Am J Cardiovasc Drugs 2005; 5:141–54.

Kapoor D, Aldred H, Clark S, et al. Clinical and biochemical assessment of hypogonadism in men with type 2 diabetes: correlations with bioavailable testosterone and visceral adiposity. Diabetes Care 2007; 30:911–17.

224 Kapoor D, Goodwin E, Channer KS, et al. Testosterone replacement therapy improves insulin resistance, glycaemic control, visceral adiposity and hypercholesterolaemia in hypogonadal men with type 2 diabetes. Eur J Endocrinol 2006; 154:899–906.)

Malkin CJ, Pugh PJ, Jones RD, et al. The effect of testosterone replacement on endogenous inflammatory cytokines and lipid profiles in hypogonadal men. J Clin Endocrinol Metab 2004; 89:3313–18.)

Heufelder AE, Saad F, Bunck MC, et al. 52-Week treatment with diet and exercise plus transdermal testosterone reverses the metabolic syndrome and improves glycaemic control in men with newly diagnosed type 2 diabetes and subnormal plasma testosterone. J Androl 2009; 30:726–33.

225 Malkin CJ, Jones RD, Jones TH, et al. Effect of testosterone on ex vivo vascular reactivity in man. Clin Sci (Lond) 2006; 111:265–74.

Malkin CJ, Jones TH, Channer KS. The effect of testosterone on insulin sensitivity in men with heart failure. Eur J Heart Fail 2007; 9:44–50.

226 Malkin CJ, Jones TH, Channer KS. The effect of testosterone on insulin sensitivity in men with heart failure. Eur J Heart Fail 2007; 9:44–50.

Low serum testosterone and increased mortality in men with coronary heart disease Volume 96, Issue 22 Heart 2010;96:1821-1825 Coronary artery disease Chris J Malkin, Peter J Pugh, Paul D Morris, Sonia Asif, T Hugh Jones, Kevin S Channer, Department of Cardiology, Royal Hallamshire Hospital, Sheffield, UK.

227 Kalin MF, Zumoff B. Sex hormones and coronary disease: a review of the clinical studies. Steroids. 1990; 55:330 –352.

228 Heart, and Stroke Facts. Dallas: American Heart Association, 1992.

Chapter Twenty-Four
229 Testosterone for Life, Abraham Morgentaler, MD, McGraw Hill, copyright, 2009, page 142.

Chapter Twenty-Six

230 Dr. Thierry Hertoghe, The Hormone Handbook 2nd Edition 2010.

231 The effects of subcutaneous hormone implants during climacteric. Maturitas. 1984 Mar; 5(3):177-84. Cardozo L, Gibb DM, Tuck SM, Thom MH, Studd JW, Cooper DJ.

232 Transdermal testosterone therapy improves well-being, mood, and sexual function in premenopausal women. Menopause. 2003 Sep-Oct; 10(5):390-8. Goldstat R, Briganti E, Tran J, Wolfe R, Davis SR.

233 Seidman, S.N. and Rabkin, J.G.: Testosterone replacement therapy for hypogonadal men with SSRI-refractory depression. J Affect Disord, 48:157, 1998.

234 Goldstat R, Briganti E, Tran J, Wolfe R and Davis S (2003) Transdermal testosterone improves mood, well-being and sexual function in premenopausal women. Menopause 10, 390–398

235 Studd JWW, Colins WP and Chakravarti S (1977b) Estradiol and testosterone implants in the treatment of psychosexual problems in postmenopausal women. Br J Obstet Gynaecol 84, 314–315.

236 Effectiveness of Compounded Bio-identical Hormone Replacement Therapy An Observational Cohort Study BMC Womens Health. 2011; 11: 27. Published online 2011 June 8. BMC Womens Health v.11; 2011 Andres D Ruiz, Kelly R Daniels, Jamie C Barner, John J Carson, and Christopher R Frei.

237 Prophylactic oophorectomy in pre-menopausal women and long term health – a review Lynne T. Shuster, Bobbie S. Gostout, Brandon R. Grossardt,, and Walter A. Rocca.
238 McKinlay JB, McKinlay SM, Brambilla D. The relative contributions of endocrine changes and social circumstances to depression in mid-aged women. J Health Soc Behav. 1987; 28:345–363.
239 Rocca WA, Grossardt BR, Geda YE, et al. Long-term risk of depressive and anxiety symptoms following early bilateral oophorectomy. Menopause. 2008 in press.
240 Sluijmer AV, Heineman MJ, De Jong FH, Evers JL. Endocrine activity of the postmenopausal ovary: the effects of pituitary down-regulation and oophorectomy. J Clin Endocrinol Metab. 1995; 80:2163–2167.
241 Burt VK, Altshuler LL, Rasgon N: Depressive symptoms in the perimenopause: prevalence, assessment, and guidelines for treatment. Harv Rev Psychiatry 1998; 6:121–132.
Menopause Core Curriculum Study Guide. Cleveland, Ohio, North American Menopause Society, 2000.
242 Research on the Menopause in the 1990s: Report of a WHO Scientific Group. World Health Organ Tech Rep Ser 1996; 866:1–107.
Stone AB, Pearlstein TB: Evaluation and treatment of changes in mood, sleep, and sexual functioning associated with menopause. Obstet Gynecol Clin North Am 1994; 21:391–403.
243 Hay AG, Bancroft J, Johnstone EC: Affective symptoms in women attending a menopause clinic. Br J Psychiatry 1994; 164:513–516.
Novaes C, Almeida O, de Melo N: Mental health among perimenopausal women attending a menopause clinic: possible association with premenstrual clinic? Climacteric 1998; 1:264–270.
Harlow BL, Cohen LS, Otto MW, Spiegelman D, Cramer DW: Prevalence and predictors of depressive symptoms in older premenopausal women: the Harvard Study of Moods and Cycles. Arch Gen Psychiatry 1999; 56:418–424.
244 Schmidt PJ, Rubinow DR: Menopause-related affective disorders: a justification for further study. Am J Psychiatry 1994; 148:844–852.

[245] Schmidt PJ, Nieman L, Danaceau MA, Tobin MB, Roca CA, Murphy JH, Rubinow DR: Estrogen replacement in perimenopause-related depression: a preliminary report. Am J Obstet Gynecol 2000; 183:414–420.

Soares CN, Almeida OP, Joffe H, Cohen LS: Efficacy of estradiol for the treatment of depressive disorders in perimenopausal women: a double-blind, randomized, placebo-controlled trial. Arch Gen Psychiatry 2001; 58:529–534.

[246] Schmidt PJ, Nieman L, Danaceau MA, Tobin MB, Roca CA, Murphy JH, Rubinow DR: Estrogen replacement in perimenopause-related depression: a preliminary report. Am J Obstet Gynecol 2000; 183:414–420.

Soares CN, Almeida OP, Joffe H, Cohen LS: Efficacy of estradiol for the treatment of depressive disorders in perimenopausal women: a double-blind, randomized, placebo-controlled trial. Arch Gen Psychiatry 2001; 58:529–534.

Rasgon NL, Altshuler LL, Fairbanks L: Estrogen-replacement therapy for depression (letter). Am J Psychiatry 2001; 158:1738.

[247] Estrogen replacement in perimenopause-related depression a preliminary report. Am J Obstet Gynecol. 2000 Aug; 183(2):414-20. Schmidt PJ, Nieman L, Danaceau MA, Tobin MB, Roca CA, Murphy JH, Rubinow DR.

[248] Shores MM, Moceri VM, Gruenewald DA, et al. Low testosterone is associated with decreased function and increased mortality risk: a preliminary study of men in a geriatric rehabilitation unit. J Am Geriatr Soc 2004; 52:2077–81.

Khaw KT, Dowsett M, Folkerd E, et al. Endogenous testosterone and mortality due to all causes, cardiovascular disease, and cancer in men: European prospective investigation into cancer in Norfolk (EPIC-Norfolk) Prospective Population Study. Circulation 2007; 116:2694–701.

Shores MM, Matsumoto AM, Sloan KL, et al. Low serum testosterone and mortality in male veterans. Arch Intern Med 2006; 166:1660–5.

Laughlin GA, Barrett-Connor E, Bergstrom J. Low serum testosterone and mortality in older men. J Clin Endocrinol Metab 2008; 93:68–75.

[249] Keating NL Diabetes and cardiovascular disease during androgen deprivation therapy: observational study of veterans with prostate cancer. J Natl Cancer Inst 2010; 102:39–46.

[250] Malavige LS Erectile dysfunction in diabetes mellitus. J Sex Med 2009; 6:1232–1247.

Wu FC Identification of late-onset hypogonadism in middle-aged and elderly men. N Engl J Med 2010; 363:123–135.

[251] Testosterone replacement therapy for hypogonadal men with ssri-refractory depression J Affect Disord. 1998 Mar; 48(2-3):157-61. Seidman SN, Rabkin JG.)

Testosterone replacement therapy improves mood in hypogonadal men--a clinical research center study. J Clin Endocrinol Metab. 1996 Oct; 81(10):3578-83. Wang C, Alexander G, Berman N, Salehian B, Davidson T, McDonald V, Steiner B, Hull L, Callegari C, Swerdloff RS.

[252] Testosterone replacement therapy improves mood in hypogonadal men--a clinical research center study. J Clin Endocrinol Metab. 1996 Oct; 81(10):3578-83. Wang C, Alexander G, Berman N, Salehian B, Davidson T, McDonald V, Steiner B, Hull L, Callegari C, Swerdloff RS.

Chapter Twenty-Seven

[253] American Diabetes Association. Checking Your Blood Glucose. http://www.diabetes.org/living-with-diabetes/treatment-and-care/blood-glucose-control/checking-your-blood-glucose.html. Accessed April 23, 2014.) (American Diabetes Association. Taking Care of Your Diabetes. http://www.diabetes.org/living-with-diabetes/recently-diagnosed/where-do-i-begin/taking-care-of-your-diabetes.html. Accessed April 23, 2014.

[254] MedlinePlus: Metabolic Syndrome

[255] Ford ES, Giles WH, Dietz WH (2002.)
Prevalence of metabolic syndrome among US adults: findings from the third National Health and Nutrition Examination Survey". JAMA 287 (3): 356–359.

[256] Kapoor D, Goodwin E, Channer KS, et al. Testosterone replacement therapy improves insulin resistance, glycaemic control, visceral adiposity and hypercholesterolaemia in hypogonadal men with type 2 diabetes. Eur J Endocrinol 2006; 154:899–906.

Malkin CJ, Pugh PJ, Jones RD, et al. The effect of testosterone replacement on endogenous inflammatory cytokines and lipid profiles in hypogonadal men. J Clin Endocrinol Metab 2004; 89:3313–18.

Heufelder AE, Saad F, Bunck MC, et al. 52-Week treatment with diet and exercise plus transdermal testosterone reverses the metabolic syndrome and improves glycaemic control in men with newly diagnosed type 2 diabetes and subnormal plasma testosterone. J Androl 2009; 30:726–33.

[257] Low Testosterone Associated With Obesity and the Metabolic Syndrome Contributes to Sexual Dysfunction and Cardiovascular Disease Risk in Men With Type 2 Diabetes CARE,VOLUME 34, JULY 2011 Christina Wang, MD, Graham Jackson, MD, T. Hugh Jones, MD, Alvin M. Matsumoto, MD, Ajay Nehra, MD, Michael A. Perelman, PHD, Ronald S. Swerdloff, MD, Abdul Traish, PHD, Michael Zitzmann, MD and Glenn Cunningham, MD.

[258] Progesterone and its derivatives are neuroprotective agents in experimental diabetic neuropathy a multimodal analysis. Neuroscience. 2007 Feb 23; 144(4):1293-304. Epub 2006 Dec 20. Leonelli E, Bianchi R, Cavaletti G, Caruso D, Crippa D, Garcia-Segura LM, Lauria G, Magnaghi V, Roglio I, Melcangi RC.

[259] Progesterone inhibits human infragenicular arterial smooth muscle cell proliferation induced by high glucose and insulin concentrations. J Vasc Surg. 2002 Oct; 36(4):833-8. Carmody BJ, Arora S, Wakefield MC, Weber M, Fox CJ, Sidawy AN.

[260] Low Testosterone Associated With Obesity and the Metabolic Syndrome Contributes to Sexual Dysfunction and Cardiovascular Disease Risk in Men With Type 2 Diabetes CARE,VOLUME 34, JULY 2011 Christina Wang, MD, Graham Jackson, MD, T. Hugh Jones, MD, Alvin M. Matsumoto, MD, Ajay Nehra, MD, Michael A. Perelman, PHD, Ronald S. Swerdloff, MD, Abdul Traish, PHD, Michael Zitzmann, MD and Glenn Cunningham, MD.

[261] Laaksonen DE The metabolic syndrome and smoking in relation to hypogonadism in middle-aged men: a prospective cohort study. J Clin Endocrinol Metab 2005; 90:712–719.

Corona GType 2 diabetes mellitus and testosterone: a meta-analysis study. Int J Androl. 24 October 2010.

[262] Corona GType 2 diabetes mellitus and testosterone: a meta-analysis study. Int J Androl. 24 October 2010.

Laaksonen DE Testosterone and sex hormone-binding globulin predict the metabolic syndrome and diabetes in middle-aged men. Diabetes Care 2004; 27:1036–10416,8.

[263] Corona GType 2 diabetes mellitus and testosterone: a meta-analysis study. Int J Androl. 24 October 2010

[264] Diaz-Arjonilla M Obesity, low testosterone levels and erectile dysfunction. Int J Impot Res 2009; 21:89–98.

[265] Lindau ST Sexuality among middle-aged and older adults with diagnosed and undiagnosed diabetes: a national, population-based study. Diabetes Care 2010; 33:2202Rosen RC, Wing RR, Schneider S, et al. Erectile dysfunction in type 2 diabetic men: relationship to exercise fitness and cardiovascular risk factors in the Look AHEAD trial. J Sex Med 2009; 6:1414–1422.

[266] Fedele D Erectile dysfunction in type 1 and type 2 diabetics in Italy. On behalf of Gruppo Italiano Studio Deficit Erettile nei Diabetici. Int J Epidemiol 2000; 29:524–531.

[267] Jones TH Testosterone replacement in hypogonadal men with type 2 diabetes and/or metabolic syndrome (The TIMES2 Study). Diabetes Care 2011; 34:828–837.

[268] Boloña ER Testosterone use in men with sexual dysfunction: a systematic review and meta-analysis of randomized placebo-controlled trials. Mayo Clin Proc 2007; 82:20–28.

[269] Isidori AM Effects of testosterone on sexual function in men: results of a meta-analysis. Clin Endocrinol (Oxf) 2005; 63:381–394.

Hatzichristou D Efficacy of tadalafil once daily in men with diabetes mellitus and erectile dysfunction. Diabet Med 2008; 25:138–146.

Rochira V Sildenafil improves sleep-related erections in hypogonadal men: evidence from a randomized, placebo-controlled, crossover study of a synergic role for both testosterone and sildenafil on penile erections. J Androl 2006; 27:165–175.

[270] Shores MM Low serum testosterone and mortality in male veterans. Arch Intern Med 2006; 166:1660–1665.

Low Testosterone Associated With Obesity and the Metabolic Syndrome Contributes to Sexual Dysfunction and Cardiovascular Disease Risk in Men With Type 2 Diabetes CARE,VOLUME 34, JULY 2011 Christina Wang, MD, Graham Jackson, MD, T. Hugh Jones, MD, Alvin M. Matsumoto, MD, Ajay Nehra, MD, Michael A. Perelman, PHD, Ronald S. Swerdloff, MD, Abdul Traish, PHD, Michael Zitzmann, MD and Glenn Cunningham, MD)

Androgen Deprivation Therapy, Insulin Resistance, and Cardiovascular Mortality An Inconvenient Truth Shehzad Basaria   Article first published 2 JAN 2013 2008 American Society of Andrology Journal of Andrology Volume 29, Issue 5, pages 534–539, September-October 2008.

[271] Malkin CJ Testosterone therapy in men with moderate severity heart failure: a double-blind randomized placebo controlled trial. Eur Heart J 2006; 27:57–64.

Caminiti G Effect of long-acting testosterone treatment on functional exercise capacity, skeletal muscle performance, insulin resistance, and baroreflex sensitivity in elderly patients with chronic heart failure: a double-blind, placebo-controlled, randomized study. J Am Coll Cardiol 2009; 54:919–927.

[272] Basaria S Adverse events associated with testosterone administration. N Engl J Med 2010; 363:109–122.

Srinivas-Shankar U Effects of testosterone on muscle strength, physical function, body composition, and quality of life in intermediate-frail and frail elderly men: a randomized, double-blind, placebo-controlled study. J Clin Endocrinol Metab 2010; 95:639–65050,51)

[273] Isidori AM Effects of testosterone on sexual function in men: results of a meta-analysis. Clin Endocrinol (Oxf) 2005; 63:381–394.

Heufelder AE Fifty-two-week treatment with diet and exercise plus transdermal testosterone reverses the metabolic syndrome and improves glycemic control in men with newly diagnosed type 2 diabetes and subnormal plasma testosterone. J Androl 2009; 30:726–733.

Kalinchenko SY Effects of testosterone supplementation on markers of the metabolic syndrome and inflammation in hypogonadal men with the metabolic syndrome: the double-blinded placebo-controlled Moscow study. Clin Endocrinol (Oxf) 2010; 73:602.

Malkin CJ. The effect of testosterone on insulin sensitivity in men with heart failure. Eur J Heart Fail 2007; 9:44–50.

Jones TH The effects of testosterone on risk factors for, and the mediators of, the atherosclerotic process. Atherosclerosis 2009; 207:318–327.

Kapoor D The effect of testosterone replacement therapy on adipocytokines and C-reactive protein in hypogonadal men with type 2 diabetes. Eur J Endocrinol 2007; 156:595–602.

Low Testosterone Associated With Obesity and the Metabolic Syndrome Contributes to Sexual Dysfunction and Cardiovascular Disease Risk in Men With Type 2 Diabetes CARE,VOLUME 34, JULY 2011 Christina Wang, MD, Graham Jackson,

MD, T. Hugh Jones, MD, Alvin M. Matsumoto, MD, Ajay Nehra, MD, Michael A. Perelman, PHD, Ronald S. Swerdloff, MD, Abdul Traish, PHD, Michael Zitzmann, MD and Glenn Cunningham, MD)

[274] Low Testosterone Associated With Obesity and the Metabolic Syndrome Contributes to Sexual Dysfunction and Cardiovascular Disease Risk in Men With Type 2 Diabetes CARE,VOLUME 34, JULY 2011 Christina Wang, MD, Graham Jackson, MD, T. Hugh Jones, MD, Alvin M. Matsumoto, MD, Ajay Nehra, MD, Michael A. Perelman, PHD, Ronald S. Swerdloff, MD, Abdul Traish, PHD, Michael Zitzmann, MD and Glenn Cunningham, MD)

[275] Basaria S., Dobs AS. Hypogonadism and androgen replacement therapy in elderly men. Am J Med. 2001; 110: 563–572.

Haffner SM, Shaten J., Stern MP, Smith GD, Kuller L. Low levels of sex hormone-binding globulin and testosterone predict the development of non-insulin-dependent diabetes mellitus in men. MRFIT Research Group. Multiple Risk Factor Intervention Trial. Am J Epidemiol. 1996; 143: 889–897.

Muller M., Grobbee DE, den Tonkelaar I., Lamberts SW, van Der Schouw YT. Endogenous sex hormones and metabolic syndrome in aging men. J Clin Endocrinol Metab. 2005; 90: 2618–2623.

[276] Satariano WA, Ragland KE, van den Eeden SK. Cause of death in men diagnosed with prostate carcinoma. Cancer. 1998;83: 1180–1188.

Lu-Yao G., Stukel TA, Yao SL. Changing patterns in competing causes of death in men with prostate cancer: a population based study. J Urol. 2004; 171: 2285–2290.

[277] Smith MR. Androgen deprivation therapy for prostate cancer: new concepts and concerns. Curr Opin Endocrinol Diabetes Obes. 2007; 14: 247–254.

Haffner SM, Valdez RA, Mykkanen L., Stern MP, Katz MS. Decreased testosterone and dehydroepiandrosterone sulfate concentrations are associated with increased insulin and glucose concentrations in nondiabetic men. Metabolism. 1994; 43: 599–603.

Laaksonen DE, Niskanen L., Punnonen K., Nyyssönen K., Tuomainen TP, Valkonen VP, Salonen R., Salonen JT. Testosterone and sex hormone-binding globulin predict the metabolic syndrome and diabetes in middle-aged men. Diabetes Care. 2004; 27: 1036–1041.

Muller M., Grobbee DE, den Tonkelaar I., Lamberts SW, van Der Schouw YT. Endogenous sex hormones and metabolic syndrome in aging men. J Clin Endocrinol Metab. 2005; 90: 2618–2623.

Pitteloud N., Hardin M., Dwyer AA, Valassi E., Yialamas M., Elahi D., Hayes FJ. Increasing insulin resistance is associated with a decrease in Leydig cell testosterone secretion in men. J Clin Endocrinol Metab. 2005; 90: 2636–2641.

[278] Marin P., Holmang S., Jonsson L., Sjöström L., Kvist H., Holm G., Lindstedt G., Björntorp P.. The effects of testosterone treatment on body composition and metabolism in middle-aged obese men. Int J Obes Relat Metab Disord. 1992; 16: 991–997.

Androgen Deprivation Therapy, Insulin Resistance, and Cardiovascular Mortality An Inconvenient Truth Shehzad Basaria Article first published 2 JAN 2013 2008 American Society of Andrology Journal of Andrology Volume 29, Issue 5, pages 534–539, September-October 2008.

[280] Haffner SM, Valdez RA, Morales PA, Hazuda HP, Stern MP: Decreased sex hormone-binding globulin predicts noninsulin-dependent diabetes mellitus in women but not in men. J Clin Endocrinol Metab 77:56–60, 1993.

[281] Holmäng A, Larsson BM, Brzezinska Z, Björntorp P: Effects of short-term testosterone exposure on insulin sensitivity of muscles in female rats. Am J Physiol 262:E851–E855, 1992.

Matthews DR, Hosker JP, Rudenski AS, Naylor BA, Treacher DF, Turner RC: Homeostasis model assessment: insulin resistance and beta–cell function from fasting plasma glucose and insulin concentrations in man. Diabetologia 28:412–419, 1985.

World Health Organization: Definition, Diagnosis and Classification of Diabetes Mellitus and its Complications: Report of a WHO Consultation. Part 1: Diagnosis and Classification of Diabetes Mellitus Geneva, World Health Org., 1999.

Holmäng A, Svedberg J, Jennische E, Björntorp P: Effects of testosterone on muscle insulin sensitivity and morphology in female rats. Am J Physiol 259:E555–E560, 1990.

Tremblay RR, Dube JY: Plasma concentrations of free and non-TeBG bound testosterone in women on oral contraceptives. Contraception 10:599–605, 1974).

[282] Insulin resistance, secretion, and elimination in postmenopausal women receiving oral or transdermal hormone replacement therapy. Metabolism. 1993 Jul; 42(7):846-53. Godsland IF, Gangar K, Walton C, Cust MP, Whitehead MI, Wynn V, Stevenson JC. Source: Wynn Institute for Metabolic Research, London, England, UK.

[283] Morley JE: Androgens and aging. Maturitas 38:61–73, 2001.

Laughlin GA, Barrett-Connor E, Kritz-Silverstein D, von Mühlen D: Hysterectomy, oophorectomy, and endogenous sex hormone levels in older women: the Rancho Bernardo Study. J Clin Endocrinol Metab 85:645–651, 2000.

Phillips GB, Tuck CH, Jing TY, Boden-Albala B, Lin IF, Dahodwala N, Sacco RL: Association of hyperandrogenemia and hyperestrogenemia with type 2 diabetes in Hispanic postmenopausal women. Diabetes Care 23:74–79, 2000)

Endogenous Sex Hormones and the Development of Type 2 Diabetes in Older Men and Women: the Rancho Bernardo Study Diabetes Care January 2002 Jee-Young Oh, MD, Elizabeth Barrett-Connor, MD, Nicole M. Wedick, MS and Deborah L. Wingard, PHD Division of Epidemiology, Department of Family and Preventive Medicine, University of California, San Diego, California.

[284] Haffner SM, Karhapää P, Mykkänen L, Laakso M: Insulin resistance, body fat distribution, and sex hormones in men. Diabetes 43:212–219, 1994.

Endogenous Sex Hormones and the Development of Type 2 Diabetes in Older Men and Women: the Rancho Bernardo Study Diabetes Care January 2002 Jee-Young Oh, MD, Elizabeth Barrett-Connor, MD, Nicole M. Wedick, MS and Deborah L. Wingard, PHD Division of Epidemiology, Department of Family and Preventive Medicine, University of California, San Diego, California.

[285] American Diabetes Association: Screening for diabetes. Diabetes Care 24(Suppl. 1):S21–S24, 2001

Reaven PD, Barrett-Connor EL, Browner DK: Abnormal glucose tolerance and hypertension. Diabetes Care 13:119–125, 1990

Endogenous Sex Hormones and the Development of Type 2 Diabetes in Older Men and Women: the Rancho Bernardo Study Diabetes Care January 2002 Jee-Young Oh, MD, Elizabeth Barrett-Connor, MD, Nicole M. Wedick, MS and Deborah L. Wingard, PHD Division of Epidemiology, Department of Family and Preventive Medicine, University of California, San Diego, California.

[286] Phillips GB, Pinkernell BH, Jing TY. The association of hypotestosteronemia with coronary artery disease in men. Arterioscler Thromb. 1994; 14: 701–706.

[287] van den Beld AW, Bots ML, Janssen JA, Pols HA, Lamberts SW, Grobbee DE. Endogenous hormones and carotid atherosclerosis in elderly men. Am J Epidemiol. 2003; 157: 25–31.

[288] Hak AE, Witteman JC, de Jong FH, Geerlings MI, Hofman A, Pols HA. Low levels of endogenous androgens increase the risk of atherosclerosis in elderly men: the Rotterdam study. J Clin Endocrinol Metab. 2002; 87: 3632–3639.

[289] Huggins C, Hodges CV. Studies on prostatic cancer, I: the effect of castration, of estrogen and of androgen injection on serum phosphatases in metastatic carcinoma of the prostate: 1941. J Urol. 2002; 168: 9–12.

[290] Liverman CT, Blazer DG, eds. Testosterone and Aging. Washington, DC: Institute of Medicine, National Academies Press; 2004.

Eaton NE, Reeves GK, Appleby PN, Key TJ. Endogenous sex hormones and prostate cancer: a quantitative review of prospective studies. Br J Cancer. 1999; 80: 930–934.

[291] Endogenous Testosterone and Mortality Due to All Causes, Cardiovascular Disease, and Cancer in Men European Prospective Investigation Into Cancer in Norfolk (EPIC-Norfolk) Prospective Population Study Epidemiology Received June 1, 2007 Kay-Tee Khaw, MBBChir, FRCP; Mitch Dowsett, PhD; Elizabeth Folkerd, PhD;

Sheila Bingham, PhD; Nicholas Wareham, MBBS, PhD; Robert Luben, BSc; Ailsa Welch, PhD; Nicholas Day, PhD.

[292] National Health and Nutrition Examination Survey (NHANES) 2003–2004 data.

[293] Testosterone Concentrations in Diabetic and Nondiabetic Obese Men Sandeep Dhindsa, MD, Michael G. Miller, PHARMD, Cecilia L. McWhirter, MS, Donald E. Mager, PHARMD, PHD, Husam Ghanim, PHD, Ajay Chaudhuri, MD, and Paresh Dandona, MD Diabetes Care. 2010 June; 33(6): 1186–1192.

[294] Testosterone Concentrations in Diabetic and Nondiabetic Obese Men Sandeep Dhindsa, MD, Michael G. Miller, PHARMD, Cecilia L. McWhirter, MS, Donald E. Mager, PHARMD, PHD, Husam Ghanim, PHD, Ajay Chaudhuri, MD, and Paresh Dandona, MD Diabetes Care. 2010 June; 33(6): 1186–1192.

Dhindsa S, Prabhakar S, Sethi M, Bandyopadhyay A, Chaudhuri A, Dandona P.: Frequent occurrence of hypogonadotropic hypogonadism in type 2 diabetes. J Clin Endocrinol Metab 2004; 89:5462–5468.

Dhindsa S, Bhatia V, Dhindsa G, Chaudhuri A, Gollapudi GM, Dandona P.: The effects of hypogonadism on body composition and bone mineral density in type 2 diabetic patients. Diabetes Care 2007; 30:1860–1861.

Kapoor D, Aldred H, Clark S, Channer KS, Jones TH.: Clinical and biochemical assessment of hypogonadism in men with type 2 diabetes: correlations with bioavailable testosterone and visceral adiposity. Diabetes Care 2007; 30:911–917.

Grossmann M, Thomas MC, Panagiotopoulos S, Sharpe K, Macisaac RJ, Clarke S, Zajac JD, Jerums G.: Low testosterone levels are common and associated with insulin resistance in men with diabetes. J Clin Endocrinol Metab 2008; 93:1834–1840.

Tomar R, Dhindsa S, Chaudhuri A, Mohanty P, Garg R, Dandona P.: Contrasting testosterone concentrations in type 1 and type 2 diabetes. Diabetes Care 2006; 29:1120–1122.

Glass AR, Swerdloff RS, Bray GA, Dahms WT, Atkinson RL.: Low serum testosterone and sex-hormone-binding-globulin in massively obese men. J Clin Endocrinol Metab 1977; 45:1211–1219.

Mulligan T, Frick MF, Zuraw QC, Stemhagen A, McWhirter C.: Prevalence of hypogonadism in males aged at least 45 years: the HIM study. Int J Clin Pract 2006; 60:762–769.

Bhasin S, Cunningham GR, Hayes FJ, Matsumoto AM, Snyder PJ, Swerdloff RS, Montori VM.: Testosterone therapy in adult men with androgen deficiency syndromes: an endocrine society clinical practice guideline. J Clin Endocrinol Metab 2006; 91:1995–2010.

Vermeulen A, Verdonck L, Kaufman JM.: A critical evaluation of simple methods for the estimation of free testosterone in serum. J Clin Endocrinol Metab 1999; 84:3666–3672.10. Vermeulen A, Kaufman JM, Deslypere JP, Thomas G.: Attenuated luteinizing hormone (LH) pulse amplitude but normal LH pulse frequency, and its relation to plasma androgens in hypogonadism of obese men. J Clin Endocrinol Metab 1993; 76:1140–1146.

Zumoff B, Strain GW, Miller LK, Rosner W, Senie R, Seres DS, Rosenfeld RS.: Plasma free and non-sex-hormone-binding-globulin-bound testosterone are decreased in obese men in proportion to their degree of obesity. J Clin Endocrinol Metab 1990; 71:929–931.

Giagulli VA, Kaufman JM, Vermeulen A.: Pathogenesis of the decreased androgen levels in obese men. J Clin Endocrinol Metab 1994; 79:997–1000.

Hofstra J, Loves S, van Wageningen B, Ruinemans-Koerts J, Jansen I, de Boer H.: High prevalence of hypogonadotropic hypogonadism in men referred for obesity treatment. Neth J Med 2008; 66:103–109.

Ogden CL, Carroll MD, Curtin LR, McDowell MA, Tabak CJ, Flegal KM.: Prevalence of overweight and obesity in the United States, 1999–2004. JAMA 2006; 295:1549–1555.

Selvin E, Feinleib M, Zhang L, Rohrmann S, Rifai N, Nelson WG, Dobs A, Basaria S, Golden SH, Platz EA.: Androgens and diabetes in men: results from the Third National Health and Nutrition Examination Survey (NHANES III). Diabetes Care 2007; 30:234–238.

Brüning JC, Gautam D, Burks DJ, Gillette J, Schubert M, Orban PC, Klein R, Krone W, Müller-Wieland D, Kahn CR.: Role of brain insulin receptor in control of body weight and reproduction. Science 2000; 289:2122–2125.

Jensen TK, Andersson AM, Jørgensen N, Andersen AG, Carlsen E, Petersen JH, Skakkebaek NE.: Body mass index in relation to semen quality and reproductive hormones among 1,558 Danish men. Fertil Steril 2004; 82:863–870.

Dandona P, Aljada A, Bandyopadhyay A.: Inflammation: the link between insulin resistance, obesity and diabetes. Trends Immunol 2004; 25:4–7.

Chandel A, Dhindsa S, Topiwala S, Chaudhuri A, Dandona P.: Testosterone concentration in young patients with diabetes. Diabetes Care 2008; 31:2013–2017.

Ding EL, Song Y, Manson JE, Hunter DJ, Lee CC, Rifai N, Buring JE, Gaziano JM, Liu S.: Sex hormone-binding globulin and risk of type 2 diabetes in women and men. N Engl J Med 2009; 361:1152–1163.

Kapoor D, Clarke S, Channer KS, Jones TH.: Erectile dysfunction is associated with low bioactive testosterone levels and visceral adiposity in men with type 2 diabetes. Int J Androl 2007; 30:500–507.

Nielsen TL, Hagen C, Wraae K, Brixen K, Petersen PH, Haug E, Larsen R, Andersen M.: Visceral and subcutaneous adipose tissue assessed by magnetic resonance imaging in relation to circulating androgens, sex hormone-binding globulin, and luteinizing hormone in young men. J Clin Endocrinol Metab 2007; 92:2696–2705.

Caronia L, Dwyer A, Hayden D, Pitteloud N, Hayes F.: Abrupt decrease in testosterone following an oral glucose load in men. Abstract presented at ENDO 09, 10–13 June 2009, Washington, DC, OR42-2.

Chapter Twenty-Eight

[295] Conway A., Boylan L., Howe C., Ross G. & Handelsman D. (1988) Randomised clinical trial of testosterone replacement therapy in hypogonadal men.)

[296] Handelsman D., Conway A. & Boylan L. (1990) Pharmacokinetics and Pharmacodynamics of testosterone pellets in man.

[297] Salmimies P., Kockott G., Price K., Vogt H. & Schill W. (1982) Effects of testosterone replacement on sexual behaviour in hypogonad men.

[298] Herbst K, Bhasin S. Testosterone action on skeletal muscle. Curr Opin Clin Nutr Metab Care 2004; 7(3):271–7.

[299] Handelsman D., Conway A. & Boylan L. (1990) Pharmacokinetics and Pharmacodynamics of testosterone pellets in man.

[300] Morgentaler A. Commentary: guidelines for male testosterone therapy: a clinician's perspective. J Clin Endocrinol Metab 2007; 92(2):416–7.

[301] Hormones in Wellness and Disease Prevention: Common Practices, Current State of the Evidence, and Questions for the Future Erika T. Schwartz, MD, Kent Holtorf, MD 10 West 74 Street, Suite 1A, New York, NY 10023, USA 23456 Hawthorne Boulevard, Suite 160, Torrance, CA 90505, USA Corresponding author. E-mail address: erika@drerika.com (E. Schwartz). Prim Care Clin Office Pract 35 (2008) 669–705 primarycare.theclinics.com 2008 Elsevier Inc.

[302] Winters J. Current status of testosterone replacement therapy in men. Arch Fam Med 1999; 8:257–63.

[303] Mulligan T, Frick M, Zuraw Q, et al. Prevalence of hypogonadism in males aged at least 45 years: the HIM study. Int J Clin Pract 2006; 60(7):762–9.

[304] "Effect of castration on the morphology of the motor end-plates of the rat levator ani muscle" European Journal of Cellular Biology, 1982; 26(2): 284-288.

[305] Davidson J, Camargo C. Effects of androgen on sexual behavior in hypogonadal men. J Clin Endocrinol Metab 1979; 48:149–61.

Shabsigh R, Kaufman J, Steidle C, et al. Randomized study of testosterone gel as adjunctive therapy to sildenafil in hypogonadal men with erectile dysfunction who do not respond to sildenafil alone. The Journal of Urology 008; 179(5): S97–102.

Saad F, Grahl AS, Aversa A, et al. Effects of testosterone on erectile function: implications for the therapy of erectile dysfunction. BJU Int 2007; 99(5): 988–92.

Greco EA, Spera G, Aversa A. Combining testosterone and PDE5 inhibitors in erectile dysfunction: basic rationale and clinical evidences. Eur Urol 2006; 50(5):940–7.

Hormones in Wellness and Disease Prevention: Common Practices, Current State of the Evidence, and Questions for the Future Erika T. Schwartz, MD, Kent Holtorf, MD 10 West 74 Street, Suite 1A, New York, NY 10023, USA 23456 Hawthorne Boulevard, Suite 160, Torrance, CA 90505, USA Corresponding author. E-mail address: erika@drerika.com (E. Schwartz). Prim Care Clin Office Pract 35 (2008) 669–705 primarycare.theclinics.com 2008 Elsevier Inc.

[306] Vanderschueren-Lodewey M. (1994) Growth Hormone Deficiency and Its Treatment. NovoCare, Copenhagen, Denmark.

[307] Harman S. Testosterone in older men after the Institute of Medicine report: Where do we go from here? Climacteric 2006; 77(5):1319–26.

[308] Phillips G. Relationship between serum sex hormones and the glucose-insulin–lipid defect in men with obesity. Metabolism 1993; 42(1):116–20.

[309] Hormones in Wellness and Disease Prevention: Common Practices, Current State of the Evidence, and Questions for the Future Erika T. Schwartz, MD, Kent Holtorf, MD 10 West 74 Street, Suite 1A, New York, NY 10023, USA 23456 Hawthorne Boulevard, Suite 160, Torrance, CA 90505, USA Corresponding author. E-mail address: erika@drerika.com (E. Schwartz). Prim Care Clin Office Pract 35 (2008) 669–705 primarycare.theclinics.com 2008 Elsevier Inc.

[310] Huggins C, Hodges CV. Studies on prostatic cancer I: the effects of castration, of estrogen and of androgen injection on serum phosphotases in metastatic carcinoma of the prostate. Cancer Res 1941; 1:293–7.

Huggins C, Stevens RE, Hodges CV. Studies on prostatic cancer II: the effects of castration on advanced carcinoma of the prostate gland. Arch Surg 1941; 43: 209–23.

[311] Ferrucci L, Maggio M, Bandinelli S, et al. Low testosterone predicts anemia in older adults. Arch Intern Med 2006; 166:1380–8.

Hormones in Wellness and Disease Prevention: Common Practices, Current State of the Evidence, and Questions for the Future Erika T. Schwartz, MD, Kent Holtorf, MD 10 West 74 Street, Suite 1A, New York, NY 10023, USA 23456 Hawthorne

Boulevard, Suite 160, Torrance, CA 90505, USA Corresponding author. E-mail address: erika@drerika.com (E. Schwartz). Prim Care Clin Office Pract 35 (2008) 669–705 primarycare.theclinics.com 2008 Elsevier Inc.)

[312] Testosterone replacement therapy – perceptions of recipients and partners ISSUES AND INNOVATIONS IN NURSING PRACTICE Trisha L. Dunning, MEd PhD AM RN FRCNA Director, Endocrinology and Diabetes Nursing Research, St Vincent's Hospital Melbourne, Endocrinology and Diabetes; and Professor, Faculty of Medicine, Dentistry and Health Sciences, University of Melbourne, Melbourne, Victoria, Australia Glenn M. Ward, BSc MBBS DPhil FRACP FRCPath Physician in Charge of the Diabetes Clinics, St Vincent's Hospital Melbourne, Endocrinology and Diabetes; and Associate Professor, Faculty of Medicine, Dentistry and Health Sciences, University of Melbourne, Melbourne, Victoria, Australia Submitted for publication 18 July 2003 Accepted for publication 9 January 2004.

[313] Testosterone replacement therapy – perceptions of recipients and partners ISSUES AND INNOVATIONS IN NURSING PRACTICE Trisha L. Dunning, MEd PhD AM RN FRCNA Director, Endocrinology and Diabetes Nursing Research, St Vincent's Hospital Melbourne, Endocrinology and Diabetes; and Professor, Faculty of Medicine, Dentistry and Health Sciences, University of Melbourne, Melbourne, Victoria, Australia Glenn M. Ward, BSc MBBS DPhil FRACP FRCPath Physician in Charge of the Diabetes Clinics, St Vincent's Hospital Melbourne, Endocrinology and Diabetes; and Associate Professor, Faculty of Medicine, Dentistry and Health Sciences, University of Melbourne, Melbourne, Victoria, Australia Submitted for publication 18 July 2003 Accepted for publication 9 January 2004.

[314] Fibromyalgia Network--Sullivan PF, *et al.* Psychological Medicine 32:881-888, 2002.

[315] Hudson JL, Goldenberg DL, Pope HG, Keck PE, Schlesinger L. Comorbidity of fibromyalgia with medical and psychiatric disorders. Am J Med 1992; 92: 363-367.

Triadafilopoulos G, Simms RW, Goldenberg DL. Bowel dysfunction in fibromyalgia syndrome. Dig Dis Sci 1991; 36: 59- 64.

[316] Combination Therapy in Fibromyalgia Current Pharmaceutical Design, 2006, 12, 11-16 11 1381-6128/06 2006 Bentham Science Publishers Ltd. A.H. Clayton and S.G. West Department of Psychiatric Medicine, University of Virginia, Charlottesville, VA.

[317] The 18 Tender Point Locations of Fibromyalgia on "The Three Graces" Masterpiece. Reprinted from ARTHRITIS & RHEUMATISM Journal, copyright 1990. Adapted from our "Patient Guide" brochure and used by permission of the American College of Rheumatology.

[318] Fibromyalgia Network.

[319] Moldofsky H. Sleep and fibrositis syndrome. Rheum Dis ClinNorth Am 1989; 15(1): 91-103.

Harding SM. Sleep in fibromyalgia patients: subjective and objective findings. Am J Med Sci 1998; 315: 367-37.

[320] Moldofsky H, Scarisbrick P. Introduction of neurasthenic musculoskeletal pain syndrome by selective sleep stage deprivation. Psychosom Med 1975; 37: 341-345.

[321] Neeck G, Crofford IJ. Neuroendocrine perturbations in fibromyalgia and chronic fatigue syndrome. Rheum Dis Clin North Am 2000; 26: 989-1002.

[322] Korszun A, Young EA, Engleberg NC, Masterson L, Dawson EC, Spindler K, et al . Follicular phase hypothalamic-pituitary-gonodal axis dysfunction in women with fibromyalgia and chronic fatigue syndrome. J Rheumatol 2000; 27: 6.

Neeck G, Riedel W. Hormonal perturbations in fibromyalgia syndrome. Ann N Y Acad Sci 1999; 876: 325-339.

Combination Therapy in Fibromyalgia Current Pharmaceutical Design, 2006, 12, 11-16 11 1381-6128/06 2006 Bentham Science Publishers Ltd. A.H. Clayton and S.G. West Department of Psychiatric Medicine, University of Virginia, Charlottesville, VA.

[323] Canaris GJ, Manowitz NR, Mayor G, et al. The Colorado thyroid disease prevalence study. Arch Intern Med 2000; 160:526–34.

Hormones in Wellness and Disease Prevention: Common Practices, Current State of the Evidence, and Questions for the Future Erika T. Schwartz, MD , Kent Holtorf, MD, 10 West 74 Street, Suite 1A, New York, NY 10023, USA 23456 Hawthorne Boulevard, Suite 160, Torrance, CA 90505, USA Corresponding author. E-mail address: erika@drerika.com (E. Schwartz). Prim Care Clin Office Pract 35 (2008) 669–705 primarycare.theclinics.

[324] Rossouw JE, Anderson GL, Prentice RL, LaCroix AZ, Kooperberg C, Stefanick ML, et al. Risks and benefits of estrogen plus progestin in healthy postmenopausal women: principal results from the Women's Health Initiative randomized controlled trial. JAMA 2002; 288(3): 321-333.

Chapter Thirty

[325] Scragg JL, Jones RD, Channer KS, et al. Testosterone is a potent inhibitor of L-type Ca(2+) channels. Biochem Biophys Res Commun 2004; 318:503–6.

Malkin CJ, Pugh PJ, Morris PD, et al. Testosterone replacement in hypogonadal men with angina improves ischaemic threshold and quality of life. Heart 2004; 90:871–6.

The Dark Side of Testosterone Deficiency III. Cardiovascular Disease Abdulmaged M. Traish, Farid Saad, Robert J. Feeley, Andre Guay Article first published online: 2 JAN 2013 Journal of Andrology Volume 30, Issue 5, pages 477–494, September-October 2009.

[326] The Dark Side of Testosterone Deficiency III. Cardiovascular Disease Abdulmaged M. Traish, Farid Saad, Robert J. Feeley, Andre Guay Article first published online: 2 JAN 2013 Journal of Andrology Volume 30, Issue 5, pages 477–494, September-October 2009.

[327] Phillips G., Pinkernell B., Jing T. The association of hypotestosteronemia with coronary artery disease in men. Arterioscler Thromb. 1994; 14: 701–706.

[328] Maggio M., Lauretani F., Ceda GP, Bandinelli S., Ling SM, Metter EJ, Artoni A., Carassale L., Cazzato A., Ceresini G., Guralnik JM, Basaria S., Valenti G., Ferrucci L. Relationship between low levels of anabolic hormones and 6-year mortality in older men: the aging in the Chianti Area (InCHIANTI) study. Arch Intern Med. 2007; 167: 2249–2254.

[329] Deanfield J, Donald A, Ferri C, Giannattasio C, Halcox J, Halligan S, Lerman A, Mancia G, Oliver JJ, Pessina AC, Rizzoni D, Rossi GP, Salvetti A, Schiffrin EL, Taddei S,

Webb DJ (2005). "Endothelial function and dysfunction. Part I: Methodological issues for assessment in the different vascular beds: a statement by the Working Group on Endothelin and Endothelial Factors of the European Society of Hypertension". J Hypertens 23 (1): 7–17.ndothelium.

[330] Flammer AJ, Anderson T, Celermajer DS, Creager MA, Deanfield J, Ganz P, Hamburg NM, Lüscher TF, Shechter M, Taddei S, Vita JA, Lerman A. The assessment of endothelial function: from research into clinical practice. Circulation. 2012 Aug 7; 126(6):753-67.

[331] Reis SE, Holubkov R, Smith AJC, Kelsey SF, Sharaf BL, Reichek N, Rogers WJ, Merz NB, Sopko G, Pepine CJ, "Coronary microvascular dysfunction is highly prevalent in women with chest pain in the absence of coronary artery disease: Results from the NHLBI WISE Study," Am Heart J, V. 141, No. 5 (May 2001), pp. 735-741.

[332] Davignon J, Ganz P. Role of endothelial dysfunction in atherosclerosis. Circulation. 2004 Jun 15; 109(23 Suppl 1):III27-32. Review.

Eren E1, Yilmaz N, Aydin O (2013). "Functionally Defective High-Density Lipoprotein and Paraoxonase: A Couple for Endothelial Dysfunction in Atherosclerosis". CHOLESTEROL 2013.

[333] Ruilope LM, Redón J, Schmieder R. Cardiovascular risk reduction by reversing endothelial dysfunction: ARBs, ACE inhibitors, or both? Expectations from the ONTARGET Trial Programme. Vasc Health Risk Manag. 2007; 3(1):1-9.

Briasoulis A, Tousoulis D, Androulakis ES, Papageorgiou N, Latsios G, Stefanadis C. Endothelial dysfunction and atherosclerosis: focus on novel therapeutic approaches. Recent Pat Cardiovasc Drug Discov. 2012 Apr; 7(1):21-32. Review.

[334] Kang SM, Jang Y., Kim JY, Chung N., Cho SY, Chae JS, Lee JH. Effect of oral administration of testosterone on brachial arterial vasoreactivity in men with coronary artery disease. Am J Cardiol. 2002; 89: 862–864.

[335] Khaw K., Dowsett M., Folkerd E., Bingham S., Wareham N., Luben R., Welch A., Day N.. Endogenous testosterone and mortality due to all causes, cardiovascular disease, and cancer in men: European prospective investigation into cancer in Norfolk (EPIC-Norfolk) prospective population study. Circulation. 2007; 116: 2694–2701.

[336] Traish AM, Saad F., Guay AT. The dark side of testosterone deficiency: II. Type 2 diabetes and insulin resistance. J Androl. 2009b; 30(1): 23–32.

Ginsberg HN. Insulin resistance and cardiovascular disease. J Clin Investig. 2000; 106: 453–458.

Haffner SM. Sex hormones, obesity, fat distribution, type 2diabetes and insulin resistance: epidemiological and clinical correlation. Int J Obes Relat Metab Disord. 2000; (suppl 2): S56–S58.

Haffner SM, Agostino RD Jr, Saad MF, O'Leary DH, Savage PJ, Rewers M., Selby J., Bergman RN, Mykkänen L.. Carotid artery atherosclerosis in type-2 diabetic and nondiabetic subjects with and without symptomatic coronary artery disease (The Insulin Resistance Atherosclerosis Study). Am J Cardiol. 2000; 85: 1395–1400.

Reaven GM, Lithell H., Landsberg L. Hypertension and associated metabolic abnormalities—the role of insulin resistance and the sympathoadrenal system. N Engl J Med. 1996; 334: 374–381.

Calles-Escandon J., Mirza SA, Sobel BE, Schneider DJ. Induction of hyperinsulinemia combined with hyperglycemia and hypertriglyceridemia increases plasminogen activator inhibitor 1 in blood in normal human subjects. Diabetes. 1998; 47: 290–293.

Sobel BE. Insulin resistance and thrombosis: a cardiologist's view. Am J Cardiol. 1999; 84: 37J–41J.

[337] Shores MM, Matsumoto AM, Sloan KL, Kivlahan DR. Low serum testosterone and mortality in male veterans. Arch Int Med. 2006; 166: 1660–1665.

[338] Carrero JJ, Qureshi AR, Parini P., Arver S., Lindholm B., Bárány P., Heimbürger O., Stenvinkel P.. Low serum testosterone increases mortality risk among male dialysis patients. J Am Soc Nephrol. 2009; 20: 613–620.

[339] Araujo AB, Kupelian V., Page ST, Handelsman DJ, Bremner WJ, McKinlay JB. Sex steroids and all-cause and cause-specific mortality in men. Arch Intern Med. 2007; 167: 1252–1260.

[340] Sochorová R., Mosnárová A., Huzuláková I. The possible influence of testosterone on calcium ion transport (investigated) in guinea pig uterus. Acta Physiol Hung. 1991; 77: 19–24.

Scragg JL, Jones RD, Channer KS, et al. Testosterone is a potent inhibitor of L-type Ca(2+) channels. Biochem Biophys Res Commun 2004; 318:503–6.

Perusquía M., Navarrete E., Jasso-Kamel J., Montaño LM. Androgens induce relaxation of contractile activity in pregnant human myometrium at term: a nongenomic action on L-type calcium channels. Biol Reprod. 2005; 73: 214–221.

Hall J., Jones RD, Jones TH, Channer KS, Peers C. Selective inhibition of L-type Ca2+ channels in A7r5 cells by physiological levels of testosterone. Endocrinology. 2006; 147: 2675–2680.

Er F., Michels G., Brandt MC, Khan I., Haase H., Eicks M., Lindner M., Hoppe UC. Impact of testosterone on cardiac L-type calcium channels and Ca2+sparks: acute actions antagonize chronic effects. Cell Calcium. 2007; 41: 467–477.

Montaño LM, Calixto E., Figueroa A., Flores-Soto E., Carbajal V., Perusquía M. Relaxation of androgens on rat thoracic aorta: testosterone concentration dependent agonist/antagonist L-type Ca2+ channel activity, and 5beta-dihydrotestosterone restricted to L-type Ca2+ channel blockade. Endocrinology. 2008; 149: 2517–2526.

[341] Webb CM, Adamson DL, de Zeigler D., Collins P. Effect of acute testosterone on myocardial ischemia in men with coronary artery disease. Am J Cardiol. 1999; 83: 437–439.

Tep-Areenan P., Kendall DA, Randall MD. Mechanisms of vasorelaxation to testosterone in the rat aorta. Eur J Pharmacol. 2003; 465: 125–132.

[342] Svartberg J., vo Muhlen D., Schirmer H., Barrett-Connor E., Sundfjord J., Jorde R.. Association of endogenous testosterone with blood pressure and left ventricular mass in men. The Tromso Study. Eur J Endocrinol. 2004a; 150: 65–71.

Svartberg J., vo Muhlen D., Sundsfjord J., Jorde R. Waist circumference and testosterone levels in community dwelling men. The Tromso Study. Eur J Epidemiol. 2004b; 19: 657–663.

[343] Smith MR, Bennett S., Evans L., Kynaton H., Parmar M., Mason M., Cockcroft J., Scanlon M., Davies J. The effects of induced hypogonadism on arterial stiffness, body composition, and metabolic parameters in males with prostate cancer. J Clin Endocrinol Metab. 2001; 86: 4261–4267.

[344] The Dark Side of Testosterone Deficiency III. Cardiovascular Disease Abdulmaged M. Traish, Farid Saad, Robert J. Feeley, Andre GuayArticle first published online: 2 JAN 2013 Journal of Andrology Volume 30, Issue 5, pages 477–494, September-October 2009.

[345] Mårin P., Holmang S., Gustafsson C., Jonsson L., Kvist H., Elander A., Eldh J., Sjostrom L., Holm G., Bjorntorp P.. Androgen treatment of abdominally obese men. Obes Res. 1993; 1: 245–251.

[346346] Zitzmann M., Nieschlag E. Androgen receptor gene CAG repeat length and body mass index modulate the safety of long term intramuscular testosterone undecanoae therapy in hypogonadal men. J Clin Endocrinol Metab. 2007; 92: 3844–3853.

[347] Anderson FH, Francis RM, Faulkner K. Androgen supplementation in eugonadal men with osteoporosis-effects of 6 months of treatment on bone mineral density and cardiovascular risk factors. Bone. 1996; 18: 171–177.

[348] Phillips GB, Jing TY, Resnick LM, Barbagallo M., Laragh JH, Sealey JE. Sex hormones and hemostatic risk factors for coronary heart disease in men with hypertension. J Hypertens. 1993; 11: 699–702.

[349] The Dark Side of Testosterone Deficiency III. Cardiovascular Disease Abdulmaged M. Traish, Farid Saad, Robert J. Feeley, Andre Guay Article first published online: 2 JAN 2013 Journal of Andrology Volume 30, Issue 5, pages 477–494, September-October 2009.

Chapter Thirty-One

[350] Published in the June 11, 1997 issue of *the Journal of the American Medical Association*.

[351] The Hordaland Homocysteine Study: a community-based study of homocysteine, its determinants, and associations with disease. Refsum H[1], Nurk E, Smith AD, Ueland PM, Gjesdal CG, Bjelland I, Tverdal A, Tell GS, Nygård O, Vollset SE.

Chapter Thirty-Two

[352] Androgen insufficiency in women diagnostic and therapeutic implications Oxford Journals Medicine Human Reproduction Update Volume 10, Issue 5 Pp. 421-432.

[353] Burger et al. (1984) reported that in postmenopausal women with poorly controlled hot flushes despite standard estrogen therapy, the addition of a testosterone implant improved the control of the hot flushes.

Burger HG, Hailes J and Menelaus M (1984) The management of persistent symptoms with estradiol-testosterone implants: clinical, lipid and hormonal results. Maturitas 6, 351–358.

Stay Young and Sexy with Bio-identical Hormone Replacement page 110 Jonathon Wright, MD and Simon, JA Testosterone therapy in women: its role in the management of hypoactive sexual desire disorder. International Journal of Impotence Research 2007; 19; 458-463.

What You Must Know About Women's Hormones" Pamela Wartian Smith, MD., MPH Square One Publishers copyright 2010.

Testosterone for Life Abraham Morgentaler, MD McGraw Hill copyright 2009.) (The Savvy Woman's Guide to Testosterone Elizabeth Lee Vliet, MD, HER Place Press copyright 2005.

Chapter Thirty-Three

[354] Journal of Urol. 2000 Mar; 163(3):888-93. Report of the international consensus development conference on female sexual dysfunction: definitions and classifications. Basson R, Berman J, Burnett A, Derogatis L, Ferguson D, Fourcroy J, Goldstein I, Graziottin A, Heiman J, Laan E, Leiblum S, Padma-Nathan H, Rosen R, Segraves K, Segraves RT, Shabsigh R, Sipski M, Wagner G, Whipple B.

[355] Biddle, AK Hypoactive Sexual Disorder in Postmenopausal Women: quality of Life and Health Burden. "Value Health": 2009, Jan 12.

[356] Rosen, RC, Sexual Well-Being, Happiness, and Satisfaction, in Women: The Case for a New Conceptual Paradigm. "J. Sexual Marital Therapy": 2008; 34(4) 291-297.

[357] Hypoactive Sexual Desire Disorder: Understanding the Impact on Midlife Women, Sheryl A. Kingsberg, PhD "Menopause Matters."

[358] Stay Young and Sexy with Bio-identical Hormone Replacement page 110 Jonathon Wright, MD and Simon, JA Testosterone therapy in women: its role in the management of hypoactive sexual desire disorder. International Journal of Impotence Research 2007; 19; 458-463.

[359] Nair KS, DHEA in elderly women and DHEA or testosterone in elderly men. New England Journal of Medicine 2006; 355:1647-1659.

[360] Leiblum, SR, Hypoactive Sexual Desire Disorder I Postmenopausal Women: US results from the Women's International Study of Health and Sexuality "Menopause", 2006; 13(1):46-56.

[361] Scarabin PY, Alhene-Ge;as M, Plu-Bureau G, Taisne P, Agher R, Aiach M. Effects of oral and tansdermal estrogen/progesterone regimens of blood coagulation and fibrinolysis in postmenopausal women. A randomized controlled trial. Artherioscler Thromb Vasc Biol. 1997; 17:3071-3078.

Scarabin PY, Oger E, Plu-Bureau G. Different associations of oral and transdermal oestrogen-replacement therapy with venous thromboembolism risk. Lancet. 2003; 362:428-432.

Chapter Thirty-Four

[362] Christian Wilde (2003). *Hidden Causes of Heart Attack and Stroke: Inflammation, Cardiology's New Frontier.* Abigon Press. pp. 182–183. ISBN 0-9724959-0-8.

[363] Nordestgaard BG, Chapman MJ, Ray K, Borén J, Andreotti F, Watts GF, Ginsberg H, Amarenco P, Catapano A, Descamps OS, Fisher E, Kovanen PT, Kuivenhoven JA, Lesnik P, Masana L, Reiner Z, Taskinen MR, Tokgözoglu L, Tybjærg-Hansen A (December 2010). "Lipoprotein(a) as a cardiovascular risk factor: current status". *Eur. Heart J.* 31 (23): 2844–53. doi:10.1093/eurheartj/ehq386. PMC 3295201. PMID 20965889.

[364] Takagi H, Umemoto T (January 2012). "Atorvastatin decreases lipoprotein(a): A meta-analysis of randomized trials". *Int. J. Cardiol.* 154 (2): 183–6. doi:10.1016/j.ijcard.2011.09.060. PMID 21996415.

[365] Ryan, George M; Julius Torelli (2005). *Beyond cholesterol: 7 life-saving heart disease tests that your doctor may not give you.* New York: St. Martin's Griffin. p.91. ISBN 0-312-34863-0.

Chapter Thirty-Five

[366] http://www.health.com/health/gallery/0,,20537878,00.html

[367] Headache Classification Subcommittee of the International Headache Society (2004). "The International Classification of Headache Disorders: 2nd edition." *Cephalalgia* 24 (Suppl 1): 9–160.

[368] Headache Classification Subcommittee of the International Headache Society (2004). "The International Classification of Headache Disorders: 2nd edition". *Cephalalgia* 24 (Suppl 1): 9–160.

[369] The American Migraine Study II.

[370] Piane, M; Lulli, P; Farinelli, I; Simeoni, S; De Filippis, S; Patacchioli, FR; Martelletti, P (December 2007). "Genetics of migraine and pharmacogenomics: some considerations". *The journal of headache and pain* 8 (6): 334–9.) About two-thirds of cases run in families.

Bartleson JD, Cutrer FM (May 2010). "Migraine update. Diagnosis and treatment". *Minn Med* 93 (5): 36–41.) Changing hormone levels may also play a role, as migraines affect slightly more boys than girls before puberty, but about two to three times more women than men.

Lay CL, Broner SW (May 2009). "Migraine in women". *Neurologic Clinics* 27 (2): 503–11.

Stovner LJ, Zwart JA, Hagen K, Terwindt GM, Pascual J (April 2006). "Epidemiology of headache in Europe." *European Journal of Neurology* 13 (4): 333–45.

[371] Bartleson JD, Cutrer FM (May 2010). "Migraine update. Diagnosis and treatment". *Minn Med* 93 (5): 36–41.

[372] Dodick DW, Gargus JJ (August 2008). "Why migraines strike". *Sci. Am.* 299 (2): 56–63.

Chapter Thirty-Six

[373] The Role of Androgens and Estrogens on Healthy Aging and Longevity J Gerontol A Biol Sci Med Sci. Nov 2012; 67(11): 1140–1152. Published online Mar 26, 2012. Astrid M. Horstman E. Lichar Dillon, Randall J. Urban, and Melinda Sheffield-Moore.

[374] http://www.webmd.com/healthy-aging/sarcopenia-with-aging

Chapter Thirty-Seven

[375] Ageing, hormones, body composition, metabolic effects. World J Urol. 2002 May; 20(1):23-7. Vermeulen A.

[376] Finkelstein, J.S., Klibanski, A., Neer, R.M., et al.: Osteoporosis in men with idiopathic hypogonadotropic hypogonadism. Ann Intern Med, 106:354, 1987.

[377] Stanley, H.L., Schmitt, B.P., Poses, R.M. and Diess, W.P.: Does hypogonadism contribute to the occurrence of a minimal trauma hip fracture in elderly men? J Am Geriatr Soc, 39:766, 1991.

[378] Androgen insufficiency in women diagnostic and therapeutic implications Oxford Journals Medicine Human Reproduction Update Volume 10, Issue 5 Pp. 421-432.

[379] Davis SR, McCloud PI, Strauss BJG and Burger HG (1995) Testosterone enhances estradiol's effects on postmenopausal bone density and sexuality. Maturitas 21, 227–236.)

Androgen insufficiency in women diagnostic and therapeutic implications Oxford Journals Medicine Human Reproduction Update Volume 10, Issue 5 Pp. 421-432.

[380] Testosterone enhances estradiol's effects on postmenopausal bone density and sexuality Maturitas 1995 Apr;21(3):227-36Susan R. Davis, Philip McCloud, Boyd J.G. Strauss, Henry Burger.

[381] Miller BE, De Souza MJ, Slade K, Luciano AA. Sublingual administration of micronized estradiol and progesterone, with and without micronized testosterone: effect on biochemical markers of bone metabolism and bone mineral density. Menopause. 2007; 7:318-326.

[382] Heshmati HM, Khosla S, Robins SP, Geller N, McAlister CA, Riggs BL. Endogenous residual estrogen levels determine bone resorption even in late postmenopausal women. J Bone Miner Res 1997; 12: Suppl 1:S121-S121 abstract.

[383] Tomkinson A, Reeve J, Shaw RW, Noble BS. The death of osteocytes via apoptosis accompanies estrogen withdrawal in human bone. J Clin Endocrinol Metab 1997; 82:3128-3135.

[384] Lanyon LE. Osteocytes, strain detection, bone modeling and remodeling. Calcif Tissue Int 1993; 53: Suppl 1:S102-S106.

[385] Dunstan CR, Evans RA, Hills E, Wong SYP, Higgs RJED. Bone death in hip fracture in the elderly. Calcif Tissue Int 1990; 47:270-275.

[386] Cummings SR, Browner WS, Bauer D, et al. Endogenous hormones and the risk of hip and vertebral fractures among older women. Study of Osteoporotic Fractures Research Group. New England Journal of Medicine 1998; 339:733-738.

[387] Cooper, C, and Campion G, Hip fractures in the elderly: a worldwide projection, Osteoporosis International, 1992; 2:285-289.

[388] Tenenhouse A, Joseph L, Kreiger N, et al. Estimation of the prevalence of low bone density in Canadian women and men using a population-specific DXA reference standard: the Canadian Mulitcentre Ostoporosis Study (CaMos). Osteoporos Int. 2000; 11:897-904.

[389] Grypas MD, Marie PJ. Effects of low doses of strontium on bone quality and quantity in rats. Bone 1990; 11:313-319.

[390] NHLBI Women's Health Initiative. http://www.nhlbi.nih.gov/whi/whywhi.htm. 2006.

[391] National Osteoporosis Foundation. Fast Facts. 20006;http//www.nof.or/osteoporosis/diseasefacts.htm. 2006.

[392] Rudman, D, et al, Relations of endogenous anabolic hormones and physical activity to bone mineral density and lean body mass in elderly men, Journal of Clinical Endocrinology, 1994; 40: 653-661.

[393] Estradiol, testosterone, and the risk for hip fractures in elderly men from the Framingham study. Am J Med. 2006 May; 119(5):426-33. Amin S, Zhang Y, Felson DT, Sawin CT, Hannan MT, Wilson PW, Kiel DP.

[394] Finkelstein, J.S., Klibanski, A., Neer, R.M., Dopplet, S.H., Rosenthal, D.I., Segre, G.V. and Crowley, W.F.: Increases in bone density during treatment of men with idiopathic hypogonadotropic hypogonadism. J Clin Endocrinol Metab, 69:776, 1989.

[395] Behre, H.M., Kliesch, S., Leifke, E., Link, T.M. and Nieschlag, E.: Long-term effect of testosterone therapy on bone mineral density in hypogonadal men. J Clin Endocrinol Metab, 82:2386, 1997.

[396] Leifke, E., Korner, H.C., Link, T.M., Behre, H.M., Peters, P.E. and Nieschlag, E.: Effects of testosterone replacement on cortical and trabecular bone mineral density, vertebral body area and paraspinal muscle area in hypogonadal men. Eur J Endocrinol, 138:51, 1998.

[397] Anderson GL, Limacher M, Assaf AR, et al. Effects of conjugated equine estrogen in postmenopausal women with hysterectomy: the Women's Health Initiative randomized controlled trial. JAMA. 2004; 291:1701-1712.

Cauley JA, Robbins J, Chen Z, et al. Effects of estrogen plus progestin on risk of fracture and bone mineral density: the Women's Health Initiative randomized trial. JAMA. 2003; 290:1872-1874.

[398] Prior JC. Progesterone as a bone-trophic hormone. Endocrine Review. 1990; 11:386-398.

[399] Felson DT, Zhang Y, Hanan MT, Kiel DP, Wison PW, Anderson JJ. The effect of postmenopausal estrogen therapy on bone density in elderly women. New England Journal of Medicine. 1993; 329:1141-1146.

[400] Orwoll ES, Nelson HD, Does estrogen adequately protect postmenopausal women against osteoporosis: an iconoclastic perspective. Journal of Clinical Endocrinology and Metaboism. 1999; 84:1872-1874.

Michaelsson K, Baron JA, Farahmand BY, et al. Hormone replacement therapy and risk of hip fracture; population based-control study. The Swedish Hip Fracture Study Group. BMJ. 1998; 316:1858-1863.

[401] Schairer C Lubin J, Troisi R, Sturgeon S, Brinton L, Hoover R. Estrogen-progestin replacement and risk of breast cancer. JAMA. 2000; 284:691-694.

[402] The Writing Group for the PEPI Trial. Effects of estrogen or estrogen/progestin regimens on heart disease risk factors in postmenopausal women. The Postmenopausal Estrogen/Progestin Interventions (PEPI) Trial. JAMA. 1995; 273:199-208.

[403] Hosking D, Chilvers CE, Christiansen C, et al. Prevention of bone loss with alendronate in postmenopausal women under 60 years of age. Early Postmenopausal Intervention Cohort Study Group. N Engl J of Med. 1998; 338:485-592.

Rosen CJ. Clinical practice. Postmenopausal osteoporosis. N Engl J of Med. 2005; 353:595-603.

[404] Basu N, Reid DM. Bisphosphonate-associated osteonecrosis of the jaw. Menopause Int. 2007; 13:56-59.

[405] Heckbert SR, Ii G, Cummings SR, Smith NL, Psaty BM. Use of alendronate and risk of incident atrial fibrillation in women. Arch Intern Med. 2008; 168:826-831.

Miranda J. Osteoporosis drugs increase risk of heart problems. CHEST 2008. Vol Philadelphia, PA: American College of Chest Physicians; 2008.

Chapter Thirty-Eight

[406] http://www.webmd.com/urinary-incontinence-oab/picture-of-the-prostate

[407] American Cancer Society American Cancer Society Guidelines for the early detection of cancer Cited: September 2011. Cancer.org. Retrieved on 2013-01-21.

[408] Suzuki, K et al., "Endocrine environment of benign prostatic hyperplasia: prostate size and volume are correlated with serum estrogen concentration," Scandinavian Journal of Urology and Nephrology, 1995; 29:65-69.

Gann, PH. Et al., "A prospective study of plasma hormone levels, nonhormonal factors, and development of benin prostatic hyperplasia," The Prostate, 1995; 26:40-49.

[409] NEJM. 2009; 360:1310-191.

[410] Available at ttp://www.nlm.nih.gov/medlineplus/ency/article/ 000381.htm. Access 6.15.10.

[411] Nutr Res Pract. 2009.

[412] HerbalGram. 1998; 43:49-53.) (Minerva Urol Nephrol. 1987 Jan; 39(1):45-50.

[413] J. of Urology. Dec. 2001; 166:2034-38.

[414] Trends Endocrin. Metab. 2003. Nov; 14(9):423.

[415] BJU Int. 2000 May; 85(7):842-6.) (In Vivo. 2005 Jan-Feb; 19(1):293-300.

[416] Nutr Res Pract. 2009 Winter; Department of Food Service Management and Nutrition, Sangmyung University, Hongji-dong, Jongro-gu, Seoul 110-743, Korea.)

Available at: http://www.helhetsdoktorn.nu/EFLA940Pumpkin02-04.pdf. Accessed 6.13.10.

[417] Ann Intern Med 1997; 127:169-70.

[418] J. Nat. Cancer Inst. 87(23):1767-76. 2005.

Current Topics in Nutraceutical Research Vol. 2, No.3 2004 pp. 127-136.

Carcinogenesis 1997 18:1847-50.

Am J Epidemiol 2002 155:1023-32.

[419] Clinc. Cancer. Res. July 1, 2006.

[420] From: http://lpi.oregonstate.edu/ss05/zinc.html. Accessed 6.13.10.

J Natl Cancer Inst. 2003 Jul 2; 95(13):1004-7.

[421] P. Nat. Acad. Sciences. May 28, 2002. Vol. 99 N. 11.

[422] DMD Fast Forward. Published on March 20, 2008 as doi: 10.1124/dmd. 107.0184242002. Vol. 99 N. 11.

[423] Newamx.com. Their phone number is 800-500-4325.

Chapter Forty-One

[424] Utian WH. Effect of hysterectomy, oophorectomy and estrogen therapy on libido. Int J Gynecol Obstet. 1975; 13:97-100.

[425] Simon JA, Abdallah RT. Testosterone therapy in women: its role in the management of hypoactive sexual desire disorder. Int J Impot Res. 2007; 19:458-463.

[426] www.mayoclinic.org/diseases-conditions/low-sex-drive-in-women

[427] "The effect of androgen on nitric oxide synthase in the male reproductive tract of the rat" Fertility and Sterility, 1995; 63(5): 1101-1107.

[428] World Health Organization. Contraceptive efficacy of testosterone-induced azoospermia and oligozoopermia in normal men. Fertil Steril, 65:821, 1996.

[429] Testosterone Replacement Therapy Wayne J.G. Hellstrom, M.D. Tulane University Medical Center, New Orleans, LA Previously published in the Digital Urology Journal The Scientific World JOURNAL 2004.

Chapter Forty-Four

[430] Schmidt J. Perspectives of estrogen treatment in skin aging. Exp Dermatol. 2005; 14:156.

[431] Sator PG, Schmidt JB, Rabe T, Zouboulis CC. Skin aging and sex hormones in women—clinical perspectives for intervention by hormone replacement therapy. Exp Dermatol. 2004'13 Suppl 4"36-40.

[432] Hudson T. Women's health update: women and skin conditions. Townsend Letter for Doctors & Patients. May 2003.

[433] Wildt L, Sir-Peterman T. Oestrogen and age estimations of perimenopausal women. Lancet. 1999; 354:224.

[434] Schmidt J. Perspectives of estrogen treatment in skin aging. Exp Dermatol. 2005; 14:156.

Punnnonen R, Soderstrom KO. The effect of oral estriol succinate therapy on the endometrial morphology in postmenopausal women: the significance of fractionation of the dose. Eur J Obstet Gynecol Reprod Biol. 1983; 14:217-224.

Punnonen R, Vaajalahti P, Teisala K. Local oestriol treatment improves the structure of elastic fibers in the skin of postmenopausal women. Ann Chir Gynaecol Suppl. 1987; 202:39-41.

Schmidt JB, Lindmaier A, Spona J. Hormone receptors in pubic skin of premenopausal and postmenopausal females. Gynecol Obstet Invest. 1999; 30:97-100.)

Grossman N. Study on the hyaluronic acid-protein complex, the molecular size of hyaluronic acid and the exchangeability of chloride in skin of mice before and after oestrogen treatment. Acta Pharmacol Toxicol (Copenh).

Grosman N, Hvidberg E, Schou J. The effect of oestrogenic treatment on the acid mucopolysaccharide pattern in skin of mice. Acta Pharmacol Toxicol (Copenh).

[435] Schmidt JB, Binder M, Demschik G, Reiner A. Treatment of skin aging with topical estrogens. Int J Dermatol. 1996; 35:669-674.

[436] Stay Young & Sexy with Bio-identical Hormone Replacement: The Science Explained by Dr. Jonathan V. Wright, Lane Lenard, PhD, SmartPublications, copyright 2010.

Chapter Forty-Five

[437] The protective role of pregnancy in breast cancer Breast Cancer Res. 2005; 7(3): 131–142. Published online 2005 April 7. Jose Russo, Raquel Moral, Gabriela A Balogh, Daniel Mailo, and Irma H Russo.

Greenlee RT, Murray T, Boldin S, Wingo P. Cancer statistics 2000. CA Cancer J Clin. 2000; 50:7–33.

MacMahon B, Cole P, Lin TM, Lowe CR, Mirra AP, Ravnihar B, Salber EJ, Valaoras VG, Yuasa S. Age at first birth and breast cancer risk. Bull WHO. 1970; 43:209–221.

Lambe M, Hsieh CC, Chan HW, Ekbom A, Trichopoulos D, Adami HO. Parity, age at first and last birth, and risk of breast cancer: a population-based study in Sweden. Breast Cancer Res Treat. 1996; 38:305–311.

Kelsey JL, Gammon MD, John EM. Reproductive factors and breast cancer. Epidemiol Rev. 1993; 15:36–47. (359)Russo J, Tay LK, Russo IH. Differentiation of the mammary gland and susceptibility to carcinogenesis. Breast Cancer Res Treat. 1982; 2:5–73.

Moon RC, Pike MC, Siiteri PK, Welsch CW, Eds Banbury Report 8 Hormones and Breast Cancer. Cold Spring Harbor, NY: Cold Spring Harbor Laboratory; 1981. Influence of pregnancy and lactation on experimental mammary carcinogenesis; pp. 353–361.

Sinha DK, Pazik JE, Dao TL. Prevention of mammary carcinogenesis in rats by pregnancy: effect of full-term and interrupted pregnancy. Br J Cancer. 1988; 57:390–394.

Yang J, Yoshizawa K, Nandi S, Tsubura A. Protective effects of pregnancy and lactation against N-methyl-N-nitrosourea-induced mammary carcinomas in female Lewis rats. Carcinogenesis. 1999; 20:623–628. doi: 10.1093/carcin/20.4.623.

Welsch CW. Host factors affecting the growth of carcinogen-induced rat mammary carcinomas: a review and tribute to Charles Brenton Huggins. Cancer Res. 1985; 45:3415–3443.

Russo J, Russo IH. Influence of differentiation and cell kinetics on the susceptibility of the rat mammary gland to carcinogenesis. Cancer Res. 1980; 40:2677–2687.

Swanson SM, Whitaker LM, Stockard CR, Myers RB, Oelschlager D, Grizzle WE, Juliana MM, Grubbs CJ. Hormone levels and mammary epithelial cell proliferation in rats treated with a regimen of estradiol and progesterone that mimics the preventive effect of pregnancy against mammary cancer. Anti-cancer Res. 1997; 17:4639–4645.

Rajkumar L, Guzman RC, Yang J, Thordarson G, Talamantes F, Nandi S. Short-term exposure to pregnancy levels of estrogen prevents mammary carcinogenesis. Proc Natl Acad Sci USA. 2001; 98:11755–11759. doi: 10.1073/pnas.201393798.

Chapter Forty-Six

[438] Ferrucci L, Corsi A, Lauretani F, et al. The origins of age-related proinflammatory state. Blood. 2005; 105(6):2294–2299.

Maggio M, Guralnik JM, Longo DL, Ferrucci L. Interleukin-6 in aging and chronic disease: a magnificent pathway. J Gerontol A Biol Sci Med Sci. 2006; 61(6):575–584.

Stenholm S, Maggio M, Lauretani F, et al. Anabolic and catabolic biomarkers as predictors of muscle strength decline: the InCHIANTI study. Rejuvenation Res. 2010; 13(1):3–11.

[439] Schaap LA, Pluijm SM, Deeg DJ, Visser M. Inflammatory markers and loss of muscle mass (sarcopenia) and strength. Am J Med. 2006; 119(6):526.e9–526.e17.

[440] Maggio M, Guralnik JM, Longo DL, Ferrucci L. Interleukin-6 in aging and chronic disease: a magnificent pathway. J Gerontol A Biol Sci Med Sci. 2006; 61(6):575–584.

[441] Khosla S, Atkinson EJ, Dunstan CR, O'Fallon WM. Effect of estrogen versus testosterone on circulating osteoprotegerin and other cytokine levels in normal elderly men. J Clin Endocrinol Metab. 2002; 87(4):1550–1554.

Malkin CJ, Pugh PJ, Jones RD, Kapoor D, Channer KS, Jones TH. The effect of testosterone replacement on endogenous inflammatory cytokines and lipid profiles in hypogonadal men. J Clin Endocrinol Metab. 2004; 89(7):3313–3318.

Yesilova Z, Ozata M, Kocar IH, et al. The effects of gonadotropin treatment on the immunological features of male patients with idiopathic hypogonadotropic hypogonadism. J Clin Endocrinol Metab. 2000; 85(1):66–70.

442 Bebo BF, Jr, Schuster JC, Vandenbark AA, Offner H. Androgens alter the cytokine profile and reduce encephalitogenicity of myelin-reactive T cells. J Immunol. 1999; 162(1):35–40.

Liva SM, Voskuhl RR. Testosterone acts directly on CD4+ T lymphocytes to increase IL-10 production. J Immunol. 2001; 167(4):2060–2067.

443 Maggio M, Ceda GP, Lauretani F, et al. SHBG, sex hormones, and inflammatory markers in older women. J Clin Endocrinol Metab. 2011; 96(4):1053–1059.

444 Estrogen and mitochondria a new paradigm for vascular protection? Mol Interv. 2006 Feb;6(1):26-35. Duckles SP, Krause DN, Stirone C, Procaccio V.

445 Mendelsohnm ME, Karas RH. The protective effects of estrogen on the cardiovascular system. New England Journal of Medicine. 1999; 340:1801-1811.

446 Khaw K, Dowsett M, Folkerd E, et al. Endogenous testosterone and mortality due to all causes, cardiovascular disease, and cancer in men. European Prospective Investigation into Cancer in Norfolk (EPIC-Norfolk) prospective population study. Circulation 2007; 116:2694–701.

447 Shores MM, Matsumoto AM, Sloan KL, et al. Low serum testosterone and mortality in male veterans. Arch Intern Med 2006; 166:1660–5.

448 Low serum testosterone and increased mortality in men with coronary heart disease Volume 96, Issue 22 Heart 2010;96:1821-1825 .1136/hrt.2010.195412 Coronary artery disease Chris J Malkin, Peter J Pugh, Paul D Morris, Sonia Asif, T Hugh Jones, Kevin S Channer Department of Cardiology, Royal Hallamshire Hospital, Sheffield, UK.

449 Bagatell CJ, Bremner WJ. Androgens in men – uses and abuses. N Engl J Med 1996; 334:707–14.

Jones RD, Nettleship JE, Kapoor D, et al. Testosterone and atherosclerosis in aging men: purported association and clinical implications. Am J Cardiovasc Drugs 2005; 5:141–54.

450 Alexandersen P, Haarbo J, Byrjalsen I, et al. Natural androgens inhibit male atherosclerosis: a study in castrated, cholesterol-fed rabbits. Circ Res 1999; 84:813–19.)

Nettleship JE, Jones TH, Channer KS, et al. Physiological testosterone replacement therapy attenuates fatty streak formation and improves high-density lipoprotein cholesterol in the Tfm mouse: an effect that is independent of the classic androgen receptor. Circulation 2007; 116:2427–34.

451 Jones RD, Nettleship JE, Kapoor D, et al. Testosterone and atherosclerosis in aging men: purported association and clinical implications. Am J Cardiovasc Drugs 2005; 5:141–54.) (Kapoor D, Aldred H, Clark S, et al. Clinical and biochemical assessment of hypogonadism in men with type 2 diabetes: correlations with bioavailable testosterone and visceral adiposity. Diabetes Care 2007; 30:911–17.

452 Kapoor D, Aldred H, Clark S, et al. Clinical and biochemical assessment of hypogonadism in men with type 2 diabetes: correlations with bioavailable testosterone and visceral adiposity. Diabetes Care 2007; 30:911–17.

Alexandersen P, Haarbo J, Byrjalsen I, et al. Natural androgens inhibit male atherosclerosis: a study in castrated, cholesterol-fed rabbits. Circ Res 1999; 84:813–19.

Nettleship JE, Jones TH, Channer KS, et al. Physiological testosterone replacement therapy attenuates fatty streak formation and improves high-density lipoprotein cholesterol in the Tfm mouse: an effect that is independent of the classic androgen receptor. Circulation 2007; 116:2427–34.

[453] Alexandersen P, Haarbo J, Byrjalsen I, et al. Natural androgens inhibit male atherosclerosis: a study in castrated, cholesterol-fed rabbits. Circ Res 1999; 84:813–19.

Nettleship JE, Jones TH, Channer KS, et al. Physiological testosterone replacement therapy attenuates fatty streak formation and improves high-density lipoprotein cholesterol in the Tfm mouse: an effect that is independent of the classic androgen receptor. Circulation 2007; 116:2427–34.

[454] Nettleship JE, Jones TH, Channer KS, et al. Physiological testosterone replacement therapy attenuates fatty streak formation and improves high-density lipoprotein cholesterol in the Tfm mouse: an effect that is independent of the classic androgen receptor. Circulation 2007; 116:2427–34.

[455] Malkin CJ, Jones TH, Channer KS. The effect of testosterone on insulin sensitivity in men with heart failure. Eur J Heart Fail 2007; 9:44–50.

Harman SM, Metter EJ, Tobin JD, et al. Longitudinal effects of aging on serum total and free testosterone levels in healthy men. Baltimore Longitudinal Study of Aging. J Clin Endocrinol Metab 2001; 86:724–31.

Shores MM, Moceri VM, Gruenewald DA, et al. Low testosterone is associated with decreased function and increased mortality risk: a preliminary study of men in a geriatric rehabilitation unit. J Am Geriatr Soc 2004; 52:2077–81.

Khaw KT, Dowsett M, Folkerd E, et al. Endogenous testosterone and mortality due to all causes, cardiovascular disease, and cancer in men: European prospective investigation into cancer in Norfolk (EPIC-Norfolk) Prospective Population Study. Circulation 2007; 116:2694–701.

[456] Heufelder AE, Saad F, Bunck MC, et al. 52-Week treatment with diet and exercise plus transdermal testosterone reverses the metabolic syndrome and improves glycaemic control in men with newly diagnosed type 2 diabetes and subnormal plasma testosterone. J Androl 2009; 30:726–33.

[457] Jones RD, Nettleship JE, Kapoor D, et al. Testosterone and atherosclerosis in aging men: purported association and clinical implications. Am J Cardiovasc Drugs 2005; 5:141–54.

Kapoor D, Aldred H, Clark S, et al. Clinical and biochemical assessment of hypogonadism in men with type 2 diabetes: correlations with bioavailable testosterone and visceral adiposity. Diabetes Care 2007; 30:911–17.

Heufelder AE, Saad F, Bunck MC, et al. 52-Week treatment with diet and exercise plus transdermal testosterone reverses the metabolic syndrome and improves glycaemic control in men with newly diagnosed type 2 diabetes and subnormal plasma testosterone. J Androl 2009; 30:726–33.

Malkin CJ, Jones RD, Jones TH, et al. Effect of testosterone on ex vivo vascular reactivity in man. Clin Sci (Lond) 2006; 111:265–74.

[458] Wang C, Nieschlag E, Swerdloff R, et al. Investigation, treatment and monitoring of late-onset hypogonadism in males: ISA, ISSAM, EAU, EAA and ASA recommendations. Eur J Endocrinol 2008; 159:507–14.

[459] Jones RD, Nettleship JE, Kapoor D, et al. Testosterone and atherosclerosis in aging men: purported association and clinical implications. Am J Cardiovasc Drugs 2005; 5:141–54.

Haddad RM, Kennedy CC, Caples SM, et al. Testosterone and cardiovascular risk in men: a systematic review and meta-analysis of randomized placebo-controlled trials. Mayo Clin Proc 2007; 82:29–39.

[460] English KM, Mandour O, Steeds RP, et al. Men with coronary artery disease have lower levels of androgens than men with normal coronary angiograms. Eur Heart J 2000; 21:890–4.

Chapter Forty-Seven

[461] Stay Young & Sexy with Bio-identical Hormone Replacement: The Science Explained by Dr. Jonathan V. Wright, Lane Lenard, PhD, SmartPublications, copyright 2010. Page 106.

Hendrix SL, Cochrane BB, Nygaard IE, et al. Effects of estrogen with and without progestin on urinary incontinence. JAMA. 2005; 293:935-948.

[462] Steinauer JE, Waetjen LE, Vittinghoff E, et al. Postmenopausal hormone therapy: does it cause incontinence? Obset Gynecol. 2005; 106:940-945.

Grady D, Brown JS, Vittinghoff E, Applegate W, Varner E, Snyder T. Postmenopausal hormones and incontinence: the Heart and Estrogen/Progestin Replacement Study. Obstet Gynecol. 2001; 97:116-120.

[463] Hunskaar S, Burgio K, Diokno A, Herzog AR, Hjalmas K, Lapitan MC. Epidemiology and natural history of urinary incontinence in women. Urology. 2003; 62:16-23.

Melville JL, Katon W, Delany K, Newton K. Urinary incontinence in US women: a population-based study. Arch Intern Med. 2005; 165:537-542.

Brown JS, Grady D, Ouslander JG, Herzog AR, Varner RE, Posner SF. Prevalence of urinary incontinence and associated risk factors in postmenopausal women. Heart & Estrogen/Progestin Replacement Study (HERS) Research Group. Obstetric Gyencology. 1999; 94:66-70.

[464] Melville JL, Delaney K, Newton W. Incontinence severity and major depression in incontinent women. Obstet Gynecol. 2005; 106:585-592.

[465] Klutke JJ, Bergman A, Hormonal influence on the urinary tract. Urol Clin North Am. 1995: 22:629-639.

Tsai E, Yang C, Wu C, Lee J. Bladder neck circulation by Doppler ultrasonography in postmenopausal women with urinary stress incontinence. Obstet Gynecol. 2001; 98:52-56.

[466] Orlander JD, Jick SS, Dean AD, Jick H. Urinary tract infections and estrogen use in women. Journal of the American Geriatric Society. 1992; 40:817-820.

Chapter Forty-Eight

[467] van Pottelbergh I., Braeckman L., de Bacquer D., de Backer G., Kaufman J. Potential contribution of testosterone and estradiol in the determination of cholesterol and lipoprotein profile in healthy middle-aged men. Atherosclerosis. 2003; 166: 95–102.

[468] Dobrzycki S., Serwatka W., Nadlewski S., Korecki J., Jackowski R., Paruk J., Ladny J.R., Hirnle T.. An assessment of correlations between endogenous sex hormone levels and the extensiveness of coronary heart disease and the ejection fraction of the left ventricle in males. J Med Invest. 2003; 50: 162–169.

[469] Low Serum Testosterone and Mortality in Older Men Gail A. Laughlin, Elizabeth Barrett-Connor, and Jaclyn Bergstrom J Clin Endocrinol Metab. 2008 January; 93(1): 68–75. Published online 2007 October 2.

[470] Njolstad I, Arnesen E, Lund-Larsen PG. Smoking, serum lipids, blood pressure, and sex differences in myocardial infarction. A 12-year follow-up of the Finnmark Study. Circulation 1996; 93:450–6.

[471] Bagatell CJ, Bremner WJ. Androgens in men – uses and abuses. N Engl J Med 1996; 334:707–14.

Chapter Forty-Nine

[472] Progestins and progesterone in hormone replacement therapy and the risk of breast cancer Carlo Campagnoli, Françoise Clavel-Chapelon, Rudolf Kaaks, Clementina Peris, and Franco Berrino, J Steroid Biochem Mol Biol. Author manuscript; available in PMC 2007 September 25. Published in final edited form as: J Steroid Biochem Mol Biol. 2005 July; 96(2): 95–108.

[473] Chlebowski RT, Hendrix SL, Langer RD, Stefanick ML, Gass M, Lane D, Rodabough RJ, Gilligan MA, Cyr MG, Thomson CA, Khandekar J, Petrovitch H, McTiernan A. Influence of estrogen plus progestin on breast cancer and mammography in healthy postmenopausal women: the Women's Health Initiative Randomized Trial. JAMA. 2003; 289(24):3243–3253.

Hulley S, Furberg C, Barrett-Connor E, Cauley J, Grady D, Haskell W, Knopp R, Lowery M, Satterfield S, Schrott H, Vittinghoff E, Hunninghake D. Noncardiovascular disease outcomes during 6.8 years of hormone therapy: Heart and Estrogen/progestin Replacement Study follow-up (HERS II) JAMA. 2002; 288(1):58–66.

[474] Fournier A, Berrino F, Riboli E, Avenel V, Clavel-Chapelon F. Breast cancer risk in relation to different types of hormone replacement therapy in the E3N-EPIC cohort. Int J Cancer. 2005; 114:448–454.

[475] Hormone Therapy Linked To Greater Risk Of Ovarian Cancer, Danish Study Wednesday 15 July 2009.

Chapter Fifty

[476] 17β-Estradiol, Its Metabolites, and Progesterone Inhibit Cardiac Fibroblast Growth Accepted October 22, 1997. Raghvendra K. Dubey, Delbert G. Gillespie, Edwin K. Jackson, Paul J. Keller.

[477] Heart, and Stroke Facts. Dallas: American Heart Association, 1992.

[478] Kalin MF, Zumoff B. Sex hormones and coronary disease: a review of the clinical studies. Steroids. 1990; 55: 330 –352.

[479] Kalin MF, Zumoff B. Sex hormones and coronary disease: a review of the clinical studies. Steroids. 1990; 55: 330 –352.

[480] Kalin MF, Zumoff B. Sex hormones and coronary disease: a review of the clinical studies. Steroids. 1990; 55: 330 –352.

Heart, and Stroke Facts. Dallas: American Heart Association, 1992.

[481] Heart, and Stroke Facts. Dallas: American Heart Association, 1992.

[482] Oparil S, Levine RL, Chen YF. Sex hormones and the vasculature. In: Sowers JR, Walsh M, eds. Endocrinology of the Vasculature. Totwa, N.J.: Humana Press; 1996: 225 –237.

[483] Oparil S, Levine RL, Chen YF. Sex hormones and the vasculature. In: Sowers JR, Walsh M, eds. Endocrinology of the Vasculature. Totwa, N.J.: Humana Press; 1996: 225 –237.

[484] Krasinski K, Spyridopoulos I, Asahara T, van der Zee R, Isner JM, Losordo DW. Estradiol accelerates functional endothelial recovery after arterial injury. Circulation. 1997; 95: 1768 –1772.

[485] Oparil S, Levine RL, Chen YF. Sex hormones and the vasculature. In: Sowers JR, Walsh M, eds. Endocrinology of the Vasculature. Totwa, N.J.: Humana Press; 1996: 225 –237.

Rosselli M, Keller PJ, Kern F, Hahn AWA, Dubey RK. Estradiol inhibits mitogen-induced proliferation and migration of human aortic smooth muscle cells: implications for cardiovascular disease in women (abstract). Circulation. 1994; 90: I –87.

[486] Dubey RK, Jackson EK, Rupprecht H, Sterzel RB. Factors controlling growth and matrix production in vascular smooth muscle and glomerular mesangial cells. Curr Opin Nephrol Hypertens. 1997; 6:88 –105.

[487] Oparil S, Levine RL, Chen YF. Sex hormones and the vasculature. In: Sowers JR, Walsh M, eds. Endocrinology of the Vasculature. Totwa, N.J.: Humana Press; 1996: 225 –237.

Oparil S, Levine R, Chen S-J, Durand J, Chen YF. Sexually dimorphic response of the balloon-injured rat carotid artery to hormone treatment. Circulation. 1997; 95: 1301 –1307.

Foegh ML, Asotra S, Howell MH, Ramwell PW. Estradiol inhibition of arterial neointimal hyperplasia after balloon injury. J Vasc Surg. 1994; 19: 722 –726.

[488] 17β-Estradiol, Its Metabolites, and Progesterone Inhibit Cardiac Fibroblast Growth Accepted October 22, 1997. Raghvendra K. Dubey, Delbert G. Gillespie, Edwin K. Jackson, Paul J. Keller.

[489] Foegh ML, Asotra S, Howell MH, Ramwell PW. Estradiol inhibition of arterial neointimal hyperplasia after balloon injury. J Vasc Surg. 1994; 19:722 –726.

[490] Imthurn B, Rosselli M, Jaeger AW, Keller PJ, Dubey RK. Differential effects of hormone-replacement therapy on endogenous nitric oxide (nitrite/nitrate) levels in postmenopausal women substituted with 17β-estradiol valerate and cyproterone acetate or medroxyprogesterone acetate. J Clin Endocrinol Metab. 1997; 82:388 –394.

Levine RL, Chen SJ, Durand J, Chen YF, Oparil S. Medroxyprogesterone attenuates estrogen-mediated inhibition of neointima formation after balloon injury of the rat carotid artery. Circulation. 1996; 94:2221 –2227.

[491] Levine RL, Chen SJ, Durand J, Chen YF, Oparil S. Medroxyprogesterone attenuates estrogen-mediated inhibition of neointima formation after balloon injury of the rat carotid artery. Circulation. 1996; 94:2221 –2227.

[492] Hersh AL, Stefanick ML, Stafford RS. National use of postmenopausal hormone therapy: annual trends and response to recent evidence. JAMA. 2004; 291(1):47---53.

Wysowski DK, Governale LA. Use of menopausal hormones in the United States, 1992 through June, 2003. Pharmacoepidemiol Drug Saf. 2005; 14(3):171---176.

Tsai SA, Stefanick ML, Stafford RS. Trends in menopausal hormone therapy use of US office-based physicians, 2000---2009. Menopause. 2011; 18(4):385---392.

[493] Anderson GL, Limacher M, Assaf AR, et al. Effects of conjugated equine estrogen in postmenopausal women with hysterectomy: the Women's Health Initiative randomized controlled trial. JAMA. 2004; 291(14):1701---1712.

LaCroix AZ, Chlebowski RT, Manson JE, et al. Health outcomes after stopping conjugated equine estrogens among postmenopausal women with prior hysterectomy: a randomized controlled trial. JAMA.2011; 305(13):1305---1314.

[494] Silverman BG, Kokia ES. Use of hormone replacement therapy, 1998---2007: sustained impact of the Women's Health Initiative findings. Ann Pharmacother.2009; 43(2):251---258.

Taylor HS, Manson JE. Update in hormone therapy use in menopause. J Clin Endocrinol Metab. 2011; 96(2):255---264.

Steinkellner AR, Denison SE, Eldridge SL, Lenzi LL, Chen W, Bowlin SJ. A decade of postmenopausal hormone therapy prescribing in the United States: long-term effects of the Women's Health Initiative.Menopause. 2012; 19(6):616---621.

Sprague BL, Trentham-Dietz A, Cronin KA. A sustained decline in postmenopausal hormone use: results from the National Health and Nutrition Examination Survey, 1999---2010. Obstet Gynecol. 2012; 120(3):595---603.

Chubaty A, Shandro MT, Schuurmans N, Yuksel N. Practice patterns with hormone therapy after surgical menopause. Maturitas. 2011; 69(1):69---73.

[495] Progesterone inhibits human infragenicular arterial smooth muscle cell proliferation induced by high glucose and insulin concentrations. J Vasc Surg. 2002 Oct; 36(4):833-8. Carmody BJ, Arora S, Wakefield MC, Weber M, Fox CJ, Sidawy AN.

[496] Neuroactive steroids: A therapeutic approach to maintain peripheral nerve integrity during neurodegenerative events. J Mol Neurosci. 2006; 28(1):65-76. Leonelli E1, Ballabio M, Consoli A, Roglio I, Magnaghi V, Melcangi RC.

[497] Testosterone Syndrome, The Critical Factor for Energy, Health, and Sexuality—Reversing the Male Menopause, Eugene Shippen, MD and William Fryer, Publisher M. Evans, Copyright 2007.

[498] Suzuki, K, et al., "Endocrine environment of benign prostatic hyperplasia: prostate size and volume are correlated with serum estrogen concentration, Scandinavian Journal of Urology and Nephrology, 1995; 29:65-68.

Chapter Fifty-One

[499] Stay Young & Sexy with Bio-identical Hormone Replacement: The Science Explained by Dr. Jonathan V. Wright, Lane Lenard, PhD, SmartPublications, copyright 2010.

[500] Cowan LD, Gordis L, Tonascia JA, Jones GS. Breast cancer incidence in women with a history of progesterone deficiency. American Journal of Epidemiology. 1981:114:209-217.

Printed in Great Britain
by Amazon

79867225R00215